Physicochemical Properties of Nanomaterials

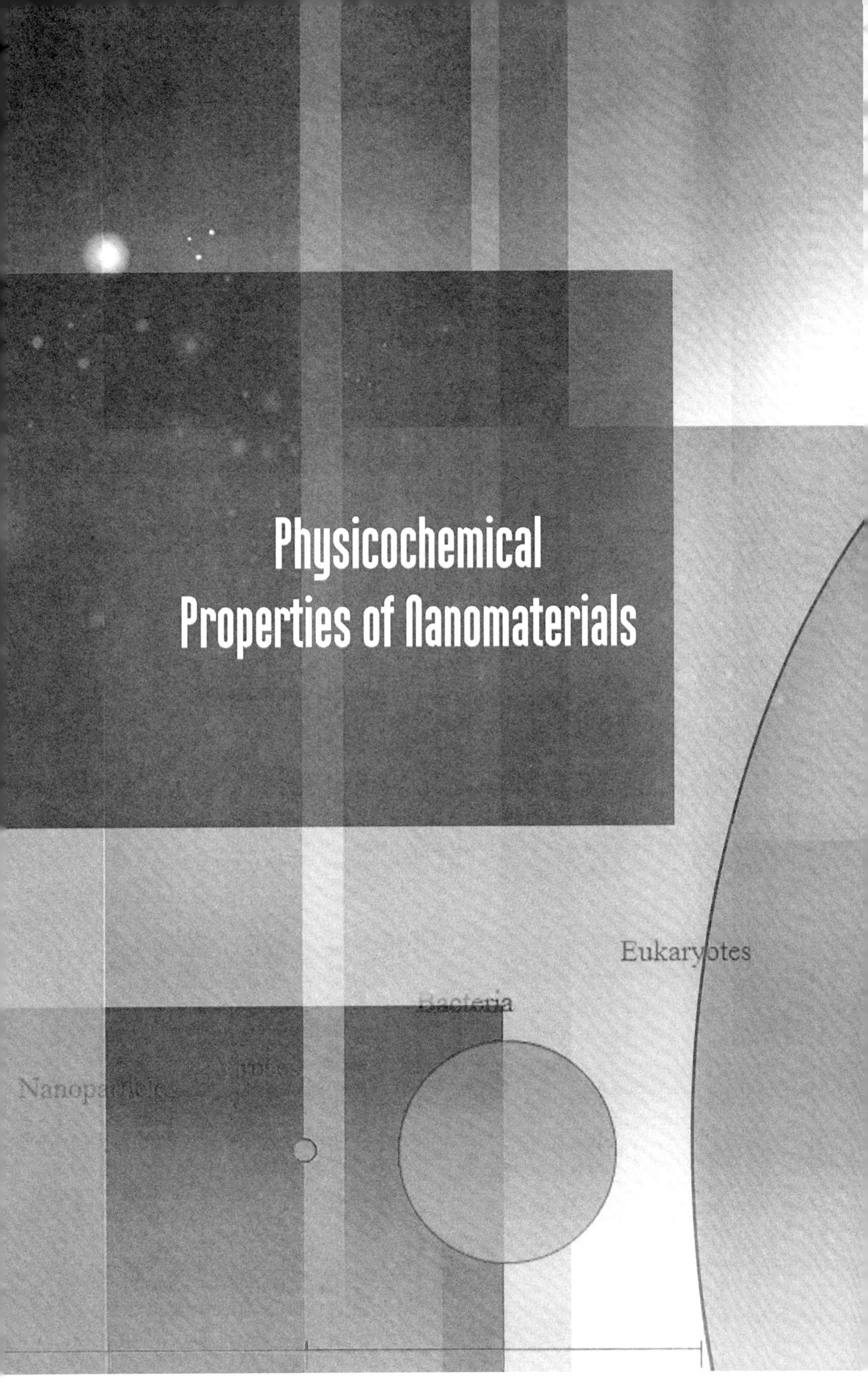

Physicochemical Properties of Nanomaterials

edited by

Richard C. Pleus | Vladimir Murashov

Pan Stanford Publishing

Published by

Pan Stanford Publishing Pte. Ltd.
Penthouse Level, Suntec Tower 3
8 Temasek Boulevard
Singapore 038988

Email: editorial@panstanford.com
Web: www.panstanford.com

British Library Cataloguing-in-Publication Data
A catalogue record for this book is available from the British Library.

Physicochemical Properties of Nanomaterials

ISBN 978-981-4774-80-2 (Hardcover)
ISBN 978-1-351-16860-1 (eBook)

Contents

Preface

What I want to talk about is the problem of manipulating and controlling things on a small scale.

—Richard P. Feynman
(http://www.zyvex.com/nanotech/feynman.html)

One has not to more than look out the window of a Boeing 787 Dreamliner as it flies across the globe to demonstrate the great progress that has been achieved in developing the productive use of engineered nanomaterials (ENMs). It also reminds us in health fields of the need to protect our workers, consumers, and the environment. Yet, more work needs to be done for their adequate characterization.

We enter yet another age of emerging technologies, manipulating and controlling things at a small scale to achieve properties unattainable with earlier technologies. While we are making progress in all areas of nanotechnology, science marches on. It is incumbent upon us to reduce uncertainty of the benefits and negative consequences of scientific discoveries leading to these emerging technologies.

This book brings together the use of physicochemical properties from scientists, experts in key areas of health and environment disciplines. They have been conducting experiments, writing, reviewing, and reading in this key area. They demonstrate how physicochemical characterization is key in their work.

Subtle changes in physicochemical properties can influence ENM toxicity and behavior in the environment, and so they can be used to help control potential ENM risks. This book illuminates the effort to understand these properties and how they may affect ENM deployment in existing or future materials and products.

We aim to further push (i) researchers, journal editors, and grant reviewers to ensure that adequate research-level physicochemical characterization is an integral part of any scientific study and reporting and (ii) standard-developing organizations to finalize the development of risk-assessment-level physicochemical characterization methods so that new ENMs are manufactured and utilized safely.

The static physical shape of nanoparticles can lead to biological interactions that are not observed for traditional chemicals. For example, the long-fiber paradigm in toxicology is based on the inability of macrophages (a type of white blood cell that engulfs and digests foreign objects, cell debris, and cancer cells) to engulf long fibers, which leads to macrophages' death and starts a chain of reactions causing adverse health effects. These toxicological effects were observed for long, rigid nanofibers and for microscale fibers, such as asbestos fibers, but not for traditional chemicals.

Physicochemical characterization of nanomaterials and other novel materials for safety and health characterization has two fundamental components. First, adequate research-level physicochemical characterization of nanomaterials and experimental setup in research studies is a basic and fundamental requirement of scientific research, ensuring that research results are reproducible and meaningful. Second, adequate risk-assessment-level physicochemical characterization for use in safety testing requires robust and feasible methods. While research-level physicochemical characterization methods have reached the point where adequate characterization can and should be conducted as part of research experiments, risk-assessment-level physicochemical characterization methods are still being developed.

This book has covered the essential components of physicochemical properties of ENMs. Adequate material characterization in the scientific literature is a key concern for human and environmental health testing. How are we, as scientists, going to be able to compare results from one study to the next or trust that the research of today can be applied to research 20 years from now? The most logical approach is to carefully characterize any tested material.

One key step toward understanding the benefits and liabilities is to clearly and accurately—to the extent possible—describe what materials we are studying. Characterizing physicochemical properties of ENMs is fundamental to knowing what we work with and what leads to their beneficial and adverse effects. This book starts with what we believe is the scientific discipline where physicochemical properties are key and have been so for decades: pharmacology (Chapter 2). Pharmacology has perhaps the longest history of interest in physicochemical properties of pharmaceutical agents. Pharmacologists have used physicochemical properties to design drugs to bind, interconnect, activate, and deactivate specific biomolecules on and in cells. The concept of intermolecular interactions expands the history underpinnings of physicochemical properties. Chapter 3 provides a context on the chemical properties of molecules (e.g., molecular weight, Henry's law) and the chemical properties of particles (e.g., density, dissolution rate). The list of physicochemical properties of nanomaterials is then applied in environmental, consumer product, and workplace safety. There is considerable overlap on what scientists from different disciplines and countries believe are the parameters of greatest importance. Chapter 4 defines those parameters and provides analytical approaches to reliably measure the parameters.

The book migrates from the hard sciences to those of applying scientific knowledge to practical issues of safety. The men and women who regularly are near or handling materials are the first and have the possibility of having the highest exposure. Chapter 5 provides current information on how physicochemical properties of nanomaterials may affect human health if released inadvertently into the workplace. The key physicochemical properties for nanomaterial risk are presented for occupational risk assessments. Chapter 6 provides the preparation of environmental samples and tools to measure physicochemical properties, including mass-based, surface area–based, ICP-MS-based, thermal, and X-ray analysis approaches. Physicochemical properties are then used (Chapter 7) to organize ENMs for risk assessment. The conceptual framework is built on categorization—classifying EMNs for environmental, health risk assessment, and occupational exposures. Chapter 8 describes the use of physicochemical properties of nanomaterials in the context of environmental regulations. Chapter 9, the last chapter, explains how ENMs are used in medicine. ENMs offer themselves as novel tools in the fight for health and warding off disease.

As we all are well informed, this new technology has its potential downsides as well. On the basis of where we are today, ENMs are new and complex. This book is an attempt to encompass the state of the science regarding physicochemical characterization of ENMs.

From the beginning, the theme was "let's get it right the first time." That has led to industry, government, and nongovernmental organizations all working together to provide scientific guidance and standardization to this field.

In summary, we have attempted to raise the importance of understanding, collecting, and using physicochemical properties of ENMs in reducing their risks. We start with a science that has long held the importance of understanding these properties to develop medications that purposely bind with targets to achieve desired health effect. We have other scientists who focus the attention of these parameters for other key areas in risk assessment and management of nanomaterials. We hope that you find this book valuable and informative and include physicochemical information in your work and published papers.

Richard C. Pleus*
Vladimir Murashov
2018

---

*Disclaimer: The findings and conclusions in this book are those of the authors and do not necessarily represent the views of the National Institute for Occupational Safety and Health (NIOSH).

Acknowledgments

This book would not be possible without our authors' generous contribution of their technical expertise.

We thank Mr. Gavin Bell for his excellent assistance in all phases of this book's development.

We also thank our colleagues Dr. Laurie Locascio, Ms. Martha Marrapese, Esq., and Mr. Steve Brown for the inspiration, rigorous scientific interaction, and friendship that they have offered over the years.

Finally, we thank all of our colleagues worldwide who have dedicated their careers to developing and implementing nanomaterials in as safe a manner as possible.

Chapter 1

Introduction

Richard C. Pleus[a,*] and Vladimir Murashov[b]

[a]*Intertox, Inc. Seattle, WA 98121, USA*

[b]*National Institute for Occupational Safety and Health (NIOSH), Washington, DC, 20201, USA*

rcpleus@intertox.com, vmurashov@cdc.gov

Throughout human history, our society has long encountered the combination of promise, risk, and uncertainty that accompanies emerging technologies. Nanotechnology is a recent example of an emerging technology which brought about engineered nanomaterials (ENMs) offering the potential to improve existing products or to develop new products that are technically superior to existing ones. As we all are well informed, this new technology has its potential downsides as well. Based on where we are today, ENMs are "new" and complex. This book is an attempt to encompass the state of the science regarding physicochemical characterization of ENMs. We believe subtle changes in physicochemical properties can influence ENM toxicity and behavior in the environment, and so can be used

*Disclaimer: The findings and conclusions in this report are those of the authors and do not necessarily represent the views of the National Institute for Occupational Safety and Health.

Physicochemical Properties of Nanomaterials
Edited by Richard C. Pleus and Vladimir Murashov

ISBN 978-981-4774-80-2 (Hardcover), 978-1-351-16860-1 (eBook)
www.panstanford.com

to help control potential ENM risks. This book aims to illuminate the effort to understand these properties and how they may affect ENM deployment in existing or future materials and products.

With this book, we aim to further push (i) researchers, journal editors, and grant reviewers to ensure that adequate "research level" physicochemical characterization is an integral part of any scientific study and reporting and (ii) standards-developing organizations to finalize the development of "risk assessment level" physicochemical characterization methods so that new ENMs are manufactured and utilized safely.

We are interested in physicochemical properties because science has shown that those properties are key to how chemical agents can affect the health, both positively and negatively, of humans and the environment. As Toews et al. state in Chapter 2, ". . . Paul Ehrlich made the prophetic statement, in Latin, that 'corpora non agunt nisis fixate' – 'entities do not act unless attached'."

Physicochemical properties of nanomaterials are critical determinants of their biological activity, including adverse health effects in people and the environment. Their adequate characterization in toxicity studies and risk assessments continue to draw attention and criticism even now after almost 20 years since governments around the world initiated national programs aimed at commercializing nanotechnology and nanomaterials. This book presents the state of the science in this critical field.

With the advent of commercial interest in nanotechnology, there was a strong incentive in the health science community to learn from the past in bringing new chemicals on the market and develop guidance on best practices or standards for nanomaterials. The theme was "let's get it right the first time." That has led to industry, government, and nongovernmental organizations all working together to provide scientific guidance and standardization to this field.

The International Organization for Standardization (ISO) started the Technical Committee 229 Nanotechnologies (TC 229), perhaps the first international standard setting organization for nanotechnology, in 2005. Other organizations, including the Organisation for Economic Co-operation and Development (OECD) and ASTM International, worked diligently to assist in developing standards to protect human and environmental health.

The focus of ISO/TC 229 is to develop standards in the field of nanotechnologies that includes either or both of the following [1]:

- *Understanding and control of matter and processes at the nanoscale, typically, but not exclusively, below 100 nm in one or more dimensions where the onset of size-dependent phenomena usually enables novel applications*
- *Utilizing the properties of nanoscale materials that differ from the properties of individual atoms, molecules, and bulk matter in order to create improved materials, devices, and systems that exploit these new properties*

The various subgroups of ISO/TC 229 focus on developing standards for terminology and nomenclature; metrology and instrumentation, including specifications for reference materials; test methodologies; modeling and simulations; and science-based health, safety, and environmental practices. The first standard that this committee developed defines different basic categories of nanomaterials starting with the nano-object, which is a discrete piece of material with one, two, or three external dimensions in the nanoscale (see Table 1.1).

Pharmacology has perhaps the longest history of interest in physicochemical properties. For a drug to be effective it must hit a specific and intended target. Pharmacologists use physicochemical properties to design drugs to bind, interconnect, activate, and deactivate specific biomolecules on and in cells. The physicochemical properties of the drug were and are critical and fundamental to its action on tissue, cells, and cellular molecules. Toxicologists have followed in the footsteps of pharmacologists and have begun to investigate how the harmful actions of contaminants, industrial chemicals, or illicit drugs can be characterized by physicochemical properties.

What are some of the unique physicochemical characteristics of nano-objects? Unlike larger particles, like atoms and molecules, nano-objects exhibit discrete electronic energy levels rather than continuous bands of energies. Changes in electronic energies lead, for example, to unique optical properties, material strength, electrical conductivity, magnetic behavior, and chemical reactivity.

Table 1.1 Core definitions for nanomaterials based on ISO/TS 80004

Nanoscale	Length range approximately from 1 nm to 100 nm
Nanomaterial	Material with any external dimension in the nanoscale or having internal structure or surface structure in the nanoscale
Nano-object	Discrete piece of material with one, two, or, three external dimensions in the nanoscale
Nanoparticle	Nano-object with all external dimensions in the nanoscale where the lengths of the longest and shortest axes of the nano-object do not differ significantly
Nanoplate	Nano-object with one external dimension in the nanoscale and the two other external dimensions significantly larger
Nanofiber	Nano-object with two external dimensions in the nanoscale and the third dimension significantly larger
Engineered nanomaterial	Nanomaterial designed for specific purpose or function
Nanotechnology	Application of scientific knowledge to manipulate and control matter predominantly in the nanoscale to make use of size- and structure-dependent properties and phenomena distinct from those associated with individual atoms or molecules, or extrapolation from larger sizes of the same material

Nanoparticles, a subset of nano-objects comprising roughly spherical particles with nanoscale diameter, are in the same size range as critical elements of biological systems such as proteins and nucleic acids. For example, the size of botulinum toxin type c, a protein, is 7.4 nm. Nanoparticles also overlap in size with viruses, as average viruses are 50 to 300 nm in diameter. Thus, the science of pharmaceuticals, pharmacology, has been studying nanoscale interactions since this scientific discipline was established.

Within ISO/TC 229, Working Group (WG) 3 focuses on the health, safety, and environmental aspects of nanotechnologies. Members of this group have introduced technical documents covering ecological, occupational, and human health. It is this mission in particular that is of the greatest interest to both editors of this book. In keeping with this focus, the purpose of this text is to allow readers to engage in this mission by providing them with scientific expertise regarding how physicochemical properties affect key components of the environmental, health, and safety of nanomaterials.

We led the development of one of the first guidance documents developed by ISO/TC 229 WG 3: ISO/TR 13014, *Guidance on Physicochemical Characterization of Engineered Nanoscale Materials for Toxicologic Assessment*; this was published in 2012. In addition to being perhaps the first international guidance document on physicochemical characterization of nanomaterials in toxicity studies, this document also introduced an important abbreviation encompassing categories of nanomaterials, which have the most potential to cause adverse health effects, NOAA (nano-objects and their aggregates and agglomerates greater than 100 nm). This abbreviation has since become widely used in nanomaterial safety and health literature and guidance. The term was developed by ISO TC229 WG3 in November 2011 during a project group meeting for another nanomaterials safety and health document (ISO TS 12901-2:2014, *Occupational Risk Management Applied to Engineered Nanomaterials: Part 2; Use of the Control Banding Approach*). However, *Guidance on Physicochemical Characterization of Engineered Nanoscale Materials for Toxicologic Assessment* was the first ISO document where this abbreviation appeared in public and, therefore, is the primary source for this abbreviation.

It has been five years since *Guidance on Physicochemical Characterization of Engineered Nanoscale Materials for Toxicologic Assessment* was published, but an adequate physicochemical characterization of nanomaterials remains a high priority for enabling science-based risk assessments and risk mitigations. The collection of papers in this book by various authors is a fuller extension and exploration of that initial guidance document.

There are many ways one can categorize according to the concept of physicochemical properties. The first approach is to divide according to the two key historical categories of environmental assessment: bulk and nanoscale objects. Looking backward in time and prior to the emergence of nanotechnology into commerce, the main focus of physicochemical characterization was on what we call bulk materials. Environmental scientists did not pay much attention to the size of the molecule (not necessarily the size of a particle, such as $PM_{2.5}$) and generally prioritized assessing bulk materials. Examples include industrial chemicals, pharmaceutical agents, and their precursors. In retrospect, some large chemical molecules of historical interest are in fact nanoscale.

Material characterization in the scientific literature is a key concern for human and environmental health testing. How are we, as scientists, going to be able to compare results from one study to the next, or trust that the research of today can be applied to research 20 years from now? The most logical approach is to carefully characterize any tested material. Chapter 4 discusses the current lists of toxicologically relevant characteristics for nano-objects. There was an initial push to have publishers and editors require adequate characterization of nanomaterials for the publication of peer reviewed manuscripts. However, the energy behind that sail was short-lived, and now publishers are back to relying primarily on peer reviewers. We encourage our community to continue requiring this for many good scientific reasons.

Since in the nanoscale size range, the fundamental physical and chemical properties of materials change and become distinct from those of larger particles and those of atoms or molecules of the same substance, new methods for characterizing physicochemical properties of nanomaterials are necessary.

Like larger particles (also referred to as bulk materials) and unlike atoms and molecules, nanoparticles have a static physical particle shape and have a core and a surface. About half of all atoms in a 1 nm particle are at the surface. This number drops off to under 1% for particles larger than 100 nm. Since interactions between particles and biological systems take place at the surface, the significant fraction of surface atoms in nanoparticles translates into their increased biological activity on a per mass basis compared to larger particles. This higher fraction of surface atoms also leads to an increased "stickiness" of nanoparticles, which manifests in the tendency of nanoparticles to clump together or agglomerate, to absorb other chemicals, and to stick to the surfaces of larger objects.

The static physical shape of nanoparticles can lead to biological interactions that are not observed for traditional chemicals. For example, the long-fiber paradigm in toxicology is based on the inability of macrophages (a type of white blood cell that engulfs and digests foreign objects, cell debris, and cancer cells) to engulf long fibers such as asbestos fibers, which leads to macrophages' death and starts a chain of reactions causing adverse health effects. Similar toxicological effects were observed for long, rigid nanofibers.

As noted by Toews et al., the history of molecular interaction is long with many tales of success. Chapter 2 provides the underlying foundation of physicochemical properties. Toews et al. define classical pharmacology (and toxicology), where much work has been accomplished with bulk chemicals, in this case pharmaceutical agents. They discuss how pharmacologists think of drugs acting on biomolecules with "selectivity" and "specificity," terms that are based on the molecular formula of the chemical agent.

Chapter 3 drills down into the fundamental analysis of chemical-to-chemical interactions. Brown provides an excellent review of fundamental chemical interactions, including chemical properties of molecules (e.g., molecular weight, Henry's law) and chemical properties of particles (e.g., density, dissolution rate), and identifies the need for physicochemical characterization (e.g., for inhalation exposure, dermal exposure).

Lists of physicochemical properties of nanomaterials necessary for risk assessments in different application areas, such as environmental, consumer products, and workplace safety, are described and compared in Chapter 4. Carpinone and Roberts provide an excellent summary of key parameters and the status of the list of parameters from a global perspective. They provide fundamental information for each parameter. For example, they define, provide analytical approaches to measuring, and provide an understanding of the value of the parameters. This sets up the baseline for the remaining chapters.

We know from the history of industrialization that workers are often the most exposed population. They are the men and women who regularly are near or who handle materials. Thus, Chapter 5 provides current information on how physicochemical properties of nanomaterials, if released inadvertently into the workplace, may affect human health. Stefaniak, a researcher in occupational health and safety, reviews key physicochemical properties that are relevant for nanomaterial risk assessment in the workplace. One of the key components of this is air monitoring. Sampling air for ENMs is a unique process that requires special techniques for accurate measurements. The chapter also contains a description of some current ENMs that have been assessed.

Whereas Stefaniak begins with worker exposure and air sampling, Kidd and Westerhoff (Chapter 6) dig deeper with the tools to measure key physicochemical properties, including mass-based, surface-area-based, inductively coupled plasma mass spectrometry (ICP-MS)-based, thermal, and X-ray analysis approaches. Also key in this chapter is a discussion of the preparation of environmental samples. They provide a summary of what we know now, although as science marches on, this information will be expanded.

In Chapter 7, Shatkin and Elde provide a framework for organizing ENMs for risk assessment. The concept is simple but is building on categorization. As they write, "Categorization is the act of sorting and organizing things according to a group or class. Classifying an object gives it an identity that is recognizable and distinguishable. In other words, categorization schemes are intended to organize a group of objects." They provide a historical approach used by several global agencies. Control banding is an example they provide that has been simple to employ and effective in the workplace for assessing fiber and particle inhalation exposures during manufacturing. The authors demonstrate the use of categorization for environmental exposures, health risk assessment, and occupational exposures to ENMs across the globe.

Chapter 8 describes the physicochemical properties of nanomaterials in the context of environmental regulations. Here, Morris points out the key aspect from a regulatory perspective. In general, where there has been a regulatory interest by a country or a world agency, information on the physicochemical properties is important for the evaluation of a nanomaterial that goes into commerce. For example, during a new chemical review process by the US Environmental Protection Agency (EPA), nanomaterials are evaluated on a case-by-case basis. This evaluation includes data on the material's physicochemical properties such as data on impurities. There are likely other chemicals that are present from the manufacture of the nanoscale material. Examples include metals such as cadmium or lead, which can be used as catalysts during production of nanomaterials. Lastly, the cross-agency list of physicochemical parameters is not universal. While there is overlap for a number of agencies and nongovernmental organizations, there is not a list that is 100% consistent as to what is enough and required.

In Chapter 9, Bhaskara et al. discuss the use of ENMs in medicine. This is an exciting area of use for ENMs as they offer novel tools in the fight for health and warding off disease. As noted in Chapter 2, pharmaceutical researchers are well versed in the importance of physicochemical properties affecting the chemical agent's or medical device's performance, safety, and efficacy. The authors discuss the application of ENMs in these tools. They provide perspective of one agency, the US Food and Drug Administration (FDA), on ENMs in medicine. The first question that they consider when a new medical product comes to the FDA is whether a product contains nanotechnology or nanomaterials? The question seems rather trite compared to the progress we have made. However, as the authors point out, there is no universally accepted definition for nanomaterials. Regulatory agencies throughout the world have their own working definitions that they use for regulation of such products.

In summary, we have attempted to raise the importance of understanding, needing, and using physicochemical properties of ENMs in reducing their risks. We start with a science that has long held the importance of understanding these properties to develop medications that purposely bind with targets to achieve desired health effect. We have other scientists that focus the attention of these parameters for other key areas. We hope that you find this book valuable and informative and include physicochemical information in your work and published papers.

Reference

1. ISO. (2005). Nanotechnologies: scope. https://www.iso.org/committee/381983.html. Accessed April 5, 2017.

Chapter 2

How Physical and Chemical Information Predicts the Action of Molecules: A Historical Overview

Myron L. Toews, JoEllyn M. McMillan, and David B. Bylund

Department of Pharmacology and Experimental Neuroscience, University of Nebraska Medical Center, S. 42nd St. & Emile St., Omaha, NE 68198, USA

mtoews@unmc.edu

2.1 A Definition for Pharmacology and Toxicology

A favored broad-scope definition of the discipline of pharmacology for the authors of this chapter, who are all pharmacologists, is "the study of the interactions of chemicals with living systems." The primary goal of most of pharmacology is to understand and improve the interactions of "drugs" with "the human body" for therapeutic benefit. However, "living systems" for pharmacologists are often isolated tissues, or cells, or animal models, or most recently highly purified and isolated "drug targets." In addition, many pharmacologic

Physicochemical Properties of Nanomaterials
Edited by Richard C. Pleus and Vladimir Murashov

ISBN 978-981-4774-80-2 (Hardcover), 978-1-351-16860-1 (eBook)
www.panstanford.com

agents are designed for animal rather than human use, particularly for agriculture and for pets. One of the reasons for using the term "chemicals" rather than "drugs" in this broad-scope definition is that for many, the term "drug" is reserved for currently approved therapeutic agents and should not be applied to other chemicals unless/until they are approved. These are only a few of the reasons for choosing the terms "chemicals" and "living systems."

Toxicologists reading this chapter will no doubt immediately realize that this definition of pharmacology applies equally well to the discipline of toxicology, another aspect of "the interaction of chemicals with living systems." This is, in fact, another strong rationale for choosing this broad-scope definition. Pharmacology and toxicology are so similar and related that they are often together in the names of academic departments or in journal and monograph titles, perhaps most notably the long-standing *Annual Reviews of Pharmacology and Toxicology*. There is another compelling reason for including toxicology together with pharmacology—the fact that nearly all drugs, even those that are clinically approved, have off-target or side effects that often rise to the level of being called toxicities. Thus even clinically oriented pharmacologists not interested in toxicology per se have compelling reasons to understand the toxicity side of the interactions of drugs with humans and other living systems. For toxicologists, the term "living systems" is perhaps even broader than for pharmacologists, with our current appreciation of the toxic effects of our vast chemical repertoire on living systems such as our forests and farms, rivers and oceans, and all of the diverse living creatures that inhabit these systems.

With this shared definition and the many overlaps among the chemicals and living systems of interest between pharmacology and toxicology, this chapter attempts to define the basic principles that drive and guide these shared interactions between chemicals and living systems. The importance of chemicals of any sort becoming attached to components of living systems to mediate their effects will be described, along with the molecular nature of these chemical "attachments" and interactions. The mathematical principles governing these interactions, and how their respective equations can be utilized for convenient graphical or computer-assisted analysis and display of those interactions, will then be described in some detail. Selected informative examples of these attachments and interactions, from the realms of both pharmacology and toxicology, will be described. Finally, new insights from elegant atomic level structural and dynamics studies of how these chemical attachments occur and how they, in turn, mediate their effects on living systems will be presented. With powerful new analytic and imaging technologies continuing to be developed and applied, the potential seems at hand for a true understanding of how chemicals of all kinds interact with living systems of all kinds, with exciting advances likely for both pharmacology and toxicology.

2.2 Entities Do Not Act Unless Attached

From early studies aimed at understanding the actions of hormones and neurotransmitters and their synthetic analogs on physiological responses, Paul Ehrlich made the prophetic statement, in Latin: *corpora non agunt nisis fixate*, that is, "entities do not act unless attached" [1]. The nature of the "site" to which these entities needed to attach to initiate their actions was totally unknown at the time. However, what was beginning to be appreciated at this time was that these chemical entities were quite selective in their interactions and effects, implying that there would be some highly selective and complementary site to which these entities would attach, or bind, to bring about their differential effects.

One classic example was the ability of nicotine to mimic some but not all of the effects of acetylcholine on various organ systems and for muscarine to mimic a different set of acetylcholine effects, leading to the idea that acetylcholine must be able to attach and interact with two different kinds of targets to mediate its full panel of effects [2]. These are now known to be the well-established sets of nicotinic and muscarinic cholinergic receptors for acetylcholine [3, 4]. The other classic interactions in early studies were those for the catecholamines epinephrine and norepinephrine, which showed an even more complex pattern as more and more analogs were developed [5]. One set of compounds worked well to mimic the endogenous catecholamines in tissue A for response X, whereas other sets of compounds were better at mimicking effects in tissue B for response Y and in tissue C for response Z. Indeed, even the two endogenous catecholamines epinephrine and norepinephrine exhibited differential patterns of effects from each other. These studies implied a diverse set of interaction targets for these agents, and these are now known to be the multiple types and subtypes of adrenergic receptors, with a total of nine relatively similar yet highly selective subtypes in all [6].

Over the course of decades, these molecular targets, or receptors, were shown to be distinct biochemical molecules that exhibited the expected patterns of tissue distribution. Radiolabeled chemical probes allowed the eventual identification and purification of these receptors and studies of the diverse signaling pathways by which they mediated their effects. Molecular biology and genetics showed that each receptor subtype was coded by a distinct gene, and cloning and expression studies documented that a distinct receptor molecule could explain each of the different patterns of interactions and effects. Most recently, X-ray crystallography has revealed amazing details of the structures of these receptors and their sites for interaction and attachment of specific drugs or other agents, and fluorescence and other biophysical studies are beginning to reveal the dynamics of the changes in those structures following attachment and activation and leading to the eventual effects of those agents on living systems.

2.3 The Language of Chemical Attachment

As already mentioned above, the sites to which chemicals attach to mediate the interactions that lead to effects on living systems are referred to as receptors, indicating that these are the biomolecules that receive the chemical information from the molecules with which they attach. The term "receptor" can be defined in a limited way or in broader terms. The most common use of the term "receptor" is for those endogenous molecules whose role is to recognize and initiate responses to endogenous hormones, neurotransmitters, growth factors, and other biomolecules. Classic examples are the cholinergic and adrenergic receptors described above, the insulin receptor, the estrogen receptor, and literally hundreds of others. A broader definition of the term "receptor" is "the molecular target to which a drug attaches to mediate its effects." This broader definition of receptor for pharmacology covers the fact that many drugs interact with targets other than the endogenous receptors of the more classic and limited definition. Many drugs are enzyme inhibitors, so the receptors for those drugs would be the enzymes to which they attach and whose activity they alter. Many drugs interact with and most commonly block various ion channels in cellular membranes, and the receptors for these drugs would be their target channel proteins. Because toxic compounds can interact with a wide variety of target biomolecules in living systems, this broader definition may be most relevant. It is important to note here that the molecular interactions and mathematical equations for drug interactions with enzymes and ion channels and diverse other targets are, in general, identical to those for interactions with classic receptors. What is often called receptor theory in general applies to enzyme and ion channel modulation as well.

The generic term for all agents that interact with a classic receptor is "ligand," which itself embodies the concept of attachment to bring about actions, sharing the same root as for the ligaments that attach tendons to bones and the surgical ligatures that are used to reattach separated tissue components following surgery. In the following section, the terms "ligand" and "receptor" will be used for convenience, but it is important to remember that these same principles apply for a diverse range of chemical–chemical interactions in both pharmacology and toxicology.

The receptor pharmacology term for attachment is "binding." Drugs and other ligands bind to their receptors; receptors can be bound if they have ligands attached, or they can be unbound or empty if no ligand is attached. Similarly, ligands can be bound to their receptors, or free if they are not bound. Their interactions are studied by receptor-binding assays of various sorts. The terms "binding" and "bound" should not be taken to imply necessarily "tight" or "irreversible" binding; in fact, nearly all clinically used drugs bind in a completely and often rapidly reversible manner. They mediate their effects while they are bound, but those effects end when the ligand is no longer bound. Tighter or even irreversible binding or attachment to biomolecules may be more common in toxicological settings, and in fact some of the toxicity of those interactions may result from tight and long-term binding, leading to prolonged and toxic effects.

"Specificity" is another important term to address. The interactions of drugs with their receptors in various organs and tissues are seldom truly specific, meaning interaction with a single and presumably desired molecular target. Rather, pharmacologists are trained and encouraged to use the term "selectivity" in place of "specificity," indicating the relative ability of the drug to act on a selected receptor target and of a receptor to select those molecules which make the most appropriate molecular interactions. Though some toxic agents are known to have highly selective or even specific targets of attachment and interaction, it seems likely that toxic agents are, in general, less selective for an individual target molecule than what is commonly observed or designed for drug molecules. In fact, the toxic effects of drugs themselves are often due to their interaction with targets other than their desired therapeutic target, making a lack of specificity a common mechanism for drug toxicity.

2.3.1 Principles and Equations that Define Attachment Quantitatively

Having described the importance of attachment for chemical interactions with living systems and the most important general terminology for those attachments, we now address the quantitative nature of chemical attachment, using the term "ligand" (L) for the chemical entity and the term "receptor" (R) for its target attachment site. These quantitative aspects of interactions between ligands and receptors have been extensively covered in a recent review article by the same authors [7] and in even more detail in other sources [8]. Therefore, less detail is provided here, with an attempt to highlight aspects of greatest relevance to toxicology.

For ligands that bind reversibly to their receptors, which include the vast majority of drugs, the concentration dependence of binding is described by the law of mass action, as shown in the equations below. A ligand (L) binds to a receptor (R) with a rate constant k_{on}—the forward or association rate constant (Eq. 2.1). The extent of binding is proportional to the concentrations of L ([L]), where brackets denote "concentration of", and R ([R]). Once the RL complex is formed, it can, in turn, dissociate, regenerating a free R and a free L. The rate constant for this dissociation is k_{off}, the reverse or dissociation rate constant.

$$R + L \underset{k_{\text{off}}}{\overset{k_{\text{on}}}{\rightleftarrows}} RL \tag{2.1}$$

$$k_{\text{on}}[R][L] = k_{\text{off}}[RL] \tag{2.2}$$

$$K_{\text{D}} = \frac{k_{\text{off}}}{k_{\text{on}}} = \frac{[R][L]}{[RL]} \tag{2.3}$$

$$R_{\text{T}} = [R] + [RL] \tag{2.4}$$

$$\frac{[RL]}{[R_{\text{T}}]} = \frac{[L]}{K_{\text{D}} + [L]} = \text{FRO} \tag{2.5}$$

$$[RL] = [R_{\text{T}}] \cdot \frac{[L]}{K_{\text{D}} + [L]} \tag{2.6}$$

The extent of dissociation is determined by the concentration of the RL complex [RL] and the dissociation rate constant. If the system is allowed to achieve equilibrium, the rate of dissociation will eventually match the rate of association such that there is no change in [R], [L], or [RL] over time (Eq. 2.2). Rearranging Eq. 2.2 generates Eq. 2.3. The terms in Eq. 2.3 are defined as the equilibrium dissociation constant, K_{D}, which can be expressed or calculated as either the ratio of the two rate constants ($k_{\text{off}}/k_{\text{on}}$) or in terms of the concentrations of the interacting entities ([RL]/[R][L]). This equation quantitatively defines the amount of the RL complex in terms of the concentrations of R and L and their relative likelihood of either associating or dissociating. Note that K_{D} is an equilibrium constant, in contrast to k_{on} and k_{off}, which are rate constants, and that the equilibrium constant is defined for *dissociation*, not for *association*.

At least in the case of drug receptors, the number of binding sites is finite. The next important equation is that the total number of receptors (R_{T}) is equal to the sum of the receptors that are occupied by ligand (RL) and those that are unoccupied or free (R), as shown in Eq. 2.4. The more receptors that are already occupied by the ligand, the fewer receptors that remain free to interact with additional ligand molecules. Another consequence of this relationship is that binding to receptors is said to saturate—increasing the ligand concentration will generate more of the RL complex, but eventually, adding more ligand does not further increase the RL complex. This is because essentially all of the receptors are already occupied by the ligand and [RL] is essentially equal to R_T.

Combining Eqs. 2.3 and 2.4 leads to the fundamental equation that defines the amount of the RL complex, shown as Eq. 2.5, which defines the fraction of receptors occupied (FRO). Finally, Eq. 2.6 is another convenient rearranged form of Eq. 2.5 that defines the *concentration* of the RL complex rather than the FRO. Both equations and values are useful in assessing receptor and ligand binding. Note that the number or concentration of receptors and the ligand and K_D are sufficient to define the amount of the RL complex that mediates the effects of drugs, and presumably toxic agents also, on cells, tissues, or the intact organism.

Arguably the most important feature of these equations is that they define the K_D value as the concentration of ligand that occupies exactly 50% of the receptors—half of the receptors are occupied in the RL complex, and half are free, not bound to the receptor. This is best seen in Eq. 2.5: when [L] is equal to K_D, the right-hand side of the equality becomes L/2L, or 0.5, or 50%. The K_D value, the concentration of ligand required for 50% receptor occupancy, is the standard way in which the interaction of different ligands with a given receptor is compared and similarly the way in which the interaction of a given ligand with its perhaps multiple receptor targets is compared.

An additional important factor, alluded to briefly before, is the time that the ligand and receptor have been exposed to each other. Early in their interaction, the concentration of RL will be relatively small and hence the extent of the reverse (dissociation) reaction will be low. As the concentration of the RL complex increases, the extent of its dissociation will become greater, and at equilibrium or steady state, again, the forward and reverse reactions will become equal. For drugs, high receptor occupancy is usually the goal, and drugs are generally taken repeatedly to maintain high receptor occupancy. In contrast, for toxic agents, intervention early in the time course of the association may be important to prevent formation of complexes that mediate toxic effects.

2.3.2 Graphical Display and Analysis of Receptor Binding Interactions

The concentration dependence of forming the RL complex can be plotted in either of two ways: both plot the concentration of the free ligand on the *x* axis and the concentration of the RL complex on the *y* axis. The difference in the plots is whether the concentration axis is linear or logarithmic. Both give equivalent values, and both are useful for illustrating or determining different aspects of receptor–ligand interaction.

A plot with a linear *x* axis is shown in Fig. 2.1. This plot generates a hyperbolic curve that approaches R_T asymptotically as the concentration of L is increased. The maximal binding at high ligand concentrations is a measure of R_T, the total number of binding sites. The other important value that can be derived from this plot is the K_D value for the ligand–receptor interaction, which is the concentration that occupies 50% of the total number of binding sites. The concentration of ligand that gives 50% of maximal binding, the K_D value, is determined as shown by the arrows in Fig. 2.1.

A plot with a logarithmic *x* axis is shown in Fig. 2.2 for the same set of concentrations of the same drug as in Fig. 2.1. This plot generates a sigmoid, or S-shaped, binding curve that approaches zero binding at very low concentrations and approaches R_T at very high concentrations.

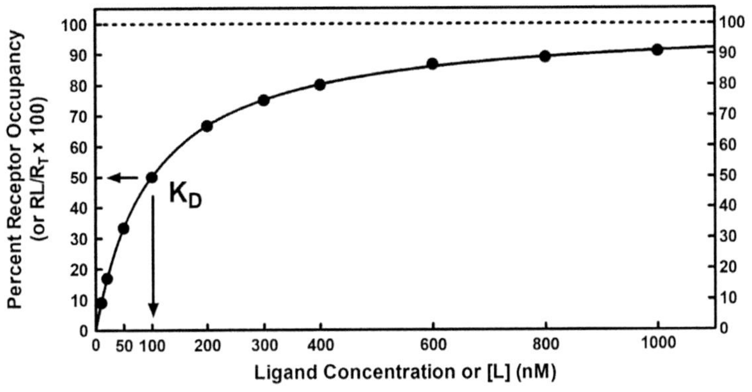

Figure 2.1 Plot of percentage receptor occupancy versus drug concentration on a linear *x* axis.

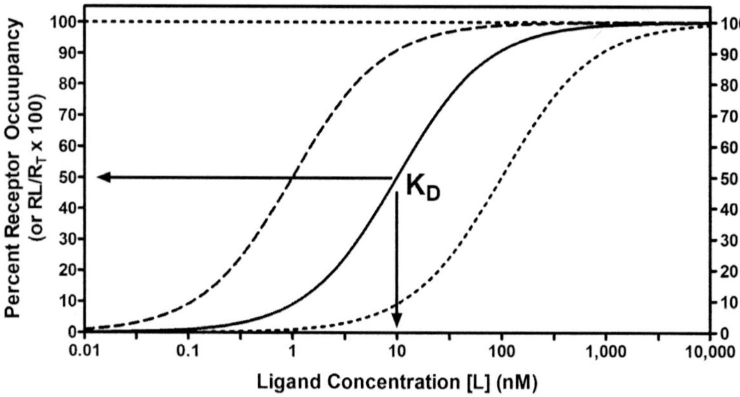

Figure 2.2 Plot of percentage receptor occupancy versus drug concentration on a logarithmic *x* axis.

Similar to the plot in Fig. 2.1, the K_D concentration of the ligand is the concentration that gives 50% of maximal receptor occupancy; however, on this plot, the K_D value is centered on the *x* axis, and the curve is symmetrical as concentrations become progressively lower or higher.

The K_D value is easier to identify with the sigmoid plot because it is centered on the *x* axis of the curve. The sigmoid plot also allows a much wider range of concentrations to be plotted, which, in turn, makes it, by far, the preferred plot for comparing binding of multiple ligands to the same receptor or the same ligand to different receptors. The curves for ligands with tenfold lower and tenfold higher K_D values are included in Fig. 2.2 to illustrate this point. This type of sigmoid plot on a logarithmic *x* axis is essentially always the way in which drug effects are plotted and analyzed.

Two additional terms, of relevance to both drug action and toxicology, are important to define. The term used for the relative K_D values of different ligands is "affinity," essentially how much the ligand and the receptor "like to be together in a complex" as opposed to "preferring not to interact." A high-affinity interaction means that 50% receptor occupancy will occur at lower ligand concentrations; note that a higher affinity for interaction corresponds to a lower numerical K_D value. Similarly, a lower-affinity interaction corresponds to a higher numerical K_D value. "Affinity" is the term for the ligand–receptor binding interaction. The corresponding term for the effects that occur in response to formation of the receptor–ligand complex is "potency"; potency defines the concentration of ligand required to mediate half of the maximal effect of the ligand. Potency is defined by EC_{50}—the concentration of the ligand for half-maximal effect. For complicated reasons that will not be discussed here, half-maximal effects of a drug or other ligand often occur at lower concentrations than those required for half-maximal receptor binding. Thus EC_{50} for the effect is often lower than the K_D for binding, and potency is often higher than affinity. This phenomenon is termed "receptor reserve" or "spare receptors," and its basis and consequences for drug action have been covered in other sources [7, 8].

2.4 Types of Drugs and Their Actions

Pharmacologists define two types of drugs at the simplest level: drugs that activate the receptor and initiate a cellular response are termed "agonists," and drugs that bind to the receptor but do not induce receptor activation are termed "antagonists." In most cases with reversible binding of the ligand to its receptor, the binding and action of antagonists are said to be competitive—the antagonist binds to essentially the same binding site as the agonist, and receptors occupied by the antagonist cannot bind the agonist simultaneously. Because the antagonist does not activate the receptor, it competitively inhibits the response to an agonist ligand by preventing the agonist ligand from binding to the receptor to initiate a response. For drug action, antagonists can be used to block receptors to prevent agonists from binding and generating responses. Because the binding of agonists is reversible, an antagonist can also be used to reduce agonist action, even if the agonist is already present. Each time an agonist molecule dissociates from the receptor, that receptor can now become occupied by the antagonist, preventing further binding of the agonist and reducing responses to the agonist, even though the agonist remains present at the same concentration. One important use of antagonist drugs is to reverse or reduce toxic side effects of agonist drug overdose. The use of the opioid receptor antagonist naloxone to prevent the toxicity of morphine or heroin overdose is perhaps a classic example.

2.4.1 Attachment Is Not Always Reversible

The descriptions, equations, and graphs given earlier are all for ligands that bind in a reversible manner to their receptors. There are also situations in which the ligand binds to its receptor in an irreversible manner, generally by formation of covalent bonds between the ligand and the receptor that prevent the ligand from dissociating. These interactions do not obey the same laws and equations as for reversible binding—the initial interaction of these agents with their receptors is defined by the same principles, but once the ligand has become irreversibly attached to the receptor, the reverse (dissociation) reaction rate becomes zero. With a high enough ligand concentration, all of the receptors can become irreversibly occupied. This irreversible receptor occupancy can lead to either sustained receptor actions or to sustained receptor blockade. Importantly, antagonists can prevent the formation of the irreversible complex if they are present before the complex forms, but they cannot reverse the formation or actions of the complex after it has formed. Though reversible and competitive interactions are, by far, the most common for pharmacology, irreversible interactions may be far more common in toxicological settings, and in fact the irreversible nature of the ligand–receptor association may well be the basis for the toxic rather than benign or therapeutic consequences of the interaction.

2.4.2 The Chemical Basis of Attachments

The chemical nature of the interactions between ligands and receptors that determine both the specificity and the affinity, or strength and duration, of the attachment are relatively well established and will be discussed briefly here, from the strongest to the weakest interaction forces. In the case of drug-related ligands binding to their clinical target receptors, the nature of these interactions and attachments is becoming clear at the atomic level of resolution from the many receptor–ligand complexes whose structures have recently been solved by X-ray crystallography [9, 10].

The strongest of the interactions between ligands and receptors are those that involve covalent bonding of the ligand to the receptor. These covalent bonds are relatively irreversible and permanent, as described above; they essentially form a new chemical entity that is composed of the atoms of the former ligand plus the receptor. Strong chemical agents or specific enzyme activity is generally required to disrupt or reverse these covalent interactions.

The second strongest are ionic bonds, or interactions between a positively or negatively charged portion of the ligand and an oppositely charged portion of the receptor. One well-established example is the interaction of the positively charged amine group of the neurotransmitter norepinephrine or structurally related agonists with a specific negatively charged carboxyl group on an aspartic residue in the binding pocket of the beta-2 adrenergic receptor, one of the adrenergic receptor subtypes [9]. These interactions are reversible, not covalent, and they can be disrupted by changes in pH or salt concentrations, which, in turn, alter the charge state of the chemical groups involved in the bond.

The next strongest are interactions termed "hydrogen bonds." These are interactions that most often occur between –OH, –SH, or –NH moieties of the ligand and the receptor. None of the interacting moieties is truly ionic or charged, but each has a relative polarity, with a greater negative charge at one end and a greater positive charge at the other end, thus allowing polar but nonionic interactions to occur. Water is also an OH-containing chemical, and some of the hydrogen bonds between ligands and receptors involve the ligand or receptor taking the place normally occupied by a paired water molecule at the interaction site. Again using beta-2 adrenergic receptor agonists as an example, their catechol ring –OH groups are known to interact with specific –OH groups on two serine amino acid residues in the receptor binding pocket [9].

Hydrophobic interactions are those that occur between different "water hating" (hydrophobic) parts of the ligand and the receptor. Alkyl groups and aromatic rings are classic examples of hydrophobic moieties; by interacting with each other, each of these hydrophobic groups is essentially protected from exposure to water, which is energetically unfavorable for stable interactions. Hydrophobic interactions between the catechol ring structure of beta-2 receptor agonists and aromatic side chains of tyrosine and tryptophan residues of the beta adrenergic receptor are the third well-established component of the binding affinity and specificity of their binding interaction [9]. Ionic interactions orient one end of the ligand, hydrogen bonds orient the other end of the ligand, and hydrophobic interactions stabilize the middle part of the ligand.

The weakest of the chemical interactions, perhaps not important individually but no doubt important in aggregates, are termed "van der Waals forces." These forces arise from transient dipolar arrangements of the electrons in otherwise nonpolar molecules. Though transient, these dipoles can contribute in important ways to the strength and stability of molecular attachments.

2.4.3 Other Attachments in Pharmacology and Physiology

The principles of attachment have been illustrated before for the area of greatest interest to pharmacologists, the binding of endogenous hormones and neurotransmitters and drug analogs of these agents to the specific receptors that mediate their effects on the body. The same kinds of chemical interaction forces lead to selective and concentration-dependent binding attachments for diverse other physiologic molecules also. A select few of these will be described here, mainly to illustrate the extent of diversity in both the ligands and the receptors for these other attachment interactions.

2.4.3.1 Attachment to enzymes

Receptors are protein molecules that exhibit selective and strong binding interactions. Another important group of proteins that specifically recognize and bind smaller molecules, similar to the way receptors do, are enzymes in or on the cell. In fact, a large group of drugs that do not bind to classic receptor proteins are enzyme inhibitors. The role of enzymes is to bind their specific substrate molecule, not to generate a signal as is the case for receptors, but rather to catalyze the chemical conversion of the substrate molecule into an altered product molecule. Enzymes are thus specific attachment sites for at least three kinds of molecules: substrates, products, and inhibitor drugs. Many enzymes bind two molecules of substrate and join them together to form a new combined product molecule. Many enzymes also bind specific cofactors that help drive their enzymatic catalysis, and these cofactors may also be chemically changed during their attachment and catalysis. A typical enzyme may thus have two to five specific attachment sites for various molecules; each of those attachment sites is a potential target for new drug development. More importantly for this treatise, each of those attachment sites for physiologic molecules is also a potential site for attachment and modification of enzyme activity by diverse toxic agents.

2.4.3.2 Attachment to channels and transporters

The third major group of proteins that are targets for endogenous molecules, drugs, and toxic compounds are a large group of membrane-localized channels and transporters. The physiological role of these channels and transporters is to control the movement of molecules from one side of the membrane to the other, in turn controlling the concentrations of those molecules inside and outside of the cell and among various intracellular compartments. Most of the channels regulate the flow of ions across cell membranes, including H^+, Na^+, K^+, and Ca^{2+} as cations and Cl^- and HCO_3^- as anions. Drugs can bind to the inside of these channels to prevent ligands from passing through the channel; alternatively drugs can bind to other parts of the channel molecule to either increase or decrease the frequency or duration of opening of the channels and movement of the selective ion. These ion channels are also known targets for attachment and modulation of action by toxic agents as well.

Note that ion channels that are regulated by ligand binding to specific regulatory sites on those channels are classified as receptors, the ligand-gated ion channel family of receptors. The channels discussed here, in contrast, are not regulated by ligand binding, but most often by the chemical and electrical gradients and membrane potential across the membrane containing these channels.

Transporters, in contrast to channels, use cellular energy to drive the movement of molecules across cell membranes. Some transporters move ions against their concentration gradients, but many transporters move much larger molecules into or out of cells or subcellular compartments. A clinically important example is a group of drug transporters that contribute to resistance to antibiotics and anticancer drugs, in particular, by pumping those drug molecules out of the cell and away from their site of action inside the cell. Similar to the case with channels, both drugs and toxic agents can block the pore of these transporters or can bind to other sites to modulate the activity of the transporter without directly blocking the site for interaction with the molecule being transported.

2.4.3.3 Attachment to antibodies

Antibodies provide perhaps the most striking examples of both specificity and high-affinity attachment of two molecules in a physiology-pathology context. Each antibody is generated and selected from a large pool of potential antibody molecules when the body is exposed to foreign chemicals, called antigens, which can range from proteins down to quite small molecules. The same chemical forces that guide the binding of ligands to receptors are involved in the binding of antigens to their own specific antibodies. In the body, the goal of antibody action is to bind, inactivate, and eliminate the foreign molecule or toxin. In the laboratory, the high specificity and affinity of antibody attachment to a single specific molecule or part of a molecule has made a variety of immunoassays of great importance for identifying and quantifying specific cellular or toxic agents in a research or analytical setting.

2.4.3.4 Attachment to nucleic acids

In addition to proteins, both DNA and RNA can also serve as attachment sites for a variety of proteins and/or small molecules, for endogenous physiologic regulation, for pharmacologic manipulation by drug molecules, or for toxic effects of exogenous molecules. Because DNA and RNA control cell growth and genetic differences among individuals that regulate normal physiology as well as disease and are transmitted to future generations during cell division and reproduction, the interaction of toxins with DNA or RNA can often have longer-term consequences than for interactions and alterations of proteins. Understanding attachments to specific subsets of RNAs is likely to become increasingly important with our rapidly advancing understanding of RNAs other than the best-known messenger RNAs, including noncoding but regulatory RNAs such as micro-RNAs (miRNAs) and long noncoding RNAs (lncRNAs) and others.

2.4.3.5 Attachment via chelation

A final example of the complexity of attachments among cellular molecules is hemoglobin, which is a target of great physiologic, pathologic, and toxicologic importance. Hemoglobin is a large and complex protein whose physiologic role is to transport oxygen from the lungs to cells throughout the body. The protein component is globin, and four globin molecules interact with each other to form a tetrameric protein complex. Each of these globin moieties, in turn, specifically interacts with one molecule of heme, a small molecule that specifically binds iron by a process termed "chelation." Each heme attached to each globin molecule of the tetramer binds one iron atom at the center of the heme ring. Finally, this heme iron is responsible for the binding of one oxygen molecule for delivery to cells. Thus oxygen is attached to iron, which is attached to heme, which is attached to globin, with four of these hemoglobin molecules joined together as a tetramer. The existence of this tetrameric complex generates complex kinetics and affinities that are different for each of the four heme moieties, with the binding state of each heme, in turn, affecting the properties of the other three. This example is particularly relevant to toxicology, because hemoglobin can not only bind and release oxygen but can also bind carbon monoxide in the setting of carbon monoxide poisoning. Carbon monoxide binds to heme with very high affinity, which, in turn, reduces the ability of hemoglobin to bind oxygen and deprives cells of this essential molecule, potentially leading to death. Treatment of carbon monoxide poisoning is by moving the victim to fresh air and providing supplemental oxygen therapy, thus removing or reducing the amount of carbon monoxide bound and restoring the oxygen binding capacity and function of hemoglobin.

2.4.4 Diverse Receptors for Toxic Agents

Several examples of attachments relevant to toxicology have been included in the sections before. A few more examples of well-established attachments of toxic agents, or mediated by those agents, are provided. These well-established examples of attachment of toxic compounds to target sites may generate useful insights for thinking about potential mechanisms for toxicities of the newly developing nanoscale molecules that are the focus of this volume.

2.4.4.1 Toxins that attach to receptors

Beginning with receptors, there are, in fact, several toxins that attach themselves to receptors, and some of these are actually useful as drugs or in receptor research. Three of these toxins target nicotinic acetylcholine receptors to block their ion channel activity, and all three have actually been adapted to take advantage of their toxic mechanism for clinical benefit. Bungarotoxin is a component of the venom of an elapid snake, the Taiwanese banded krait, that attaches irreversibly to nicotinic receptors [11]. For the snake, this toxin causes paralysis, respiratory failure, and death in the victim. Bungarotoxin is not used clinically, but it has been and continues to be an important experimental tool for studying the properties of cholinergic receptors. Botulinum toxin is derived from the bacterium *Clostridium botulinum* and it also binds and blocks nicotinic receptors [12], but specifically at presynaptic sites of neuromuscular synapses, decreasing the release of acetylcholine. Although it is one of the most potent biotoxins known, it has been adapted for clinical use in treating a wide variety of disease conditions, including chronic migraine, and is perhaps best known for its cosmetic use in tightening skin to reduce wrinkles and frown lines. Curare is a third example of a nicotinic receptor-targeted toxin [11], synthesized by a variety of plant species. In this case, its clinical use is in muscle paralysis for anesthesia and surgery.

Dioxin (2,3,7,8-tetrachlorodibenzodioxin, TCDD) is one of the most studied toxic agents. It is a by-product generated during incineration, paper bleaching, and manufacture of chlorinated phenols. TCDD is primarily released during the combustion of fossil fuels and wood, and it is a ubiquitous environmental contaminant. Dioxin interacts with a receptor called the aryl hydrocarbon receptor" or Ah receptor [13, 14]. Binding of dioxin to this receptor is necessary, though it is not alone sufficient to bring about a chain of events leading to enzyme induction, immunotoxicity, reproductive and endocrine effects, developmental toxicity, tumor promotion, and other effects. Immunotoxicity and effects on the reproductive system are among the most sensitive responses. The Ah receptor functions as a transcriptional enhancer, interacting with other regulatory proteins such as heat shock proteins, kinases, translocases, and DNA-binding species, which, in turn, regulate the transcription and translation of genetic information into proteins. This is the same mechanism as for all of the physiologically and pharmacologically important steroid hormones, such as estradiol, testosterone, and the anti-inflammatory glucocorticosteroids, and the Ah receptor is a member of this larger steroid hormone receptor or nuclear transcription factor receptor family. Thus, dioxin is a toxin that appears to function much like a hormone, initiating a cascade of events that is dependent upon the environment of each cell and tissue.

2.4.4.2 Toxins that attach to enzymes

Downstream of receptors are a diverse set of signal transduction molecules that relay the effects of receptor occupancy to proper actions inside the cell. A relatively large number of bacteria have developed toxins that act by specific attachments to endogenous mammalian molecules. Prominent among these for pharmacologists are the cholera and pertussis toxins [15–17], both of which modify specific heterotrimeric guanosine-5'-triphosphate (GTP)-binding switch proteins termed "G proteins" that are physiologically regulated by the G protein-coupled receptor (GPCR) family of hormone and neurotransmitter receptors, which includes the beta adrenergic receptor for norepinephrine mentioned before. Both of these toxins are enzyme proteins that attach an adenosine diphosphate (ADP)-ribose moiety derived from NAD+ to one of two G protein families that, in turn, regulate adenylyl cyclase enzyme activity and cyclic adenosine monophosphate (AMP) generation. Cholera toxin ADP-ribosylates the G_S protein that stimulates cyclic AMP generation, causing it to be irreversibly activated and to produce cyclic AMP continuously. In the gut, where cholera bacteria localize, this increase in cyclic AMP increases fluid entry into the intestines, leading to a watery diarrhea that makes the mammalian host feel ill but that also promotes the elimination and dissemination of the cholera bacteria into the environment for spread to other hosts and victims. Pertussis toxin, in contrast, ADP-ribosylates the G_i proteins that normally inhibit cyclic AMP formation and prevents their action. Without G_i-mediated inhibition, cyclic AMP again increases, in this case in the airways that pertussis bacteria colonize. Elevated cyclic AMP again drives fluid secretion, in this case into the airways; the victim coughs excessively to clear the airway fluid, leading again to dissemination of the bacteria into the environment for further rounds of infection. These are excellent examples of toxins that attach noncovalently and then act as enzymes to covalently attach ADP-ribose to the cellular target. Their target is the enzymatic activity of a G protein that is only one step downstream from the receptors themselves.

Acetaminophen is an example of a drug that binds and inhibits the activity of the cyclooxygenase enzymes to mediate its analgesic and antipyretic effects for clinical benefit. However, acetaminophen is metabolized by cytochrome P450 to a reactive metabolite termed *N*-acetyl-p-benzoquinone imine, or NAPQI, and this metabolite binds to sulfhydryl groups on essential liver cell proteins [18] and can lead to cell necrosis and death. This is a serious concern with the use of acetaminophen, particularly when young children take massive overdoses thinking of it as candy. Fortunately the sulfhydryl modification is preventable with the use of other nontoxic sulfhydryl reagents such as *N*-acetylcysteine so that acetaminophen toxicity can be ameliorated if it is treated before irreversible liver damage occurs.

2.4.4.3 Toxins that attach to ion channels or transporters

Some of the receptor-targeted toxin examples given before are also examples of targeting ion channels, because they target the ligand-gated ion channel receptor for acetylcholine. Ciguatoxins produced by marine dinoflagellates and concentrated in tropical predatory fish cause central and peripheral neurotoxicity in those who eat contaminated fish. They act by inhibition of voltage-gated sodium channels [19] rather than the ligand-gated channels that are classified as receptors. Symptoms develop within a few hours after eating contaminated fish and include nausea, vomiting, diarrhea, cramps, excessive sweating, headache, and many others. Ciguatera poisoning is rarely fatal, and symptoms usually clear in one to four weeks. It is perhaps surprising that these toxins have not been converted into useful sodium channel drug agents.

2.4.4.4 Toxins that attach to DNA

Nitrogen mustards are vesicants and alkylating agents developed for use in warfare. They act by rapidly attaching to cell proteins but also to DNA and other molecules, causing skin, eye, and respiratory tract injury [20, 21]. Covalent and irreversible attachment to purine bases in DNA leads to guanine cross-linking, which is the basis for their use as anticancer drugs for clinical benefit. Aflatoxin B1 is an example of a well-studied carcinogen that acts by attaching to and altering DNA [22]. It is a mycotoxin produced by the mold *Aspergillus flavus* that can be a contaminant of agricultural commodities and can cause hepatocellular carcinoma in individuals exposed to the mold. Aflatoxin B1 is metabolized by liver cytochrome P450 enzymes to a reactive epoxide that binds to and forms adducts on guanine bases in DNA that, in turn, cause guanine to thymine transversion mutations, specifically in the tumor suppressor *p53* gene.

2.4.4.5 Toxins that generate attachments

Many foreign proteins and other agents are, of course, toxic because they are recognized by the immune system as foreign molecules, leading to the production of antibodies to bind and block their effects. Halothane is an anesthetic gas used clinically, and it can induce severe hepatotoxicity with repeated exposure in patients. Halothane is metabolized by liver cytochrome P450 enzymes to the reactive intermediate trifluoroacetyl chloride, which then binds covalently to hepatocyte macromolecules [23] that, in turn, act as sensitizing neoantigens, evoking an immune-mediated response and the development of antibodies. Upon subsequent exposures these antibodies can attack self-proteins in the liver, leading to severe hepatotoxicity that can be life-threatening. Thus attachment to an enzyme and catalytic conversion to a new product, then product attachment to additional protein targets, and finally antibody generation and their attachment to the patient's own proteins, are all involved in the complex toxicity of this clinically important agent.

2.4.4.6 Metal ion attachment, chelation, and toxicity

A wide variety of metal ions are known to be toxic. In these cases, it is their attachment to specific cellular targets that mediates their toxic effects. Equally important is the role of specific attachments in remediating their toxicity. Just as heme physiologically chelates iron, a variety of other chelating agents with relative selectivity for one or more monovalent or divalent ions have been developed. These chelating agents can be added to the toxic setting such that the toxic metal ions bind preferentially to the chelating agent, thus reducing or eliminating their toxic attachments to various important physiologic targets. Desferoxamine is an example of a chelator used for treating hemochromatosis [24], a disease of iron accumulation. Dimercaptosuccinic acid (DMSA) and calcium-disodium ethylenediaminetetraacetic acid (EDTA) are used for treatment of lead poisoning [25, 26]. Thus the same principles of attachment are involved in both the toxicity of these metal ions and in the treatment and reversal of that toxicity. The same principles of competitive binding that were described for ligand–receptor interactions apply to the competition between the cellular target and the clinical chelating agent in terms of the amount of the therapeutic antidote that will be necessary to prevent the toxic interaction from continuing.

2.4.5 What about Attachment in the Case of Particle Toxicity?

The attachment examples given before, both for pharmacologic and for toxicologic agents, have all been for chemical agents in solution. However, a wide variety of particulate agents are known to be toxic and to cause a variety of diseases. These include agents such as diesel exhaust particles, agricultural dusts, fly ash and other smoke components, cement dust, and many others. In some cases, such as agricultural dusts, the toxicity can be explained at least in part by soluble chemicals that are adsorbed onto the dust particles [27]. But in other cases, the particles themselves are strongly implicated as the toxic agent [28]. How do such particles interact with cells and tissues to cause toxicity? Is it via the same sorts of specific chemical attachments as for the other toxins above? Or do cells somehow sense the physical presence of a particle, perhaps without a specific chemical attachment? Or perhaps both of these mechanisms, and others, are all involved.

Asbestos toxicity provides a potentially useful starting point for thinking about the toxicity of non-soluble particulates [29]. Asbestos fibers are phagocytosed by alveolar macrophages and mesothelial cells following interaction with integrins, which serve as the initial attachment site for the fibers. Phagocytosis of these fibers then induces proinflammatory cytokine and chemokine release. However, the presence of high amounts of iron attached to these asbestos fibers is also involved, inducing production of reactive oxygen species that drive further cellular responses. Thus both the fibers themselves and the iron attached to the fibers contribute to the induction of fibrogenesis, mesothelioma, and bronchogenic carcinoma that are the hallmarks of asbestos toxicity.

What are the mechanisms for nanoparticle toxicity in particular? Is it the particles themselves that drive cellular toxicity? Or is it the chemical composition of the particles? Or will adsorption of other environmental molecules onto nanoparticles prove to be major component of their toxicity? These questions are the focus of the remaining chapters in this volume. And is it not truly intriguing that nanoparticles, just like so many of the toxins described above, are being extensively studied by pharmacologists for use as nanomedicines for drug delivery and therapeutic benefit, even as toxicologists are studying the basis for their toxic effects and how to prevent or treat them? Yet again, pharmacology and toxicology are moving this field forward, side by side.

References

1. Ehrlich, P. (1913). Address in pathology, on chemiotherapy: delivered before the Seventeenth International Congress of Medicine. *Br. Med. J.*, **2**, 353–359.
2. Dale, H. H. (1914). The action of certain esters and ethers of choline, and their relation to muscarine. *J. Pharmacol. Exp. Ther.*, **6**, 174–190.
3. Caulfield, M. P., and Birdsall, N. J. (1998). International union of pharmacology. XVII. Classification of muscarinic acetylcholine receptors. *Pharmacol. Rev.*, **50**, 279–290.

4. Lukas, R. J., Changeux, J. P., Le Novere, N., Albuquerque, E. X., Balfour, D. J., Berg, D. K., Bertrand, D., Chiappinelli, V. A., Clarke, P. B., Collins, A. C., Dani, J. A., Grady, S. R., Kellar, K. J., Lindstrom, J. M., Marks, M. J., Quik, M., Taylor, P. W., and Wonnacott, S. (1999). International union of pharmacology. XX. Current status of the nomenclature for nicotinic acetylcholine receptors and their subunits. *Pharmacol. Rev.*, **51**, 397–401.

5. Ahlquist, R. P. (1948). Comparative effects of sympathomimetic amines on the vasomotor resistance of the kidney, mesentery and leg. *Fed. Proc.*, **7**, 202.

6. Bylund, D. B., Eikenberg, D. C., Hieble, J. P., Langer, S. Z., Lefkowitz, R. J., Minneman, K. P., Molinoff, P. B., Ruffolo, R. R., Jr., and Trendelenburg, U. (1994). International union of pharmacology nomenclature of adrenoceptors. *Pharmacol. Rev.*, **46**, 121–136.

7. Bylund, D. B., and Toews, M. L. (2014). Quantitative versus qualitative data: the numerical dimensions of drug action. *Biochem. Pharmacol.*, **87**, 25–39. doi: 10.1016/j.bcp.2013.07.027.

8. Limbird, L. E. (1985). *Cell Surface Receptors: A Short Course on Theory and Methods* (Springer, New York).

9. Chan, H. C., Filipek, S., and Yuan, S. (2016). The principles of ligand specificity on beta-2-adrenergic receptor. *Sci. Rep.*, **6**, 34736. doi: 10.1038/srep34736.

10. Soriano-Ursua, M. A., Trujillo-Ferrara, J. G., Correa-Basurto, J., and Vilar, S. (2013). Recent structural advances of beta1 and beta2 adrenoceptors yield keys for ligand recognition and drug design. *J. Med. Chem.*, **56**, 8207–8223. doi: 10.1021/jm400471z.

11. Kudryavtsev, D., Shelukhina, I., Vulfius, C., Makarieva, T., Stonik, V., Zhmak, M., Ivanov, I., Kasheverov, I., Utkin, Y., and Tsetlin, V. (2015). Natural compounds interacting with nicotinic acetylcholine receptors: from low-molecular weight ones to peptides and proteins. *Toxins (Basel)*, **7**, 1683–1701. doi: 10.3390/toxins7051683.

12. Pirazzini, M., Rossetto, O., Eleopra, R., and Montecucco, C. (2017). Botulinum neurotoxins: biology, pharmacology, and toxicology. *Pharmacol. Rev.*, **69**, 200–235. doi: 10.1124/pr.116.012658.

13. Bock, K. W. (2016). Toward elucidation of dioxin-mediated chloracne and ah receptor functions. *Biochem. Pharmacol.*, **112**, 1–5. doi: 10.1016/j.bcp.2016.01.010.

14. Beischlag, T. V., Luis Morales, J., Hollingshead, B. D., and Perdew, G. H. (2008). The aryl hydrocarbon receptor complex and the control of gene expression. *Crit. Rev. Eukaryot. Gene Expr.*, **18**, 207–250.

15. Verheugd, P., Butepage, M., Eckei, L., and Luscher, B. (2016). Players in ADP-ribosylation: readers and erasers. *Curr. Protein Pept. Sci.*, **17**, 654–667.

16. Thiagarajah, J. R., and Verkman, A. S. (2005). New drug targets for cholera therapy. *Trends Pharmacol. Sci.*, **26**, 172–175. doi: 10.1016/j.tips.2005.02.003.

17. Carbonetti, N. H. (2015). Contribution of pertussis toxin to the pathogenesis of pertussis disease. *Pathog. Dis.*, **73**, ftv073. doi: 10.1093/femspd/ftv073.

18. Lancaster, E. M., Hiatt, J. R., and Zarrinpar, A. (2015). Acetaminophen hepatotoxicity: an updated review. *Arch. Toxicol.*, **89**, 193–199. doi: 10.1007/s00204-014-1432-2.

19. Dickey, R. W., and Plakas, S. M. (2010). Ciguatera: a public health perspective. *Toxicon*, **56**, 123–136. doi: 10.1016/j.toxicon.2009.09.008.

20. Malaviya, R., Sunil, V. R., Venosa, A., Vayas, K. N., Heck, D. E., Laskin, J. D., and Laskin, D. L. (2016). Inflammatory mechanisms of pulmonary injury induced by mustards. *Toxicol. Lett.*, **244**, 2–7. doi: 10.1016/j.toxlet.2015.10.011.

21. Einhorn, J. (1985). Nitrogen mustard: the origin of chemotherapy for cancer. *Int. J. Radiat. Oncol. Biol. Phys.*, **11**, 1375–1378.

22. Kew, M. C. (2013). Aflatoxins as a cause of hepatocellular carcinoma. *J. Gastrointestin. Liver Dis.*, **22**, 305–310.

23. Safari, S., Motavaf, M., Seyed Siamdoust, S. A., and Alavian, S. M. (2014). Hepatotoxicity of halogenated inhalational anesthetics. *Iran. Red Crescent Med. J.*, **16**, e20153. doi: 10.5812/ircmj.20153.

24. Beutler, E., Hoffbrand, A. V., and Cook, J. D. (2003). Iron deficiency and overload. *Hematology Am. Soc. Hematol. Educ. Program*, 40–61.

25. Andersen, O., and Aaseth, J. (2016). A review of pitfalls and progress in chelation treatment of metal poisonings. *J. Trace Elem. Med. Biol.*, **38**, 74–80. doi: 10.1016/j.jtemb.2016.03.013.

26. Flora, S. J., and Pachauri, V. (2010). Chelation in metal intoxication. *Int. J. Environ. Res. Public Health*, **7**, 2745–2788. doi: 10.3390/ijerph7072745.

27. Dodmane, P. R., Schulte, N. A., Heires, A. J., Band, H., Romberger, D. J., and Toews, M. L. (2011). Airway epithelial epidermal growth factor receptor mediates hogbarn dust-induced cytokine release but not Ca^{2+} response. *Am. J. Respir. Cell Mol. Biol.*, **45**, 882–888. doi: 10.1165/rcmb.2010-0419OC.

28. Sayan, M., and Mossman, B. T. (2016). The NLRP3 inflammasome in pathogenic particle and fibre-associated lung inflammation and diseases. *Part. Fibre Toxicol.*, **13**, 51. doi: 10.1186/s12989-016-0162-4.

29. Liu, G., Cheresh, P., and Kamp, D. W. (2013). Molecular basis of asbestos-induced lung disease. *Annu. Rev. Pathol.*, **8**, 161–187. doi: 10.1146/annurev-pathol-020712-163942.

Chapter 3

Physicochemical Characterization: From Molecules to Particles

Scott C. Brown
The Chemours Company, 1007 Market Street, Wilmington, DE 19899, USA
scott.c.brown@chemours.com

In this chapter, the concept of physicochemical characterization and its application to chemical substances is further introduced. The origins of physicochemical properties in molecules and particles are highlighted from a materials interaction perspective. Similarities, differences, and nuances are noted when characterizing molecules present as a continuous phase versus as particulate species. The physicochemical characterization of nanomaterials is discussed in comparison to more traditional chemicals from a fit-for-purpose perspective highlighting similarities and differences based on modern knowledge. Current and future challenges in characterizing molecules and nanoscale materials for EHS purposes are also highlighted.

Physicochemical Properties of Nanomaterials
Edited by Richard C. Pleus and Vladimir Murashov

ISBN 978-981-4774-80-2 (Hardcover), 978-1-351-16860-1 (eBook)
www.panstanford.com

3.1 Introduction

Physicochemical characterization covers a broad spectrum of techniques and methods that aid in probing the interrelationship of chemistry and physical phenomena. The methods range from fundamental studies on subatomic particles to applied methods that probe the collective behavior of molecules, macromolecular, and (larger) particulate systems. For the purpose of this chapter, physicochemical characterization will be focused on molecules and particulate systems and their interaction with and distribution within biotic and abiotic systems. Less attention will be paid to factors resulting in intrinsic physical hazards (e.g., flammability and corrosivity) and chemical reactivity.

The physicochemical characterization of chemical substances is an essential part in the journey to understand and predict the impact of molecules and particles for human health and environmental applications. However, ensuring that characterization efforts are suitable and meaningful is not always straightforward due to the vast range of potential measurements, approaches, nuances, and varying interpretations of the data. Because of this, characterization needs to be approached in an interactive manner with careful attention to the necessary detail.

Moving from molecular to particulate systems adds complexity, greatly increasing sources of error and uncertainty, in addition to adding to the fundamental considerations. To deconvolute the most practical and meaningful path forward for characterizing the physicochemical properties of materials, an understanding of how the applied methods are confounded by other physicochemical properties and system variables is required, while keeping the overall purpose of the analysis in mind. For this reason, many confounding factors are noted throughout this chapter in order to highlight pertinent uncertainties.

3.2 Origins of Physicochemical Properties

Physicochemical properties—in both molecules and particles—originate from subatomic processes that give rise to intramolecular charges and electromagnetic fields that ultimately define how molecules and particles interact amongst themselves and with each other. In essence, the majority of relevant physicochemical properties can be attributed to the forces between molecules and between surfaces, either at present or through a series of past events (nonequilibrium processes). For instance, the boiling points (BPs) of liquids can be calculated from charge fluctuation (or van der Waals and hydrogen bonding) forces; and the shape of particles can be understood by following the balance between pertinent molecular interactions versus thermal and shear force histories during particle synthesis. It is important to note that history is an important concept when dealing with the physicochemical characterization of solids and multiphase systems. When processes are not fully reversible—or at least within the time frame of the experiment—then attention to detail on the sequence and content of historical events is often critical. The inability to rely on equilibrium phenomena and the need for explicit attention to phenomena such as order of interaction is a key distinguishing point when attempting to predict the behavior of particles versus molecules. The origin of this phenomena is based on nuances between particles and molecular interactions.

Chapter 2 highlighted the importance of molecular interactions in pharmacology and toxicology. In addition to interactions with biomolecules that define what a molecule might do in vivo, molecular interactions also define the phase behavior and likely environmental partitioning and exposure routes. Due to the importance of intermolecular and interparticle phenomena on the physicochemical properties of matter, they are briefly detailed later to provide perspective of the hierarchical and interwoven relationship between subatomic processes to molecular and larger particle-level interactions. It is important to realize that the same basic forces that dictate the behavior of gases and liquids also control particulate systems; however, nuances and considerations for the later are significantly more complicated. The major interactions that describe the association of molecules, their interconnection and their somewhat different treatment and manifestations for describing particulate systems are briefly described in the following sections to place context discussions in the ensuing sections of this chapter. For additional detail a number of excellent texts are available [1–7].

3.3 Intermolecular Interactions

How molecules interact depends on a number of factors, including their constituent atoms, atomic arrangement and bonding, relative proximity, concentration, and temperature. At a more fundamental level, the basis for all intermolecular interactions can be defined by the movement and partitioning of subatomic particles (e.g., electrons, protons, neutrons, and lesser known subatomic particles) that collectively give rise to electromagnetic fields and charge movements that dictate not only how molecules interact with other molecules but also how molecules interact with electromagnetic radiation. The latter phenomena enables the use of spectroscopic techniques (e.g., Raman and infrared spectroscopies) for identifying molecules and associations, which, in turn, also allows interactions with electromagnetic radiations predict the nature of interactions between particulate substances.

For descriptive purposes, intermolecular forces can be loosely categorized into three fundamental classes of interactions: (i) quantum-mechanical interactions, (ii) electrostatic interactions, and (iii) polarization interactions. These interactions are briefly detailed in the following sections and in Table 3.1. It should be noted that the classification is not intended to be rigid nor exhaustive, but merely for exemplary purposes.

3.3.1 Quantum-Mechanical Interactions

Herein we refer to quantum-mechanical interactions explicitly as interactions between subatomic particles that take place at atomic and subatomic length scales. Quantum-mechanical interactions give rise to the covalent bonding and charge transfer interactions. They also lay the basis for steric repulsion via Pauli's exclusion principle. Although the theory of quantum mechanics has been applied to describe or predict longer range electrostatic and polarization interactions, for the purpose of this chapter, those longer-range phenomena are treated as being distinct interactions. In this context, quantum-mechanical interactions result primarily in intramolecular versus intermolecular phenomena, but importantly impact intermolecular association by defining the movement of electrons and charges within a molecule and how they interact with electromagnetic radiation. As such, quantum-mechanical interactions play an important part of chemical characterization.

Table 3.1 Common types of interactions between molecules

Interaction class	Type	Dipole state	Interaction energy $w(D)$
Quantum-mechanical interactions	Covalent/ Metallic		Complicated
Electrostatic interactions	Ion–ion (coulombic)		$Q_1Q_2/(4\pi\varepsilon_0 D)$
	Ion–dipole	Fixed	$-Q\mathbf{u}\cos\theta/4\pi\varepsilon_0 D^2$
		rotating	$-Q^2\mathbf{u}^2/6(4\pi\varepsilon_0)^2kTD^4$
	Dipole–dipole (Keesom)	Fixed	$-\mathbf{u}_1\mathbf{u}_2[2\cos\theta_1\cos\theta_2 - \sin\theta_1\sin\theta_2\cos\varphi]/4\pi\varepsilon_0 D^3$
		Rotating	$-\mathbf{u}_1\mathbf{u}_2/3(4\pi\varepsilon_0)^2kTD^4$
	Hydrogen bond		Complicated
Polarization interactions	Ion–induced dipole		$-Q^2\alpha/2(4\pi\varepsilon_0)^2D^4$
	Dipole–induced dipole (Debye)	Fixed	$-\mathbf{u}\boldsymbol{\alpha}(1+3\cos^2\theta)/2\pi(4\pi\varepsilon_0)^2D^6$
		Rotating	$-\mathbf{u}^2\boldsymbol{\alpha}/(4\pi\varepsilon_0)^2D^6$
	Induced dipole–induced dipole (London, dispersion)		$-3h\nu\boldsymbol{\alpha}^2/64(\pi\varepsilon_0)^2D^6$

$w(D)$, interaction energy; Q, electric charge; **u**, electric dipole moment; $\boldsymbol{\alpha}$, electric polarization; D, distance between interacting atoms or molecules; k, Boltzmann constant; T, absolute temperature; h, Plank's constant; ν, electronic absorption (ionization) frequency; ε_0, dielectric permittivity of free space. Subscripts represent respective interacting bodies.

Note: Interaction forces are obtained by differentiating the energy $w(r)$ with respect to distance r.

Reprinted from Ref. [8], Copyright (1998), with permission from Elsevier.

Chemical characterization is distinct from physicochemical characterization. Physicochemical characterization addresses phenomena that is derived from the physical interactions between chemical constituents and not phenomena that lead to covalent or chemical bonds. Chemical bonds result in a complete change of the electron charge distributions of the participating atoms, resulting in an essential merger of the charge distributions and fields between atoms. This is in contrast to physical bonding, where the charge distributions of participating atoms are merely perturbed. Even though physical interactions are not as transformative as covalent bonding, they can be of similar strength and importantly can manifest themselves collectively and over much longer distances (e.g., several nanometers to centimeters versus angstroms). Physical interactions hold atoms and molecules together in solids and in liquids and in complex phase-segregated systems such as cellular and subcellular biological assemblies. While quantum-mechanical interactions define the nature and temporal charge distributions within a substance through subatomic processes and chemical modifications (i.e., chemical composition), larger-scale physical interactions describe the behavior of those chemical substances and serve as the primary origin of physicochemical properties. Indeed, physical interactions such as those described below are the primary regulating interactions in all environmental safety and health phenomena that do not involve chemical reactions and biological transformations.

3.3.2 Electrostatic Interactions

Electrostatic interactions originate from the coulombic force between charges and are pertinent for ions as well as for molecules exhibiting permanent dipoles. A dipole is a separation of positive and negative electrical charges that are inherent within a molecule (or molecular region) that contains no net charge. Molecules like water are polar and exhibit a dipole but do not have a net charge. In contrast, ions (e.g., dissolved chlorine from table salt in water) contain a net charge and sign.

Electrostatic interactions are by far the strongest physical interactions and can at times be stronger than covalent interactions (e.g., ionic interactions in salt crystals). These interactions define where ions and polar molecules are likely to associate and also dictate their solubility. In principle, solubility is strictly determined by the difference between the free energy of the substance as a solid and the free energy of the substance in solution. Integration of electrostatic interactions gives rise to solvation energies and self-energies that are dependent on the magnitude of charge, relative separation distances, and relevant dielectric susceptibilities. Indeed, good agreement is found between simple first principle estimations of solubility of simple ions and polar substance from purely electrostatic considerations [9]. The readers are referred to Refs. [1, 9] for a detailed discussion of the formulae and approaches to calculating solubility from electrostatic interactions for simple ionic and polar molecules.

There are four major types of electrostatic interactions that include charge–charge, charge–dipole, dipole–dipole, and hydrogen bonding. Some important notes regarding the significance of these interactions are provided next.

3.3.2.1 Charge–charge interactions

Charge–charge interactions are used to interpret the interactions of ions. These interactions are used to determine the lattice energies of traditional salt crystals together (e.g., NaCl), in addition to more complex ionic structures such as SiO_2 and TiO_2 [10]. They form the basis for understanding the movement of electrons and holes within and amongst ionic materials and also result in the unique properties of ionic liquids [11].

3.3.2.2 Charge–dipole interactions

Charge–dipole interactions are used to describe the solubility of salts and many metal oxides in nonionic polar solvents. Importantly, this interaction also describes the hydration of ions (e.g., the hydration number and hydronium ion) and serves as a molecular origin to the hydration forces between particles (discussed later). Ion–dipole interactions are strong and lead to structural solvation forces that have a number of industrial and biological implications [3]. These interactions are also result in the ionic nucleation of rain droplets in thunderclouds and provide the basis for using salts to increase BPs and suppress freezing points of important polar liquids like water.

3.3.2.3 Dipole–dipole interactions (Keesom interactions)

Dipole–dipole interactions (also known as Keesom interactions) describe the interaction of nonionic polar molecules. These interactions are not are not as strong as the ion interactions described above and usually is not strong enough to lead to any strong mutual alignment of molecules in the liquid state. Dipole–dipole interactions describe the miscibility of polar solvents and their interactions resulting in characteristic parameters like melting points (MPs), BPs, etc. Dipole–dipole interactions are also included in van der Waals interactions along with Debye and London interactions.

Hydrogen bonding is a form of dipole–dipole (Keesom) interaction where the particularly small size of the electron depleted H atom enables close approach to highly electronegative atoms such as –O, –N, and –F, resulting in a very strong field and attractive force. It is important to realize that proximity is a key determinate in the strength of interaction for all intermolecular forces. The closer the molecules, the stronger the interaction. Unlike typical dipole–dipole interactions, hydrogen bonding is strong enough to result in the structuring of molecules in liquids. The importance of the ability of intermolecular interactions to lead to structure development in liquids has practical significance when interpreting interparticle interactions. In the absence of structuring, solvation and hydration forces between particles are not believed to be possible.

3.3.3 Polarization Interactions

In all matter, thermal agitation and unavoidable quantum-mechanical uncertainties of the positions and momenta of subatomic particles lead to continuous fluctuations of charge and polarity at the subatomic level. This results in transient electric and magnetic fields that act on and react to other charges and fields. Polarization interactions arise from the induction of charge separation on molecule to form instantaneous dipoles due to the approach of one or more molecules and their corresponding electromagnetic fields. It is important to realize that polarization interactions can manifest themselves amongst all molecule types. However they are notably dominant in interactions with nonpolar molecules.

Polarization interactions are notably much weaker than their electrostatic and quantum-mechanical counterparts, but are more widespread and give rise to equally important phenomena. There are three general types of polarization interactions: ion–induced dipole, dipole–induced dipole, and induced dipole–induced dipole.

3.3.3.1 Ion–induced dipole interactions

Ion–induced dipole interactions result in the formation of an induced charge separation on the nonpolar molecule (or molecular regions) due to the approach of an ion and its electrical fields. This interaction impacts phenomena like the solubility of ions in nonpolar as well as weakly polar media.

3.3.3.2 Dipole–induced dipole interactions (Debye interactions)

Dipole–induced dipole interactions are also known as Debye interactions and like dipole–dipole interactions are a component of van der Waals interactions. Here a molecule exhibiting a dipole causes the electric fields to polarize on a nonpolar molecule (or molecular region) during approach. These are weaker interactions than dipole–dipole (Keesom) interactions, and ion–nonpolar interactions and are relatively sluggish.

3.3.3.3 Induced dipole–induced dipole interactions (London interactions)

The third type of interaction is also the most common as a permanent dipole or ion is not necessary. Induced dipole–induced dipole interactions are also known as London or dispersive interactions and are typically the major component of van der Waals interactions. These forces describe the association of all molecules and generally exceed the dipole dependent polarization interaction except for small highly polarizable molecules like water. The induced dipole–induced dipole interaction between nonpolar molecules is typically higher than the interaction between polar and nonpolar molecules, explaining immiscibility and providing one of key components of the hydrophobic force pertinent to particulates systems.

3.3.4 Complex Molecular Systems

Not all molecular interactions can be simplified into simple interactions between ions, polar molecules, and nonpolar molecules. As the size (and molecular weight [MW]) of molecules and the diversity of component properties increase, the overarching interactions between molecules become much more complex. As one moves from simple, small molecules to surfactants, to self-assembling polymer systems and biomolecules the necessary considerations and uncertainties substantially increase. As multiple regions within a molecule begin to participate in physical bonding, these differential interactions begin to alter the conformation of the host molecule as well as subsequent self-assembled macrostructures (or particles). Indeed, the collective contributions of molecular structure (shape) and constituent areas of differing intermolecular activity provides the basis for specific interactions and the foundation for the design and activity of many biomolecular systems (e.g., enzymes, antibodies). There are a number of treaties on the physicochemical characterization of complex macromolecules [3, 12–18]. It is important to realize that as molecules become more complex, of higher MW, and of lower solubility in their respective medium, their behavior becomes more particulate in nature. According to the International Organization for Standarization (ISO) a particle is defined a "minute piece of matter with defined physical boundaries" [17]. To have defined physical boundaries a substance must be phase-segregated from the continuous medium. Hence, solvated molecules do not exist as particles unless they are of sufficient MW or are self-assembled into a structure that can exist as a distinct phase. As this occurs, the collective increase in MW, the loss of independent molecular motility, and the onset of massive particulate Brownian dynamics facilitate longer range interactions across a medium defined by a blurred averaged of the constituent molecular interactions. The molecular nature of interactions in particulate systems become smeared due to increased distances at which the collective substance is "felt," in turn, because of the increased mass (and therefore electromagnetic charge density and field strength). Once this occurs, constituent molecules or interacting subunits do not have the ability optimize their own interactions—unlike when they are present individual molecules—

due to the overall particle momentum, providing further complexity. Considering these aspects, complex molecular systems can act like particles; after all particles are simply phase-segregated collections of molecules.

3.4 Particle–Molecule Interactions

Molecules interact with particles in a manner very similar to how they interact with themselves. The electrostatic, polarization, and quantum interactions that define molecular associations and behaviors also define how molecules interact with particle surfaces. However, there are nuances due to collective behavior of molecules, surface heterogeneity, competition effects, and particle structural effects. For the purpose of this chapter we will simplify molecular interactions with particles into two basic yet interconnected processes that will be important for the future discussions: adsorption and wettability.

3.4.1 Interactions Governing the Physical Adsorption of Molecules to Particle Surfaces

Adsorption is the process of a molecule migrating across a medium and adhering to a surface. The driving force for physical adsorption involves a balance between the prevailing electrostatic and electrodynamic interactions between the adsorbate molecules and the continuous phase and the surface. In many cases, unfavorable interactions between the adsorbate and the medium, often due to higher self-affinities of the medium molecules (recall the discussion on the origin of hydrophobic (desolvation) interactions in Section 3.3.3.3), can drive adsorbates to segregate or desolvate to interfaces including the surface of particles. This is often referred to as desolvation phenomena. Segregation-/desolvation-induced associations—such as those promoted by molecular hydrophobicity in water—only drive molecules to surfaces but do not necessarily keep them there. Favorable physical binding interactions between available regions of the segregated molecules and the surface need to exist to promote durable attachments. It is noted that the strongest and most efficient physical adsorption is often achieve via synergistic desolvation interactions and favorable electrodynamic or electrostatic surface anchoring. In part, this is due to the self-assembling nature of desolvating molecules as well as the additional driving force to the surface due to desolvation. It is dually notable that phase-segregated surfaces often have heterogeneous and structurally restricted active binding sites. This is due to the lack of independent thermal molecular motility of the solid surfaces. Hence, binding optimization is limited to the ability of the adsorbing molecules to optimally orient and displace solvent molecules. The inherent heterogeneity of surface sites lead to a distribution of binding affinities wherein a handful of strongly bound molecules act as anchors. Depending on solvency other molecules may self-assemble with these anchor molecules in the process of adsorption to the interface [19–21].

Because the physical adsorption of molecules has finite on and off rates, the persistence of the phenomenon is dependent on an appreciable adsorbate concentration in the continuous phase (recall binding discussions in Chapter 2). The magnitude of this dependency is typically linked to solvency of the adsorbate in the continuous phase and the strength of the binding affinity. It is worthwhile to note that the process of adsorption can in some instances increase the desolvation of the adsorbed molecule, for instance, when an ionized molecule becomes neutralized during the adsorption process, reducing the apparent polarity of the overall molecule. Also, in many real-world scenarios, multiple molecules in solution may compete for active surface adsorption sites on the particle surface. This competition between molecules for surface sites also depends on difference in binding, molecular solvency, and free concentrations in the continuous phase. Hence, physical adsorption is dynamically based on the constituents in the free continuous phase and the absorbed moieties are subject to change with changing environmental conditions.

3.4.2 Interactions Governing Particle Surface Wettability

Surface wettability is a measure of the affinity for the surface for a liquid versus the continuous phase, which is usually gas or vapor (commonly referred to as surface hydrophobicity when the solvent is water). As with adsorption phenomena, the same interactions that describe molecule–molecule associations also dictate surface wettability. For macroscopic surfaces, the wettability of surfaces is frequently described in terms of a contact angle, which is the smallest angle measured between a liquid and a flat surface through the liquid phase. A contact angle of 0° (~flat drop spread over a surface) signifies complete wetting, whereas a contact angle of 180° (~rounded droplet hardly in contact with the surface) signifies complete dewetting. Young's equation describes macroscopic contact angles as the result of a balance of overarching interfacial tensions at the liquid–vapor, solid–vapor, and liquid–solid interfaces. These interfacial tensions arise due to the fundamental molecular interactions described in Section 3.3. Often contact angles between a test surface and a series of pure test liquid of different ionic, dipole, induced-dipole, and hydrogen-bonding characteristics are used to estimate component interactions of the solid surface. Details of these methods can be found elsewhere [22, 23].

For small particles, contact angles cannot be directly measured on their surfaces however a range of methodologies exist to estimate their values [22–24]. These include film flotation, phase partitioning, pellet formation, capillary rise techniques, and critical surface pressure methodologies. It is important to note that for very small particles curvature effects can increase surface solubility, as discussed in detail by Iller [25]. It is also worth noting that surface wettability primarily involves interactions with the outermost layer of the particle surface. Hence the adsorption of molecule to the surface from the liquid phase or the partial solvation of the surface can have a significant impact on wettability. Notably, surface-active molecules are frequently used to aid in the wet-in of powders into highly cohesive solvents for this very reason. The adsorption of molecules to surfaces whereby solvent-loving molecular features are exposed to the bulk fluid results in improved wetting and solvent compatibility. As noted in the previous section, this can be a rather dynamic and environment-dependent process as adsorption and exchange are dependent on the composition in the continuous fluid phase.

3.5 Particle–Particle Interactions

In the previous section, the interactions between molecules and particles were briefly discussed. It was noted that binding sites on phase-segregated surfaces can lack conformational freedom, inhibiting the ability of free molecules to bind optimally to surfaces. These structural barriers at least for solid-phase materials add to the overall heterogeneity of surface-binding affinities for molecules to particles. Other phenomena like strain during or after particle formation can also result in changes in the apparent local electronic and magnetic fields and charge movements [26, 27].

In particle–particle interactions, molecular specificity (unless explicitly engineered in through attached molecular surface layers) is typically further lost. As two particle surfaces approach, the overall interaction is dictated by collective participation of molecules in the approaching interaction zone. The bulky nature of the particles (compared to individual molecules) and the structural confinement of surface groups—that often lack substantial conformational freedom (due to attachment and prevailing particle surface interactions)—results in more stochastic than equilibrium interactions upon contact. In particle–particle interactions near contact, shape, topology, and size become much more important than in molecule-particle interactions previously discussed. At far distances (e.g., several nanometers of separation), individual molecular contributions are further blurred and appear as part of a continuum of contributors participating in more equilibrium-like interactions typically referenced with respect to thermal energy. For small particles, the stochastic thermal fluctuations in particle movement or Brownian motion, represents the energy that needs to be overcome for either association or disassociation.

However, unlike considerations for molecules (wherein intermolecular forces are always dominant) for particle systems one must first determine the significance of intermolecular and surface interactions on the behavior of particles within the system. Interaction forces always describe a balance between the forces in question and the force that controls the movement of the molecules/particles. For molecules and small particles, movement is driven by thermal diffusion or Brownian energy; for larger-size or granular particles inertial forces and gravitational forces dominate their movement. In more simple terms, it is important to determine if the particles in question are large and act like grains of coarse sand (being driven by gravity and hydrodynamics) or as colloidal particles that are governed predominantly by the electrostatic and electrodynamic interactions previously discussed.

For colloidal particles, the predominant particle–particle interaction forces are van der Waals, electrostatic, steric, and solvation interactions. These interactions will be briefly detailed in the following sections.

3.5.1 Van der Waals Interactions

Van der Waals interactions between particles and surfaces are often dominant in many important phenomena like wetting, agglomeration, adsorption, and deposition, especially upon contact or at short separation distances (e.g., < 5nm). These interactions integrate a broad range of charge fluctuation or electrodynamic interactions and originate from the dynamic interaction of electric fields between molecules that make up the interacting particles as well as the intervening media. Between real materials, van der Waals attraction can originate from a widely varied umbrella of interactions, as indicated in Table 3.1 and previously discussed in the molecular interaction section. In principle, every charge movement that can respond to an applied electric field is a charge movement that can create transient electric fields and therefore is a component of van der Waals interactions. Consequently, hydrophobic and hydrogen-bonding forces are, in principle, van der Waals in nature (and coulombic interactions contribute to the overall van der Waals forces). London, Keesom, and Debye contributions, however, are often regarded as the classical, longer-range van der Waals components. The London, or dispersion, interaction is typically the most dominant due to the nonzero instantaneous dipole moments of all atoms and molecules. The Keesom and Debye interactions are also significant, yet they require the presence of permanent dipoles. The Keesom interaction originates from the attraction between rotating permanent dipoles, whereas the Debye contribution emanates from the interaction between rotating permanent dipoles and the polarizability of all atoms and molecules.

For most materials and colloidal systems, macroscopic continuum approaches for estimating van der Waals interactions are the most relevant. However, these methods are only valid over separation distances at which the surfaces can be treated as a continuum. In other words, the objects in question must be far enough apart such that they do not experience molecular or atomic features in their respective structures (i.e., the separation distance must be larger than the graininess of atomic packing). For most materials, separations down to ~20 Å are allowed. Upon contact a different approach to identifying the van der Waals attraction, namely the surface energy approach to adhesion, should be utilized. The latter is has similarity to the methods applied for measuring wettability.

3.5.2 Macroscopic Continuum Approach to van der Waals Attraction

From a macroscopic perspective, the van der Waals free energy is dependent on the difference between the dielectric susceptibility—or dielectric permittivity (ε)—of each of the bodies and the medium. This difference has traditionally been represented by the Hamaker constant (A) that incorporates the London, Keesom, and Debye interaction contributions.

Though it is denoted as a constant for historical reasons, it is important to recognize that the terminology is flawed due to the fact that the effective Hamaker constant can vary with separation distance. Distance-dependent variations in the Hamaker constant are largely due to retardation effects attributed from the finite velocity of electromagnetic signals and screening effects due to the presence of intervening ions. The frequencies at which charges and fields fluctuate are similar to those at which they resonate to adsorb electromagnetic energy, enabling the use of absorbance spectra for deriving Hamaker constants. This process is detailed elsewhere [1, 5, 28–30]. More simplistic estimations, such as the method proposed by Tabor and Winteron [31], use widely available parameters such as refractive indices and dielectric constants to provide reasonable estimates for some materials. Indeed, for many nonmetallic materials, Hamaker constants increase with increasing refractive index.

Table 3.2 Van der Waals attraction between different geometries

Geometry of interaction	Energy of interaction	Force of interaction
Two flat surfaces (infinite)	$\frac{A}{12\pi D^2}$	$\frac{A}{6\pi D^3}$
Spherical particle to flat surface (infinite)	$\frac{AR}{6D}$	$\frac{AR}{6D^2}$
Two spherical particles	$\frac{A}{6D}\frac{R_1R_2}{(R_1+R_2)}$	$\frac{A}{6D^2}\frac{R_1R_2}{(R_1+R_2)}$
Two crossed cylindrical rods	$\frac{A\sqrt{R_1R_2}}{6D}$	$\frac{A\sqrt{R_1R_2}}{6D^2}$
Two parallel cylindrical rods (equal length)	$\frac{AL}{12\sqrt{2}D^{2/2}}\sqrt{\frac{R_1R_2}{R_1+R_2}}$	$\frac{AL}{8\sqrt{2}D^{2/2}}\sqrt{\frac{R_1R_2}{R_1+R_2}}$

A, the Hamaker constant for the interacting materials across the medium; D, surface separation distance; R_1 and R_2, radius of the sphere and rod, respectively; L, length of rods.

Outside of retardation effects, the force and energy of interaction is largely dependent on the geometries that define the interaction zone—this is the case for all surface forces. As two bodies approach each other, the intervening area in which crosstalk can occur between electric fields from the opposing body increases (i.e., the interaction zone increases). The formulae for calculating the van der Waals interaction for some common geometries are given in Table 3.2. Note that these were derived using Dejaguin's approximation, which is valid for conditions in which the distance of significant van der Waals attraction is far less than the radius of the particles or cylinders [1], and that force is the negative differential of energy. A more detailed description of van der Waals forces, their origin and their calculation in complex systems can be found in an excellent text by Parsegian [5].

3.5.3 Electrostatic Interactions

For particle systems, "electrostatic interaction" refers specifically to either coulombic/static electric effects (interactions in air) or ion electrostatics (interaction in liquids). Electrostatic interactions typically operate over longer particle–particle separation distances than van der Waals and the other interactions that will be discussed in this chapter. Hence they tend to define the approach of particles from distant separations.

3.5.4 Coulombic/Static Electric Effects

Static electric effects impact aerosol particle deposition, powder segregation, dust generation, and static discharge (electrical arc formation) potential during powder handling. The potential for a particle to develop a charge depends on a wide range of variables. Fundamentally the electronic structure of the particulate material and its surface composition and structure will define the capacity for the particle to develop a charge, how that charge is distributed across the surface, and the persistence/capacity for the charge to be transferred or dissipated. Particles can gain electrostatic charge by electrical contact with a charged surface, through interactions with charged ions, through interaction with electromagnetic radiation, and by contact with surfaces not presenting a charge (e.g., triboelectric) along with other mechanisms. A review from thought leaders in the field provides a good overview of the mechanisms, current theories and knowledge gaps for the charging of powders through surface contact [32]. The movement and interactions between particles once charged is described by a balance of hydrodynamic drag and the coulombic force for small particles. This balance of coulombic interactions and hydrodynamics serves the basis of modern differential mobility analyzer system instruments that are capable of separating and measuring charged aerosols from roughly 1 to 1000 nm in mobility diameter.

3.5.5 Ion Electrostatics

In liquids, the presentations of electrostatic forces between particles are quite different. The ability of molecules to ionize leads to the generation of electrical fields and associated ion populations that can induce longer range interaction forces than the van der Waals interactions discussed in previous sections, but not as far reaching as the or static electric interactions above that are capable of operating over cm rather than a few nm. It is worth noting that the surface potential in aqueous system is typically on the order of millivolts, whereas charged aerosol can have surface potentials in at kilovolt levels. It is also further noted that the properties of these attractive or repulsive interactions are not adequately explained by the principles of dipole synchronization or coulombic interactions alone.

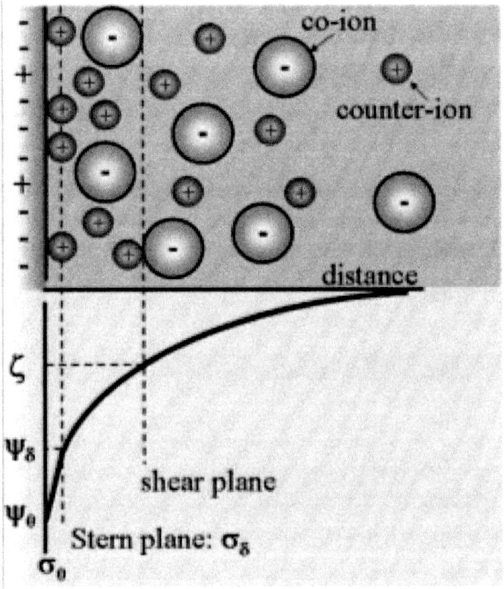

Figure 3.1 Schematic of the Stern–Grahme electrical double layer at a net negatively charged interface. Note that the zeta potential, z, is determined at the shear plane. y0 is the surface potential, and yδ is the Stern plane potential.

Instead the ion electrostatic interactions between particles in liquids are governed by surface group ionization and the adsorption and movement of ions and charged molecules in the solution environment. This can be described by the Gouy–Chapman model of the electrical double layer which postulates that counter ions exist in a diffused concentration gradient surrounding particles (Fig. 3.1). When these concentration gradients overlap an interaction zone develops where surface charge and osmotic effects combine (Fig. 3.2). Often the charges on particle surfaces are estimated by measuring a zeta potential. Note that zeta potential measurement only provides an indication of the mobility of a particle in a medium under a given electrical field using a number of assumptions. The potential provided from zeta potential measurements (see Chapter 4) is not a property of the particle surface but rather of a fluid shear plane a finite and often variable distance from the surface [33].

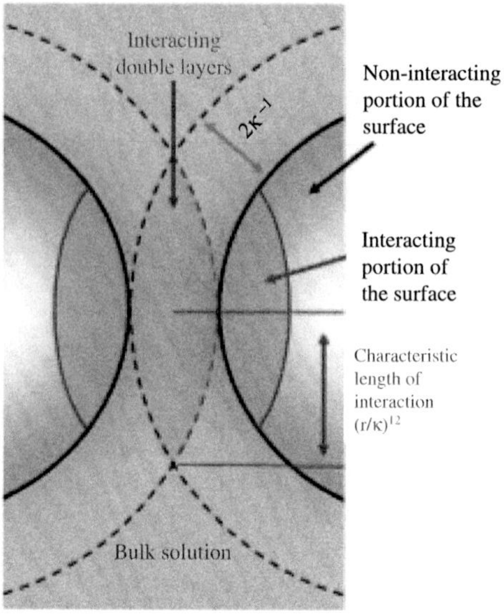

Figure 3.2 Double-layer interaction between two particles in a suspension of radius *r* and double-layer thickness κ^{-1}. Adapted from Ref. [34], Copyright (1999), with permission from Elsevier.

The presence of complex adsorbates can lead to electrostatic field- and shear-induced changes in charge due to the development of what is often referred to as a Donnan layer. A Donnan layer is essentially a deformable layer of material (e.g., biomolecules, polymers, gelatinous material) that present an external surface charge and has the potential to have internally associated ions. Hence deformation of the layer or the presentation of significant electrical field can induce surface and apparent potential changes. Donnan layers are common in biological systems and the illustration of a modified Gouy–Chapman model including a Donnan layer is shown in Fig. 3.3.

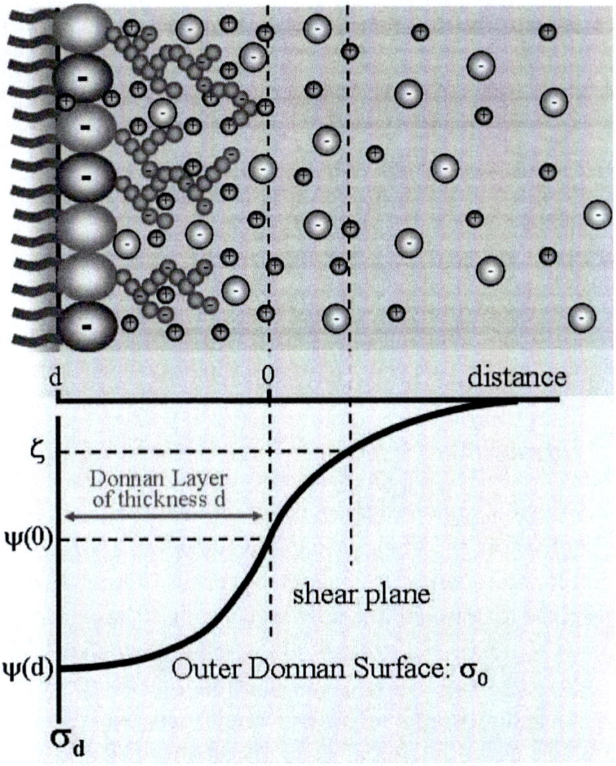

Figure 3.3 Schematic of the Ohshima–Ohki-modified Donnan double layer at a net negative interface, shown with a lipid-anchored surface. Note that the zeta potential, ζ, is determined at the shear plane. $\psi(0)$ is the outer Donnan layer surface potential, and $\psi(d)$ is the inner Donnan surface potential. Note, σ_d and σ_0 are the inner and outer Donnan surface charges, respectively.

It is outside of the scope of this chapter to go into detail regarding the estimation of electrostatic interactions. This has been the subject of nearly over a half century of research. However, it is important to note that as two charged surfaces approach one another the state of ionization and the state of adsorption of ions at the surface can change. This gives rise to further complexity and is often dealt with using range-bearing assumptions such as that of constant surface charge or constant surface potential [1]. However, charge regulation methods are also available [35]. Ion electrostatics is dealt with in detail in numerous texts. Knowledge gaps and commentary on the most useful information derived from characterization ion electrostatic properties have been enumerated by the International Union of Pure and Applied Chemistry (IUPAC). It is worth noting that the balance between ion electrostatic interactions and van der Waals interactions serves as the basis of the Derjaguin–Landau–Verwey–Overbeek (DLVO) theory that has proven useful to describe the behavior of many colloids in simple systems. The extended DLVO theory includes additional interactions and works toward describing more complicated systems. The interactions described in the following sections are included in extended DLVO treatments. DLVO interactions are also considered in Chapter 6.

3.5.6 Hydrophobic (Solvation) Interactions

In environmental and biological systems, solvation interactions dealing with water as the principle solvent are the most relevant. Hydrophobic interactions are attractive solvation interactions that occur when the major media constituent is water. These interactions result when water has a greater affinity for itself than the solid particle surfaces. Practically, these interactions begin to appear between particles when the contact angle between the particles and the liquid phase is greater than about 60°. It is noted that by nomenclature, surfaces are deemed hydrophobic when the contact angle with pure water is greater than 90°, but practically speaking, attractive interactions can develop between surfaces with lower contact angles.

The presence of hydrophobic surfaces leads to attraction between those surfaces in water. As discussed in previous sections, hydrophobic forces in the purest sense are a form of van der Waals interaction and can in some situations be described adequately through the approximations and methods mentioned previously. However, in practice, hydrophobic forces often occur over very long distances that are not predicted though electrodynamic effects alone. Indeed, Higashitani and others identified that long-range hydrophobic forces were due to dissolved gases present in the liquid phase [36]. The dissolved gas nucleated as nanobubbles on the surface of particles and those bubbles mediated the long-range interactions. In addition to gases, small amounts of hydrophobic liquids can also result in similar long-range behaviors.

It should be noted that normally hydrophilic surfaces can be rendered hydrophobic due to the adsorption of surfactants or lipids on their surfaces at low concentrations typically referred to the hemimicelle regime and that hydrophobic surfaces can be rendered hydrophilic through the same mechanism. Also the ionization of surface sites can be an important component for defining the nature of solvation interaction on surface. Charged surface are typically more hydrophilic than surfaces that are not ionized.

3.5.7 Hydration (Solvation) Interactions

Repulsive solvation forces arise in aqueous environments between particles whenever water molecules bind strongly to hydrophilic surface groups—these repulsive interactions are commonly termed "hydration interactions" and are of solvation origins. In essence, during the close approach between surfaces intervening water molecules provide a physical barrier, shielding the underlying surface from direct interaction with opposing surfaces. It is believed that the forces induced from bound water or hydration layers are a direct reflection of the energy required to dehydrate surface molecules (often hydrogen bonding functional groups) as two surfaces approach one another. Between rigid surfaces, such as hydrated crystals, these forces are often oscillatory due to what has been hypothesized to be the formation and collapse of multiple layers of ordered water molecules between the two surfaces. Essentially as hydrated rigid surfaces are brought together the water molecules will order between the surfaces to conserve space, until at a certain distance and a corresponding repulsive force maximum, at which the structure critically fails resulting in a momentary attraction for osmotic reasons until the structures reform and the cycle repeats itself. These oscillations have been measured with a periodicity of the diameter of a water molecule (0.25 nm), hence they appear to be attributed to a layer by layer restructuring and failure process [37, 38]. Hydration forces in biologically and environmentally relevant systems are thought to arise from two primary mechanisms, either from intrinsic hydrophilicity in which hydrogen bonding is involved as in the case of the ethylene oxide and sugar groups or through an induced hydrophilicity that is regulated by ion exchange in which water structure is coordinated by hydrated ions. In the latter case, strong surface associations (binding) with hydrated ions such as Na^+, Li^+, or Mg^{2+} lead to induced hydration forces; hence, this mechanism is highly dependent on the type and concentration of ionic species present [1].

Though much research has focused on hydration forces, their absolute origin remains unclear. In the case of monotonically repulsive hydration forces, a number of unconfirmed theories exist as well as experimental examples which counter the described mechanisms [39]. Much of this is likely the result of mistaken identity, since—as mentioned earlier—it is particularly difficult to measure hydration forces exclusively in such systems where steric forces can co-reside. Provocative examples of hydration forces in simulated biological systems exist. For instance, Duzgunes, Wilschut, and coworkers [40] showed that phosphatidylserine vesicles fuse in dilute $CaCl_2$ solutions but not in $MgCl_2$ solutions, which is thought to be due to the greater hydration of Mg^{2+} ions, which may prevent the surfaces from coming into sufficient close contact for fusion to occur. However, it is also becoming evident that in many biologically and environmentally relevant systems, these hydration forces do not act alone to prevent adhesion between surfaces upon close contact. Indeed, many experiments seem to indicate that steric forces could dominate repulsion in biological interactions, and that hydration forces may simply aid in this process. Hydration forces are consider to be the most important of the least understood interaction forces encountered in colloidal science and biology.

3.5.8 Steric Interactions

Steric forces originate for quantum-mechanical considerations. Pauli's exclusion principle states that two electrons cannot have the same quantum state. This leads to a very steep rise in energy when the electron shell of one atom starts to penetrate the electron shell of another. The end result is repulsion and the inability of two objects from occupying the same space at the same time.

When thermally active surface-bound moieties are confined between two interfaces leading to a decrease in entropy, an opposing force develops, known as steric repulsion. In general, the forces that arise in opposition to unfavorable changes in configuration entropy of surface bound molecules or structures fall under the umbrella of steric forces. With some respects, the hydration force visited in the previous section are believed to emanate from similar intermolecular and thermodynamic origins; however, in principle steric interactions are different, particularly since, in many cases, they are rather solvent independent. As with hydration forces, the presence of steric forces in biological and environmental interactions are almost a given. Biological surfaces are inherently rough at the nano- and the angstrom scale and their asperities are typically comprised of constructs (e.g., sugar residues, proteins), which exhibit molecular-scale thermal fluctuations.

In the classical sense, steric forces are most commonly thought of when a rigid surface coated by protruding, fluctuating polymers chains is brought in close enough proximity to an opposing rigid surface. Though this is perhaps the most common form of steric repulsion reported in the literature and described by colloidal scientists; one must recognize that there are a wide variety of steric forces which can emanate from surfaces, particularly those that are as a whole, thermally active, such as the case of the plasma membrane of living cells [1].

It is import to not that particle systems that use steric adsorbates to prevent agglomeration are also subject to the phase behavior of those adsorbates. Meaning that under conditions where the adsorbed polymers become incompatible with the medium, attraction rather than repulsion between macromolecule-coated particles occurs [4]. It is important to note that critical flocculation temperatures and other environmental conditions for polymer stabilized particles exist above or below which flocculation is eminent. These temperature and environmental conditions are frequently consistent with the theta points for the free polymer. Hence the behavior of sterically stabilized particles is often strongly influenced by the solvency of the adsorbed molecular layers.

3.6 Collective and Complex Interparticle Interactions

As seen in the previous sections, particle–particle interactions emanate from the collective electrodynamic and electrostatic interactions that exist between the molecules that make up the particles, the molecules and ions adsorbed to particle surfaces, and the molecules in the medium between the particles. Not only are the interactions important but also the geometries and the molecular structure of the approaching particles and how those surfaces dynamically interact with the intervening medium.

Although many of the component interactions are known and are understood at a fundamental level, it still remains a challenge to fully predict the interaction between particles a priori, especially with real materials. Confounding factors due to particle structure, chemical heterogeneity and the dependence on the intervening media (as well as other environmental factors) greatly complicate our predictive capabilities.

Besides particle shape and topography, particle history can also be a critical because not all interactions with particles surfaces are completely reversible (e.g., adsorption of molecules from solution) within the timescales of pertinent interactions. This stresses the need for phenomenological measurements since particle systems are confounded not only by shape, size, and surface properties but also by the distributions of these properties that describe the particle system as well as the individual history of the particles in the system. In comparison to purely molecular systems, particulate systems comprise far more confounding factors, nuances, and ill-defined parameters that further complicate and distinguishing particle interactions from purely molecular interactions.

Furthermore the particle–particle interactions in the previous section are only dominant when the motion of the interacting particles is predominantly controlled by thermal or Brownian motion. As particles grow larger or as agglomeration ensues, gravitational interactions become dominant and the pertinent interactions can shift toward inertia or flow-based phenomena. The particle Peclet number is a convenient way of determining the interaction regime of particles and is describe in the next section.

3.6.1 The Particle Peclet Number

Peclet numbers are dimensionless numbers commonly applied to identify the relative importance between advection and diffusional transport processes. Particle Peclet numbers (Pe) provide insight into the primary modes of particle association within a system. Surface and intermolecular forces dominate interactions in the diffusional transport regime while mechanical and gravitational forces dominate interactions in the advective regime. The particle Peclet number is defined as the balance between Stokes sedimentation versus the Stokes–Einstein diffusion for individual particles and is given as

$$\mathrm{Pe} = 4\pi\Delta\rho g a^4/3k_{\mathrm{B}}T, \tag{3.1}$$

where $\Delta\rho$ is the difference in density between the particle and the medium, a is the radius of the equivalent settling solid sphere, g is the gravitational acceleration constant, k_{B} is the Boltzmann constant, and T is the temperature of the system. A Pe value of 1 represents the equivalence point between Brownian motion and inertial motion dominance. Accordingly, a Pe value of much less than 1 indicates that interactions are Brownian or surface and intermolecular force interaction dominated, whereas a Pe value of more than 1 indicates that the system is in the inertial-force-dominated, orthokinetic regime where surface and intermolecular force play a negligible role. Through this comparison it can be shown that the behavior of nanoparticles is somewhat between the behavior of molecules and granular particles, that the explicit change in interaction behavior depends not only on size but also on the relative density difference between the particles and the medium, and that there does not exist a clear behavioral shift discretely observed at for particles of 100 nm in diameter—rather for many common systems the behavior between a 50 nm, 100 nm, and 300 nm particles are frequently similar. Hence, from purely fundamental interaction considerations, granular particles are more different than traditional molecules than nanoparticles. In this chapter, details into complex orthokinetic or inertia dominated interactions will not be given. The primary focus will be on surface and intermolecular force contributions to particulate behavior; however, it is noted that as Brownian motion dominated systems begin to coarsen due to agglomeration, orthokinetic phenomena will eventually need to be considered to fully capture the behavior of the particle systems [41, 42].

3.7 Principles of Physicochemical Characterization

As evident from the previous sections, the origins of physicochemical properties are both intramolecular and intermolecular. However, as the substance and the systems become more complicated in structure and the interactions become more diverse, estimations from first principles become challenging, requiring direct characterization.

Physicochemical characterization covers a broad range of properties at differing levels of complexity. For seemingly mundane parameters like particles size or even water solubility, there are a multitude of different techniques and approaches available that could be used for characterization purposes. A challenge in physicochemical characterization is choosing the identifying the most meaningful measurands and the best-possible approaches for measurement. Competent physicochemical characterization requires an understanding of (i) the purpose for characterization, (ii) the nuances and limitation of the methods involved, and (iii) the interconnection of the properties measured with other substance properties and text matrix parameters. These principles are universally applicable and need to be considered when planning and evaluating experiments.

3.8 Interactions, Dependencies, and Hierarchy

Some physicochemical properties have a strong dependency and interaction with the surrounding test environment, while others do not. Properties that are independent of the surrounding environment are termed "intrinsic," and those that are dependent on the environment are termed "extrinsic." An intrinsic property of a substance is dependent mainly on the chemical composition and molecular structure of matter (i.e., a result of chemistry and intermolecular interactions within the material). They are characteristically independent of the amount of mass and size of the constituent particles. Extrinsic properties, on the other hand, are largely dependent on system or test environment (e.g., media, temperature, volume, shear) properties. Because of the interrelationship between system properties, substance concentration, and endpoint, extrinsic properties are far more complicated to measure. Difficulties in simulating real-world conditions in the laboratory,are likely to result in complications leading to discrepancies. Hence it is typically recommended to measure extrinsic properties under multiple experimental conditions and in particular under conditions that (i) facilitate substance comparison and (ii) that more reasonably resemble real-world scenarios through appropriate media choices and timescales [1, 2]. Because of the complications in measuring extrinsic properties, intrinsic properties are typically used to identify substances and are considered characteristic properties of materials. Examples of intrinsic and extrinsic properties are found in Table 3.3.

Table 3.3 Example intrinsic and extrinsic physicochemical properties

Intrinsic properties	Extrinsic properties
Boiling point	Dissolution behavior
Melting point	Dustiness
Crystallinity	Surface and interfacial properties
Density	Active site populations
Refractive index	Available surface area
Dielectric constant	Dispersibility
Work function/band gap	System rheology

However, intrinsic and extrinsic considerations, by themselves, also do not capture full complexity of chemical substance characterization. There exists a property hierarchy wherein basic intrinsic, extrinsic, and system (surrounding environment) properties give rise to more confounded substance behaviors. Subsequently, multiple behaviors result in effects, which are generally the macroscopic phenomena of interest (e.g., exposure). This hierarchy is depicted in Fig. 3.4. It is noted that "history," "[substance] abundance," and "time" also feed into extrinsic properties as described in the present chapter. This is done to highlight the influence of history (e.g., sample preparation, processing, storage) and experimental time frame on extrinsic properties. In many cases, these parameters are not sufficiently reported. Relevant timescales and sample history are known to impact results particularly for rate and surface dependent phenomena like dissolution, agglomeration, and adsorption.

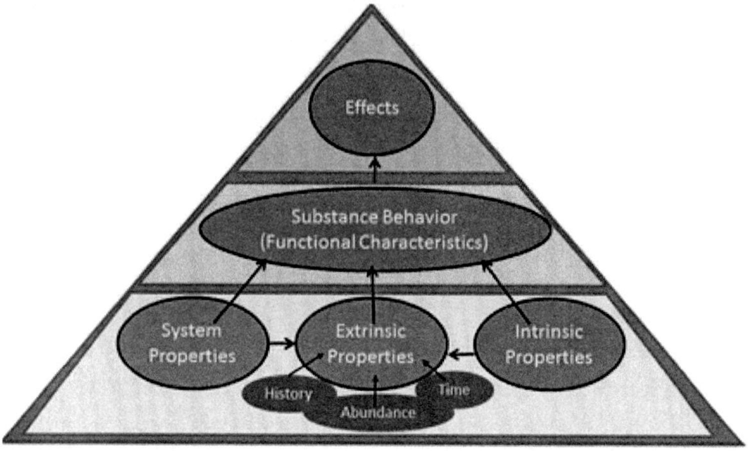

Figure 3.4 Illustration of the physicochemical property hierarchy. Basic system, intrinsic, and extrinsic properties combine to exhibit substance behaviors. Substance behaviors collectively combine to ultimately produce effects.

Although recently brought to the spotlight of physiochemical characterization for environmental, health, and, safety (EHS) purposes [42, 43], functional assays are commonly applied in industry, in the field of particle science, and have been a cornerstone of modern risk assessment for some time. Functional assays are defined as measurement strategies aimed at describing substance behaviors that are predictive of highly confounded final effects. Octanol-/water-partitioning coefficients, dustiness indexes, biochemical oxygen demand, and dissolution testing are examples of functional characteristics or substance behaviors that are currently used in risk assessment. Bulk powder flow, system rheology, and spontaneous dispersion are some functional characteristics frequently used in industry and in particle science. The underlying principle is that the isolation and characterization of key behaviors that are more closely related to important effects is a more efficient route to predicting critical phenomena than attempting to measure and characterize the myriad of basic physicochemical properties that feed into that behavior. Figure 3.5

various surface, particle, and solvent exposure properties feed into dissolution behavior.

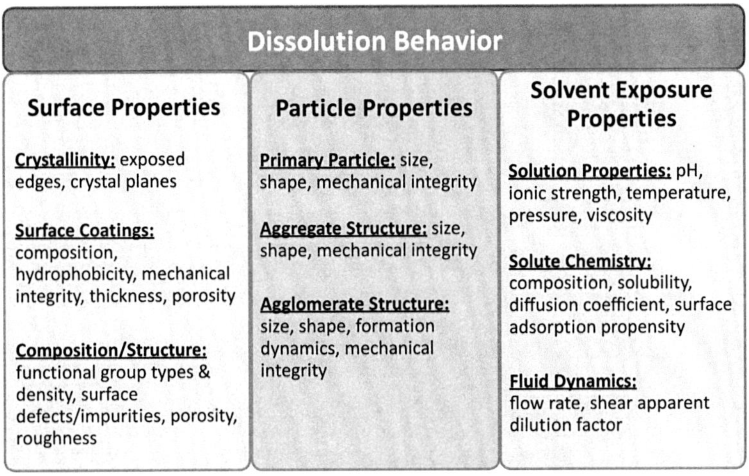

Figure 3.5 Properties that influence dissolution behavior.

As one could imagine, the direct measurement of dissolution behavior in complex environments is typically simpler and more efficient than attempting to predict the phenomena from lower- level properties. The route to identifying key behaviors is empirical and a number of statistical tools are available aid in their identification. These tools are typically enumerated in Six Sigma coursework in industry or through statistical design-of-experiments coursework in academia.

3.9 Characterizing for Purpose and Not for Endpoint: The Fit-for-Purpose Criterion

Often, multiple approaches to measure a physicochemical parameter will exist and the identification of the best option should, in part, depend on the intended purpose for the measurement with consideration of the inherent properties of the substance to be tested. The fit-for-purpose criterion is aimed at ensuring that ensuing test methods will fulfill the intended purpose in terms of scientific rigor, comparability, reliability, and practicality.

As elucidated in the preceding section, it is important that characterization is done consciously and not simply to arrive at an endpoint. The vast majority of physiochemical parameters are extrinsic in nature adding additional procedural concerns. It is not uncommon for standard protocols to be found not fit-for-purpose for certain substances. Deviations need to be identified and raised in order to continually refine and improve methods for all relevant substances. Examples of common questions used to determine if a physicochemical characterization method suitable for an intended purpose are described in Table 3.4. Due diligence on this assessment becomes more important as the test materials become more complex, as tested parameters lie higher in the property hierarchy and with the introduction of new, less familiar test methods.

Table 3.4 Common questions used to determine fit-for-purpose status

Questions	Dimension
Is the fundamental measurement suitable for the intended purpose? Are more suitable, reasonable alternatives available?	Relevance
Are the test matrix and testing timescales appropriate for the test substance and intended use of the resulting information?	Relevance
Is the method robust enough to facilitate comparisons across laboratories, as needed?	Reliability
Are the controls and calibration practices suitable and relevant for the substances of interest?	Reliability
Are sample preparation and sampling adequately addressed?	Adequacy
Have potential material incompatibilities and interferences been addressed?	Reliability
Is the test overly tedious for the intended purpose?	Practicality/ relevance
Are the assumptions applied to arrive at measure and acceptable/valid?	Relevance
Is the test substance unintentionally transformed during analysis?	Relevance

3.10 Reporting

Sufficient reporting is an essential part of characterization and ultimately will define the impact of the associated study. Reporting should be sufficient to clearly describe the substance being tested as well as the methods being used to determine physicochemical parameters. For particulate systems, emphasis needs to be placed on sufficiently describing sample preparation and sample history. Frequently, the materials and methods applied for the determination of the physicochemical properties of substances are not sufficiently detailed in reports leading to a substantial amount of uncertainty and inability to compare results or draw collective property-effect relationships. In particular, a lack of sufficient physicochemical characterization as well as insufficient reporting in nanotoxicology data was identified as significant challenges [44–50]. It is imperative that sufficient detail be provided to enable duplication of the characterization method in another laboratory as well as sufficient characterization to enable the assessment of material similarities. In addition to physicochemical properties, chemical purity is often not specified or reported, in particular in studies involving lab synthesized particles. Although guidelines for reporting may be found with standard method procedures; on occasion, those recommendations may not be fully suitable for the specific substance being evaluated. Exceptions are not uncommon and it is important to consider whether or not additional information is required to engender the reproduction of testing or to allow for substance comparisons in all scenarios.

3.11 Standard Methods and Reference Materials

To promote harmonization and aid in comparability, a number of international and national organizations serve society by providing for methods and frameworks for characterizing chemical substances developed by experts. These organizations include the Organization of Economic Co-operation and Development

(OECD), IUPAC, the ISO, ASTM International (ASTM), the United States Environmental Protection Agency (US EPA), the European Committee for Standarization (CEN), the American National Standards Institute (ANSI), the British Standards Institute (BSI), the Standards Council of Canada (SCC), Standards Australia (SAI), and others. It is noted that often, regional differences in the standards do exist (e.g., water solubility) and the methods are often continually in flux in order to adapt to new technologies, identified changes in information scope, and new, more complicated substances. When possible it is recommended to adhere to standard protocols, when available; however, an assessment of whether a protocol remains fit-for-purpose for the substance and scenario in question needs to be evaluated. Relevant reference materials as close to the test substance as possible with respect to detection sensitivity and material properties should be used when applicable and available.

3.12 Physicochemical Characterization: From Molecules to Particles

The physicochemical characterization of molecules encompasses the characterization of traditional chemicals as well as particle systems. After all, particles are composed of molecules, yet have very different interaction potentials due to their size and the type of interfaces present. As one moves for characterizing a molecule to a particle (or nanoparticle) new considerations need to be dealt with as indicated in the preceding sections, and testing strategies may require modification. However, the overall purpose of the characterization remains similar; re-emphasizing a need to maintain a focus on the end goal. With this, it is important to note that physicochemical properties by themselves are not sufficient to infer potential risk. Rather the intrinsic hazards of the chemical substance are an essential starting point that is often only modified by physicochemical parameters. Indeed, most physicochemical parameters tend to impact the fate and transport of materials, resulting in changes in exposure processes and potentially local dose.

3.13 Review of Select Physicochemical Properties: Molecules

Prior to linking the application of physiochemical parameters to their purposeful use in risk assessment, it is important to briefly describe key parameters and importantly how one or more parameters can be applied to estimate others.

3.13.1 Flammability, Corrosivity, and Oxidizing Ability

Flammability, corrosivity, and oxidizing ability are largely related to chemical reactivity and chemical characterization, albeit frequently included in the physical hazard characterization of chemicals. Flammability is the ability of a substance to burn or ignite, causing fire or combustion. Flammability is correlated with chemical composition and a variety of test protocols exist to quantify flammability through fire testing. Corrosivity is associated with the ability of a molecule to cause destruction of the human skin at the site of contact for a specific duration of time. Chemicals that do not degrade skin but do corrode steel or aluminum are also considered corrosive. Oxidizing ability is the ability of a chemical to cause or enhance the combustion of another chemical by yielding oxygen.

3.13.2 Molecular Weight

The MW of a substance is the sum of the atomic weight of all the atoms in a molecule. Macromolecules, such as polymers, may not have a single MW but rather exist as a distribution of MWs. The MW of a polymer is frequently reported as a number-average weight (the sum of the MWs of molecules divided by the number of molecules). A number of methods exist for measuring the MW distribution of a polymer system. Along with the MW of a molecule its apparent size and shape also play a role in molecular interactions.

3.13.3 Boiling Point

The BP of a liquid is the temperature at which its vapor pressure (VP) is equal to the atmospheric pressure. A liquid boils when the attractive forces between its molecules is overcome by thermal energy. In general the stronger intermolecular cohesion, the higher the BP for a molecule at a given pressure. Accordingly, the BPs of substances in a homologous series of substances generally increase in a uniform manner with increasing MW. A number of different methods are available to estimate the BP of liquids from molecular structure alone [51]. The thermal energy or heat required to overcome intermolecular attractive forces is termed the latent heat of vaporization. Most solid substances melt to a liquid phase prior to boiling; however, a few materials go directly from a solid to a gaseous state and sublime. The sublimation temperature of a substance is analogous to the BP.

Boiling and sublimation temperatures provide an indication of the volatility of a substance. These parameters can be used to estimate the VPs of substances, which provides information regarding inhalable content. A number of methods are available to determine BPs, including (i) the use of an ebulliometer, (ii) the vapor recondensation method, (iii) the distillation method, (iv) the Siwolloboff method, (v) and the photocell method.

3.13.4 Vapor Pressure

The VP of a substance is the pressure at which a liquid and its vapor are in equilibrium at a given temperature. This occurs when the rate of condensation of vapor and the rate of evaporation are equivalent.

The VP, like the BP, is an indication of the volatility of a substance. Several experimental procedures are available for its measurement including the isotensiscope technique and the gas saturation method. Since the VP of a substance is also related to electrostatic and electrodynamic interactions between pure substances, it too can be reasonably predicted by a number of methods.

3.13.5 Henry's Law Constant

Henry's law constant describes the propensity of a molecule to partition from the gas phase to the aqueous phase and vice versus. It is frequently presented as the equilibrium concentration of a particular molecule in air to its concentration in water. In this form, a higher Henry's law constant indicates a greater tendency of a molecule to volatize, indicating a dominance of thermal motion over water-molecule interactions. Low Henry's law constants are indicative of relatively strong interactions between a molecule and water [52].

3.13.6 Water Solubility

The water solubility of a substance is the maximum amount of the substance that will dissolve in a given volume of water at a specified temperature and pressure. There are a number of methods and standard techniques to determine water solubility. The two most common experimental methods are the shake-flask and generator column methods [51, 53–56]. Due to the number of extrinsic factors that can complicate water solubility measurements it is not uncommon to have significant variability, even if measured using the same substance and same method. For instance, for many substances pH of water is important and internal strain or high levels of curvature in a material can lead to supersaturation in the aqueous phase [25].

The importance of water solubility for a number of purposes has led to several methods for its estimation. As described by Yalkowsky and Banerjee, water solubility is governed by the entropy of mixing and the difference between the solute–solute, water–solute, and water–water adhesive interactions. For solid materials, additional electrostatic intermolecular interaction associated with the lattice energy of solids must also be taken into account. These estimates tend to work better for liquid substances, in particular due to the greater variability of solid constituents. For solid materials of the same substance the method of preparation of the material, its structure and surface properties can alter the observed water solubility following guideline testing protocols. Hence, a priori intermolecular interaction parameters estimates for idealized solid substances may not be sufficient for quantitative solubility predictions. Accurate estimation of water solubility is generally difficult for solid substances and typically requires direct measurement.

3.13.7 Octanol–Water Partition Coefficient

The octanol–water partition coefficient is commonly expressed as K_{ow} or as P. It is defined as the ratio of a chemical's concentration in the octanol phase to its concentration in the aqueous phase of a two-phase octanol–water system. The equation for K_{ow}, or P, is

$$K_{ow} = \frac{[\text{chemical substance}]\text{ in n} - \text{octanol}}{[\text{chemical substance}]\text{ in water}}, \tag{3.2}$$

where concentrations are given in mols/L.

The octanol–water partition coefficient is not the same as the ratio of a chemical's solubility in octanol to its solubility in water. It is important to note that both water and octanol have some mutual solubility and therefore do not exist as pure substances when present together. K_{ow} is used as a relative measure of lipophilicity. For simplification K_{ow} is often reported as its common logarithm (log K_{ow}, or log P). While a substance with a large positive log P is considered lipophilic due to a stronger interaction for the oil phase, a molecule with a negative log P has a stronger interaction with water than octanol and is hydrophilic. For reference, a chemical substance with a log P of 1 has ten times the affinity for n-octanol than it has for water, whereas a chemical substance with a log P of –1 has ten times the affinity for water than n-octanol.

For ionizable substances, log D, or the partitioning distribution coefficient is used and determination is analogous to log P, except that aqueous system parameters may be varied, resulting in changes in partitioning due to charge development. Log D is pH dependent and represents the partitioning of both ionized and nonionized species as a function of aqueous testing conditions. When a substance is not ionizable then log P and log D are equivalent. Log D for acids/bases can be readily calculated when pK_a values and log P for the nonionized form are known. Hence, log P will primarily discussed in the ensuing discussions.

Several methods for measuring the octanol–water partition coefficient exist. As with water solubility, a number of system and methodological factors can impact the outcome. Hence the advantages and disadvantages of the methods to be applied need to carefully considered with regards to the properties and form of the substance to be tested. Common methods include the shake-flask method, the slow-stir method, and the generator column method. A number of methods for estimating log K_{ow} are available and commonly include intermolecular interactions estimates. These methods have been reviewed elsewhere [57–60].

3.13.8 Acidity (pK_a)/Ionization State

Many molecules undergo ionization with pH, resulting in a change in their apparent hydrophobicity (e.g., apparent log *P*, log *D*). The pK_a of a molecule represents the pH at which 50% of its acidic sites are ionized. Molecules tend to be more lipophilic at pH values lower than their pK_a or when they are less ionized.

3.13.9 Soil/Sediment Adsorption Coefficient

The soil/sediment adsorption coefficient (soil sorption coefficient in Fig. 3.6), K_{oc}, is a measure of the tendency of a chemical to be adsorbed onto soil or sediment. K_{oc} is defined as the ratio of the amount of a substance adsorbed per unit weight of organic carbon in soils or sediments to the concentration of the chemical in solution at equilibrium:

$$K_{oc} = \frac{\mu\text{g adsorbed/g organic carbon}}{\mu\text{g/mL solution}} \tag{3.3}$$

Substances that interact strongly with organic carbon matter and less with water will have a high K_{oc}. Values of K_{oc} can range from 1 to 1×10^7.

An experimental protocol for determining K_{oc} that involves the determination of an adsorption coefficient *K* using an assumed adsorption model to calculate K_{oc} has been provided by the US EPA [56]. Other methods are available to estimate K_{oc} from empirical relationships with other properties, as reviewed by Lyman [51]. Methods also exist that predict K_{oc} from molecular connectivity indices and fragment descripts that are highly based on molecular accessibility and interaction forces [61]. Discussions on soil and sediment adsorption are available elsewhere [62].

3.13.10 Hydrogen Bonding

The capacity to hydrogen bond is recognized as an important property related to the membrane permeation of molecules. Various scales expressing hydrogen bonding have been developed [63]. The availability of hydrogen bonding groups for external bonding is an important parameter; however, deciphering availability can be complicated for larger molecules.

3.13.11 ΔE Energy [HOMO–LUMO]: Reactivity

Frontier orbital energies (highest occupied molecular orbital [HOMO], lowest unoccupied molecular orbital [LUMO]) provide an indication of chemical reactivity with nucleophiles and electrophiles which translates to the potential reactivity with biomolecules in vivo. For instance, molecules with a ΔE (difference between HOMO and LUMO energies) greater than 9 eV as calculated by semi-empirical methods have recently been shown to be much less likely to be acutely or chronically toxic to aquatic species [64, 65].

3.14 Review of Select Physicochemical Properties: Particles

Particles add to the overall complexity of analysis and add a need to be cognizant of a broader range of parameters in order to access their potential impact.

3.14.1 Dustiness

For chemical substances in powder form, dustiness is a relevant parameter that describes the propensity of a material to aerosolize by a prescribed mechanical stimulus. Dustiness testing is intended to replicate mechanisms of dust generation encountered when handling a material. In essence dustiness is a measurement of the ability of particle–particle interactions to be broken by agitation resulting in suitably fine particles or particle clusters that become airborne. As such, dustiness is impacted by a number of extrinsic and system properties that impact particle interactions, such as static charge, humidity (capillary interactions), material shape, bulk density (how the material is initially packed, that is, number of physical particle–particle bonds that may need to be broken), and particle size distribution (PSD). A number of techniques are available to measure dustiness, including the rotating-drum, continuous-drop, and single-drop methods [66–72].

3.14.2 Dissolution Rate

For particulate substances, water solubility data provides limited information since it refers to equilibrium conditions that may not be practically achievable when dealing with particulate systems given the relative timescales of dissolution and fluid turnover. Dissolution is a dynamic process driven by the affinity of a solvent to interact with a solid surface. It is highly dependent on the properties of the exposed surface as well as fluid conditions (e.g., composition, volume, flow rate, pH, solutes; see Fig. 3.5). An increase in dissolution rate for smaller sized particulates is commonly attributed to kinetic and thermodynamic considerations resulting from significantly different surface curvature, higher surface-to-volume ratios, and differences in intermolecular interactions [73]. However, in practice, a decrease in dissolution [74], no change [75], or an increase in dissolution with reduction in particle size is observed [76]. The variability in outcome is often due to differences in material properties that are incurred during synthesis, processing, or storage. By changing the levels of surface or bulk defects/impurities, by modifying the surface through coatings or by altering the surface chemistry, dissolution phenomena can be significantly altered. A number of methods exist for measuring the dissolution of particulate materials however a number of challenges remain for achieving robust comparable measurements under simulated physiological conditions [77].

3.14.3 Characteristic Primary Particle Size Distribution

Characteristic primary particle size is often misconstrued as an intrinsic property of a substance. The primary particle size of a distribution of particles represents the smallest particle size observable by microscopic means using morphological cues. Historically, primary particle size was developed as a means to understand aggregation processes during the aerosol synthesis of particles. The primary size often reflects the size of nodules that no longer have discrete interfaces and therefore technically should not be considered individual particles. Regardless, this morphological assessment is often used for identifying substances. It is stressed that the primary size is not always attainable through dispersion processes and that frequently the practical dispersible size may be orders of magnitude larger. Hence, the size distribution in many cases is not applicable for predicting transport processes. For many particle systems, particularly those where Oswald ripening occurs or simply dissolution, the primary particle size will change. The primary PSD is determined by the history of synthesis and environmental factors during the synthesis process, for some substances of the same originating droplet size, the primary particle size is distinctly different due to difference in environmental conditions during curing. Primary particle size is an apparent characteristic morphological size distribution at a given point in time and should be used with caution.

3.14.4 Dispersible Particle Size Distribution

The dispersible PSD is a measure of how finely divided a system of particles becomes under prescribed mechanical and environmental conditions. Due to the cohesive forces discussed earlier, the impact of synthesis and procurement conditions and overall sample history, the PSD can vary largely based on sample preparation (e.g., dispersion chemistry, energy input).

Unless the sample preparation and the mechanical dispersion process can be precisely controlled (or if relatively large uncertainty is acceptable), PSDs at the extremes of dispersion/mechanical energy are frequently preferred over intermediate values. Spontaneous or wet-in dispersion PSDs are applied to determine dispersion with minimal mechanical input and PSDs at plateau dispersion are applied to determine the smallest attainable PSD for a given process. Currently there is a paucity of standard protocols for these measurements.

The analysis method and type of PSD also matter when attempting to make correlations between diverse material types and for predicting phenomena. For instance, methods that measure aerodynamic diameters are preferred for predicting the deposition of aerosols. Likewise hydrodynamic diameter methods (e.g., centrifugal sedimentation) are preferred when monitoring sedimentation in liquids. Other methods such as light scattering are useful for quickly estimating PSDs but typically have more uncertainty due to proprietary methods applied by instrument manufacturers. Note that PSDs are commonly based on mass, surface area or number. Due to intrinsic assumptions the chosen basis should keep in mind the parameter that is actually measured by the technique in question and the purpose for the measurement.

3.14.5 Characteristic Particle Shape

Particle shape is a measure of the geometry of a particle. Shape analysis can be complicated and there are a number of competing definitions and methodologies to arrive at the same parameters. Due to these complications, most information to date is based on rather large distinctions between material sets. For most practical purposes, particle shape primarily refers to whether the particle exists as a platelet, a spheroid, or a rod. For rod-like particles the aspect ratio is often important indication for inhalation toxicity potential. Insoluble fiber-like particles have been associated with adverse pulmonary effects. Water-insoluble fibers of concern have been identified to have and aspect ratio (length/diameter) greater or equal to three and an overall diameter less than 100 microns with a length greater than 5 microns [78].

3.14.6 Density

Density is a measure of the mass of a substance per unit volume. Density measurement can become complicated when issues such as excluded volume and internal closed pores enter in the discussion. For liquid systems, the measurement of density simply involves filling a vessel of known volume with a liquid and determining its mass. If this is done for a particulate system, the result will be a bulk density and not the density of the individual particles. It is important to note that the bulk density of particles is more of a particle packing measurement and is sensitive to mechanical agitations. For most solid particles, helium pycnometry and buoyancy measurements are commonly applied. The determination of density for solid systems that may contain pores can be complicated and often requires the use of multiple methods.

3.14.7 Surface pK_a, Surface Charge, and Isoelectric Point

Like molecule ionizable groups on a particle surface also have a pK_a or a pH value where 50% of the sites are ionized. As with molecules, the surface wettability of particles is altered with pH. Particles with a significant surface charge at a pH tend to be more hydrophilic than when less charged. For some particulate systems the surface pK_a and surface isoelectric points have been shown to coincide.

3.14.8 Specific Surface Area

The specific surface area (SSA) of a material is a measure of the total surface area of a materials divided by its mass. The SSA of particles is typically measured via nitrogen gas adsorption applying the BET method.

3.14.9 Wetting Behavior

The wetting behavior of a solid substance is a description of its interaction with a given liquid (see Section 3.4.2). When a liquid spreads over the surface due to favorable interactions, it is said to wet the surface. There are a number of methods to determine the wetting behavior (sometimes also referred to as the surface energy) of solids and particles. These methods include contact angle measurements, capillary rise measurements, film flotation, phase partitioning, relative medium dispersibility, and vapor adsorption, amongst others. For particulate systems, packing and agglomeration can complicate and influence observed outcomes. Details on available experimental protocols and theoretical interpretations are available elsewhere [2, 22, 24, 79, 80].

3.14.10 Deposition, Heteroagglomeration, and Homoagglomeration Potential

The propensity of a particle to deposit on a surface or adhere to another particle will impact its fate and transport in biotic and abiotic systems. When a particle adheres to another particle through adhesive physical interaction it is termed "agglomeration." "Heteroagglomeration" occurs when the opposing particle is of a different substance, whereas "homoagglomeration" occurs when the opposing substance is of the same substance. Currently, there is a paucity of generally accepted protocols and proportionality constants for determining deposition, heteroagglomeration, and agglomeration potentials. Ongoing efforts by Weisner and coworkers are beginning to culminate into methodologies for determining the adhesive interactions between surfaces [43]. Historical approaches have involved measuring changes in apparent PSD or the loss of dispersed particle concentrations over time (e.g., sedimentation time, filtrate particle concentrations). Chapter 6 discusses the importance of heteroagglomeration and emerging methodologies.

3.14.11 Surface Reactivity

Surface reactivity involves the full scope of mechanisms wherein the surface of a particle either plays a direct role in the catalyst of a reaction through the momentary binding of reactants or as a mediator for the transfer of electrons or creation of free radicals. The ability of particle surfaces to enable chemical reactions by interacting with molecules in the vapor or liquid phase has been known for some time and is commonly exploited in heterogeneous catalysis. It is important to recognize that the vast majority of these processes require exceptional control of the exposed environment to avoid deactivation or poisoning of the surface. The vast majority of industrial catalysts are rapidly inactivated by uncontrolled exposure to complex environments.

However, surface reactivity in a nonspecific sense, leading to the generation of free radicals can be an important consideration. Photocatalytic activity has been an area of attention for many particulate and requires that light be absorbed (e.g., a via suitable band gap), resulting in electron–hole separation at the interface resulting in the generation of free radicals. A number of tests are available to test photocatalytic activity; however, most analyses are confounded by the incongruence of adsorption of the test molecule that is to be degraded amongst other factors. Modified electron spin resonance (ESR) methods offer an alternative testing strategy [81]. The generation of reactive oxygen species from nanoparticle surfaces in the absence of light has also been identified as a potential contributor. Riebeling et al. [82] has suggested a tiered approach for measuring this parameter. Additionally, band-gap-induced reactivity may become a concern when the band gap of a particle is in the same region as the redox potentials observed for biological function [83, 84]. Ultraviolet–visible–near infrared (UV-Vis-NIR) measurements are commonly applied for band-gap determination.

3.15 Purpose for Physicochemical Characterization

Physicochemical characterization is typically performed on chemicals to identify their physical state and how they interact with and distribute amongst and within biotic and abiotic environments. The most common physicochemical parameters for nonparticulate chemicals include melting point (MP), BP, VP, pK_a, molecular dimensions, and various phase-partitioning coefficients, including Henry's law constant, water solubility, the octanol–water partition coefficient, and the octanol–air partition coefficient [85, 86]. Notably, these physiochemical parameters are either intrinsic properties or functional characteristics. Figure 3.6 provides a context and identifies the purpose for the use of many of these parameters in risk assessments. For particulate systems, other parameters such as dustiness, dispersible PSD, surface area, and wetting behavior might be more relevant depending on the intended purpose. Similarities and differences in the physicochemical characterization for molecules and particles will be discussed in the ensuing sections with a focus on purpose. It is stressed that the following discussions are intended to provide an overview and not to be comprehensive. Additional details are provided in other chapters throughout this text.

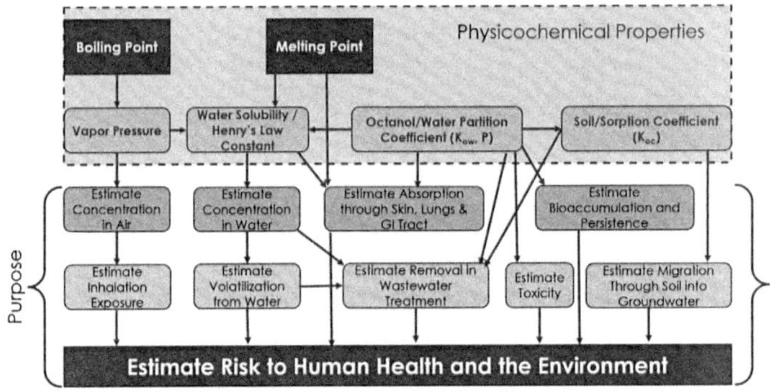

Figure 3.6 Important physicochemical properties, interrelationships, and their uses in risk assessment. Adapted from Ref. [86].

3.15.1 Estimating Inhalation Exposure

The potential for inhalation exposure for a substance relates to proportion of the given substance in the air at a size that is inhalable. For molecules, the content in air is primarily attributed to the ability of a substance to vaporize. Hence BPs, VPs, and Henry's law constant are relevant factors for estimating concentrations in air.

For particles, the dustiness of a particle system and the aerosolizable PSD are key determinants regarding whether a substance can be distributed in air at a size that is susceptible to inhalation to the lungs. The aerodynamic diameter of the particles also dictates where the particles are likely to deposit in the lungs. Inhalable particles have apparent aerodynamic diameter less than 100 microns, respirable particles have diameters less than 5–10 microns. In general, less cohesive powders of lower bulk densities and of smaller particle sizes have a greater probability to be inhaled into the lungs at lower mechanical energy inputs. The dispersible size in air and the envelope density of that assembly also impact the time frame at which a substance may remain suspended in air. This is further modified by the agglomeration behavior of the substance in air, which can greatly increase sedimentation rate and can reduce respirable fractions.

3.15.2 Estimating Concentration in Water

To determine potential concentrations in water the ability of a substance to dissolve or disperse in the liquid phase is required. For molecules, this involves an understanding of the water solubility of the substance and how the substance may volatilize and is commonly informed by water solubility data and Henry's law constant. However, for azeotropes and surface-active materials, the analysis is more complicated.

For particles, the ability to disperse in the relevant aqueous media and depending on scenario, the dissolution rate of the particles in that media may be substantially more relevant than equilibrium water solubility data. It is also import to note that surface and bulk structure of particles can influence dissolution and solubility. The adsorption of molecules to the surface of particles including ions, biomolecules, and other substances in the environment can influence both solubility and dissolution. Once dissolved, interactions between the dissolved components with macromolecules, small molecules, ions, and surfaces, along with environmental parameters can also promote re-precipitation or of the constituent dissolved components. For dispersed particles, the tendency to agglomerate and deposit on surfaces through particle interactions is important for determining the time frame at which the particles will be maintained in and travel with the aqueous phase. The particle Peclet number for individually suspended particles or clusters of particles is a useful tool for gauging sedimentation propensity.

3.15.3 Estimating Migration through Soil into Groundwater

Soils and sediment systems are highly complex, yet methods for estimating the transport of chemicals through these systems have been available for some time. For the most part transport across soil into groundwater is largely dependent on the solubility of a compound and its propensity to adsorb onto soil surfaces and organic media. Factors like the permeability of the soil and the variable progression of soil types during migration toward groundwater sources in different geographic regions, can impact transport. Principal molecular substance characteristics that impact transport are those that modify thermal mobility (i.e., MW and configuration/shape) and those that impact adsorption to surfaces (e.g., log P and K_{oc}, solubility, pK_a, hydrophilicity, MW). Log P and K_{oc} along with water solubility data have been applied for rough estimates of soil transport probability [51, 61, 62].

For particulate systems, transport through soil is largely prohibited by filtration mechanisms. For particles of small enough physical and hydrodynamic diameters and low enough Peclet numbers remain suspended and capable of flowing through the tortuous soil pore structure, the propensity of the particles to agglomerate or heteroagglomeration on the soil medium is important consideration as with molecules.

3.15.4 Estimating Removal from Wastewater Treatment

Wastewater chemical treatment processes apply physical, chemical, and biological processes to separate contaminants from water and vary by location. Common treatment processes involve the use of precipitation, flocculation, flotation, and oxidation technologies. For molecules, water solubility, Henry's law constant, pK_a, K_{oc}, and log P aid in estimating removal capacity. Water solubility provides a rough indication of the ability to oxidatively degrade a material and also can indicate ease of precipitation—albeit the chemical structure is required to utilize this relative information. K_{oc} and log P are indicators of the propensity of a molecule to adsorb into sludge or separate at interfaces for removal via skimmers. Henry's law constant provides an indication of volatilization propensity during treatment.

For particles, dominant indicators are the dispersible particle size, its relevant Peclet number and the propensity of the particles to deposit on surfaces and heteroagglomerate under wastewater treatment plant conditions. The dissolution and remediation of dissolved components are also important factors.

3.15.5 Estimate Absorption through the Skin, Eyes, Lungs, and the GI Tract

The transport across the skin, eyes, lungs, and the gastrointestinal (GI) tract involve a number of complex phenomena; however, the process largely involves diffusion-limited events modulated by the interaction of the molecules and particles with barrier membranes.

The skin is a very effective barrier designed to prevent excessive water loss as well as to protect the body from microorganisms, UV radiation, and other deleterious agents. The MW, pK_a, and log P of molecules can largely modulate transport. A low MW (<400 Da), oil-soluble liquids (log P from 0 to 6), and vapors have a greater propensity for transport. Unless the integrity of the skin is compromised particles are not anticipated to transfer.

Transport across the eyes is similar to the skin. The impact of water solubility tends to vary with substances. In general, molecule less than 500 Da can transport across the corneal epithelium, and molecules less than 10,000 Da can transport across the conjunctival epithelium. Vapors with VPs less than 0.0001 mmHg appear to be able to diffuse across. Particles generally are not capable of transport.

Transfer across the gastrointestinal tract occurs more generally for solubilized materials of less than 500 Da; however, soluble lipophilic molecules of log P from 0 to 5 and nonionized at GI tract conditions tend to have higher transfer rates. Facilitated and active transport also occurs when molecules are sufficiently similar to molecules that naturally undergo facilitated diffusion or are actively uptaken across the gut like glucose. Some particles are believed to be transported across the gut through Pyre patches or through pinocytosis; however, this transport is believed to be minimal. The impact of particle properties on transport across the gut is not well understood.

Transfer across the lungs can occur for gases, vapors and particles. Gases transport across the lung through facilitated and passive transport mechanisms. VPs less than 0.0001 mmHg facilitate improved transport. Solubility in the lung lining fluid is an important variable following principles of Graham's law. Henry's law constant in water is used to screen for gas solubility. For liquid constituents, transport across the lungs if facilitated by water solubility. Molecules of less than 400 Da tend to readily diffuse across the lung. Poorly soluble and lipophilic substances have longer in lung retention times. Respirable particulate materials (<5 microns) are transported from the lungs via phagocytosis. The dissolution of particles in the lung lining fluid, in endosomes, in lysosomes, or in interstitial fluid can facilitate molecular transport. In the case of rigid highly acicular particles, transport across the lungs into the pleural space has been suggested to occur via mechanical damage. Large particles are cleared from the lungs through the cilial escalator, where they are subsequently ingested. Stefaniak discusses the importance of physicochemical properties of particles in assessing relevant occupational inhalation metrics in Chapter 5.

3.15.6 Estimating Aquatic Toxicity

It is generally not possible to predict the toxicity of a substance by physicochemical parameters alone. Chemical composition and molecular identity are key components in toxicity assessment. However, for aquatic toxicity some general trends have been noted. As the MW increases, aquatic bioavailability and toxicity decrease. At an MW greater than approximately 1000, bioavailability is often considered negligible; however, caution must be taken to consider possible smaller breakdown products that may exert toxicity. Log P tends to correlate exponentially with acute toxicity by narcosis for nonionic organic chemicals up to a value of about log P values of ~6. Chemicals with a log P of less than 2 have tend to have low acute [87] and chronic [64] aquatic toxicity effects. Very poorly water soluble substances (<1 ppb) generally have low bioavailability and are less toxic. As noted earlier, ΔE values from frontier orbitals are showing utility for screening purposes. Molecules with calculated semi-empirical energy differences greater than 9 ev seem to be less reactive and therefore less toxic to aquatic species.

Physicochemical property trend analysis for estimating toxicity can be generally applied but needs to be approached with due caution. Knowledge of relevant pathways and exposure routes should be applied to gauge the potential impact of changes in physicochemical parameters on outcomes. In general, log P has been applied by the US EPA and other agencies to infer potential differences between chemical substances for the purpose of identifying differences in toxicity. This estimate is often based on the assumption that log P influences biodistribution and accumulation, reduces the hydrolysis and other chemical degradation pathways, and can also intensify potency for certain chemical classes.

For particles, log *P* is not a relevant metric; however, surface affinity and the propensity for biomagnification might be in some scenarios. The mode of action for the constituent molecules in a particle, or of the particle itself, for particle-initiated responses, and how physicochemical properties of the particle modulate apparent (local) dose and potency are important considerations. Toxicity is dependent on dose and potency, which can be modulated by a variety of particle parameters, depending on the mode of action. For instance, if the mode of action for a substance is related to dissolved constituent ions, and the particle dissolution rate and exposed mass and location will be key factors. If the mode of action is through surface reactivity, then the exposed particles surface area, and apparent surface reactivity will be key factors.

3.15.7 Estimate Bioaccumulation, Biomagnification, and Persistence

Bioaccumulation occurs when a substance is absorbed faster than it is cleared. This generally occurs for oil-soluble molecules. Biomagnification occurs when a substance bioaccumulates with increasing concentrations in the food chain. Log *P* is frequently used to screen for both bioaccumulation and biomagnification concerns.

The persistence of a molecule is the length of time it remains in a particular environment before it is chemically or biologically transformed or physically moved to another compartment [88]. The persistence of a chemical in the environment is often estimated in terms of its biodegradation potential.

For molecules large chemical structural databases combined with recent developments in quantitative structure property relationships are proving to be useful in identifying potentially persistent, bioaccumulative, and toxic (PBT) chemicals [89].

For particulate systems, the ability of particles to adhere to tissues is believed to be the corresponding factor. The deposition of particles in tissues inhibits their clearance in a similar manner as lipophilicity. However, trophic transfer is less established and believed to be infrequent due to the difficulties associated with the transport of particles across the gut.

3.16 Considerations and Challenges for Nanoscale Particulate Chemical Substances

Nanomaterials represent a class of chemicals in between traditional molecules and traditional particles. Although societies experience and exposure to nanomaterials has occurred for millennia, only recently have we placed a deep focus on how ultrafine particles may impact human health and the environment. The promise for nanotechnology to lead to technological advances, has also lead to concerns regarding its potential impact. To date, nanospecific effects have not been corroborated, indicating that nanomaterials tend to either behave like traditional molecules or similar to traditional particles. At a fundamental level this is consistent with predictions from interaction considerations between molecules, traditional particles, and nanoparticles and their potential impact on human health and the environment.

However, this analysis is confounded by the overall uncertainty and noise in modern nanotoxicological research and significant uncertainty remains for potential low-level chronic impacts. However, similar concerns also exist for traditional chemicals. As elucidated by Krug, many published nanotoxicology studies fail to report suitable information and are frequently of poor quality. To gain an understanding of potential effects of nanomaterials, experimental and reporting due diligence needs to be improved. Physicochemical characterization needs to be done interactively and done with purpose rather than simply as a requirement to check a box. Researchers need to become more diligent with the use of reference materials and standard protocols amongst their own experiments to afford comparability. Regulators and funding agencies also need to implement mechanisms to better encourage high-quality data and reporting. Moreover, methods for comparing the relative impact of nanomaterials to traditional chemicals are needed to ensure that the appropriate chemical substances are prioritized.

The assessment of nanomaterials has brought to the spotlight an important gap in modern risk assessment of chemicals: the lack of recognition of colloidal and surface phenomena. Integration of these concepts will require contributions across the continuum from small molecules to large particles. Standard methods and universal definitions remain lacking. The movement to functional assays and the recognition of the importance of particle history and surface interactions should aid in our overall understanding of the behavior and interactions of nanomaterials in biotic systems.

A number of efforts are under way to curate nanotoxicological data in the hopes that big data approaches may facilitate better clarity [90, 91]. However, without systematic methods for data acceptance and sufficient improved data and fit-for-purpose methodologies, these approaches may fail to offer additional meaningful correlations.

This chapter has omitted discussions around unexpected novel properties. These properties were a significant concern in the early years of nanotechnology when deviations in material properties with size were not as thoroughly explored. Today "transition" phenomena and property shifts are known to exist when the lines between molecules and particles are blurred, resulting in substantial changes in some intrinsic properties compared to the bulk substance. Advances in computational methods combined in tandem with experimentation have progressed to a point where many properties of nanoscale materials are predictable through atomistic and other theoretical modeling [92–94]. Indeed, in some instances it is more difficult to predict the properties of larger particles due to their size and associated structural uncertainties.

This being said, how changes in intrinsic properties and discretization of normally blurred phenomena (as observed in larger particles) enabled by nanoscale sizes may lead to unexpected interactions with biota and should not be fully discounted for environmental, health, and, safety (EHS) reasons. Novel and unique properties of nanoparticles need to be rationally defined and tested to determine the potential significance of their effects and when changes in intrinsic properties may require additional interrogations. However, given the state of nanotoxicological research there is a preceding need for data quality improvement prior to facilitate such advances.

As engineering at the nanoscale continues to advance, new material behaviors are expected to emerge that are far more complex than those incurred by today's simple nanomaterials that tend to just be a smaller version of familiar larger particles. To be able to predict the potential impact of next-generation complex nano-enabled materials, robust correlations between experimental and theoretical physicochemical properties and human health and environment outcomes are highly desired. Such correlations are critical for engendering safe-by-design practices intended to maintain function, while reducing risk. To facilitate robust knowledge generation and utility, the necessary standard testing methodologies, reference materials, and reporting protocols to engender comparability and data reliability must be in place and need to be incorporated in common practice.

3.17 Summary

Chapter 2 introduced the importance of attachment or interaction of molecules to biomolecules for the induction of pharmacological or toxic effects from molecules. This chapter continued the discussion from the broader context of EHS, introducing the importance of molecular and particulate interactions in transport and exposure processes. The increasing complexity and extrinsic nature of interactions moving from molecules to particles were noted, along with corresponding challenges in measurement.

As one moves from molecules to nanoparticle systems, the number of physicochemical endpoints required to determine the potential human health and environmental impact of nanomaterials increases. This is largely due to the increase in the number of factors that need to be considered to obtain the same level of knowledge, due to a fundamental increase in relevant variables and confounding factors that control their interactions. It is important to note that although the number of considerations may increase, the fundamental purpose for the physicochemical characterization for molecules and particles remains the same.

The origins of physicochemical properties in all matter were discussed, connecting basic interaction principles from molecular to particulate scale phenomena. The common origins of the interaction forces that govern molecule–molecule, molecule–particle, and particle–particle interactions were described. Complexity and confounding extrinsic and kinetic factors necessitate the use of more strategic characterization approaches for nanoparticulate systems. The philosophy of characterizing for purpose and the need for interactive characterization approaches, including functional testing, in particulate and nanomaterial research were highlighted. Parameters commonly measured for molecules were reviewed in context with their intended purpose. Parallels between molecular and particulate systems were provided along with an overview of future challenges for the physicochemical characterization of nanoparticulate systems.

References

1. Ackler, H. D., French, R. H., and Chiang, Y.-M. (1996). Comparisons of Hamaker constants for ceramic systems with intervening vacuum or water: from force laws and physical properties. *J. Colloid Interface Sci.*, **179**, 460–469.
2. Adamson, A. W., and Gast, A. P. (1997). *Physical Chemistry of Surfaces*, 6th Ed. (Wiley, New York).
3. Bach, S., and Schmidt, E. (2008). Determining the dustiness of powders--a comparison of three measuring devices. *Ann. Occup. Hyg.*, **52**, 717–725.
4. Bach, S., and Schmidt, E. (2014). Reply to the 'comment on comparison of powder dustiness methods' by Douglas Evans, Leonid Turkevich, Cynthia Roettgers, and Gregory Deye (*Ann. Occup. Hyg.*, 2014, **58**(4), 524–528). *Ann. Occup. Hyg.*, **58**, 782–783.
5. Bach, S., Eickmann, U., and Schmidt, E. (2013). Comparison of established systems for measuring the dustiness of powders with the UNC Dustiness Tester developed especially for pharmaceutical substances. *Ann. Occup. Hyg.*, **57**, 1078–1086.
6. Baker, J. R., Mihelcic, J. R., and Sabljic, A. (2001). Reliable QSAR for estimating Koc for persistent organic pollutants: correlation with molecular connectivity indices. *Chemosphere*, **45**, 213–221.
7. Baszkin, A., and Norde, W. (2000). *Physical Chemistry of Biological Interfaces* (Marcel Dekker, New York).
8. Israelachvili, J. (1998). Some thermodynamic aspects of intermolecular forces, In: *Intermolecular & Surface Forces*, 2nd Edition, p. 28.
9. Benes, K., Tong, P., and Ackerson, B. J. (2007). Sedimentation, Péclet number, and hydrodynamic screening. *Phys. Rev. E Stat. Nonlinear Soft Matter Phys.*, **76**, 056302.

10. Borm, P., Klaessig, F. C., Landry, T. D., Moudgil, B., Pauluhn, J., Thomas, K., Trottier, R., and Wood, S. (2006). Research strategies for safety evaluation of nanomaterials, part V: role of dissolution in biological fate and effects of nanoscale particles. *Toxicol. Sci.*, **90**, 23–32.

11. Bouwmeester, H., Lynch, I., Marvin, H. J., Dawson, K. A., Berges, M., Braguer, D., Byrne, H. J., Casey, A., Chambers, G., Clift, M. J., Elia, G., Fernandes, T. F., Fjellsbo, L. B., Hatto, P., Juillerat, L., Klein, C., Kreyling, W. G., Nickel, C., Riediker, M., and Stone, V. (2011). Minimal analytical characterization of engineered nanomaterials needed for hazard assessment in biological matrices. *Nanotoxicology*, **5**, 1–11.

12. Boverhof, D. R., and David, R. M. (2010). Nanomaterial characterization: considerations and needs for hazard assessment and safety evaluation. *Anal. Bioanal. Chem.*, **396**, 953–961.

13. Bozzolo, G., Noebe, R. D., and Abel, P. B. (2007). *Applied Computational Materials Modeling: Theory, Simulation and Experiment* (Springer, New York), xvi, 491 p.

14. Brown, I. D. (2002). *The Chemical Bond in Inorganic Chemistry: The Bond Valence Model* (Oxford University Press, New York).

15. Brown, S. (2014). *Inorganic Nanoparticles and Functional Testing Considerations, Categorization Strategies for Engineered Nanomaterials in a Regulatory Context*, pp. 1–3.

16. Brown, S. C., Olivieira, R. C. G., and Moudgil, B. M. (2003). Method for characterizing the wettability of filler particles, In: Kellar, J., Herpfer, M. A., and Moudgil, B. M. (eds.), *Functional Fillers and Nanoscale Minerals* (Society for Mining, Metallurgy & Exploration, New York).

17. Brown, S. C., Palazuelos, M., Sharma, P., Powers, K. W., Roberts, S. M., Grobmyer, S. R., and Moudgil, B. M. (2010). Nanoparticle characterization for cancer nanotechnology and other biological applications. *Methods Mol. Biol.*, **624**, 39–65.

18. Brown, S., and Moudgil, B. (2004). Influence of nanoscale roughness on surface wettability. *Miner. Metall. Process.*, **21**, 33–35.

19. Burello, E., and Worth, A. P. (2011). A theoretical framework for predicting the oxidative stress potential of oxide nanoparticles. *Nanotoxicology*, **5**, 228–235.

20. Chan, D. Y., Healy, T. W., Supasiti, T., and Usui, S. (2006). Electrical double layer interactions between dissimilar oxide surfaces with charge regulation and Stern-Grahame layers. *J. Colloid Interface Sci.*, **296**, 150–158.

21. Ciccotti, G., Frenkel, D., and McDonald, I. R. (1987). *Simulation of Liquids and Solids: Molecular Dynamics and Monte Carlo Methods in Statistical Mechanics* (Elsevier Science Pub. Co., New York).

22. Doucette, W. J. (2003). Quantitative structure-activity relationships for predicting soil-sediment sorption coefficients for organic chemicals. *Environ. Toxicol. Chem.*, **22**, 1771–1788.

23. Doucette, W. J., and Andren, A. W. (1987). Correlation of octanol/water partition coefficients and total molecular surface area for highly hydrophobic aromatic compounds. *Environ. Sci. Technol.*, **21**, 821–824.

24. Dunbar, B. S., Wardrip, N. J., and Hedrick, J. L. (1980). Isolation, physicochemical properties, and macromolecular composition of zona pellucida from porcine oocytes. *Biochemistry*, **19**, 356–365.

25. Dunn, W. J., Block, J. H., Pearlman, R. S., American Pharmaceutical Association, and Academy of Pharmaceutical Sciences (1986). *Partition Coefficient: Determination and Estimation* (Pergamon Press, New York).

26. Duszgunes, N., Wilschut, J., Fraley, R., and Papahadjopoulos, D. (1981). Calcium-induced and magnesium-induced fusion of mixed phosphatidylserine-phosphatidylcholine vesicles - effect of ion binding. *J. Membr. Biol.*, **59**, 115–125.

27. Evans, D. E., Turkevich, L. A., Roettgers, C. T., and Deye, G. J. (2014). Comment on comparison of powder dustiness methods. *Ann. Occup. Hyg.*, **58**, 524–528.

28. Fernandez, M., and Barnard, A. S. (2015). Identification of nanoparticle prototypes and archetypes. *ACS Nano*, **9**, 11980–11992.

29. Franklin, N. M., Rogers, N. J., Apte, S. C., Batley, G. E., Gadd, G. E., and Casey, P. S. (2007). Comparative toxicity of nanoparticulate ZnO, bulk ZnO, and ZnCl2 to a freshwater microalga (Pseudokirchneriella subcapitata): the importance of particle solubility. *Environ. Sci. Technol.*, **41**, 8484–8490.

30. French, R. H., Cannon, R. M., DeNoyer, L. K., and Chiang, Y. M. (1995). Full spectral calculation of non-retarded Hamaker constants for ceramic systems from interband transition strengths. *Solid State Ionics*, **75**, 13–33.

31. Gill, T. E., Zobeck, T. M., and Stout, J. E. (2006). Technologies for laboratory generation of dust from geological materials. *J. Hazard. Mater.*, **132**, 1–13.

32. Hendren, C. O., Lowry, G. V., Unrine, J. M., and Wiesner, M. R. (2015). A functional assay-based strategy for nanomaterial risk forecasting. *Sci. Total Environ.*, **536**, 1029–1037.

33. Hendren, C. O., Powers, C. M., Hoover, M. D., and Harper, S. L. (2015). The nanomaterial data curation initiative: a collaborative approach to assessing, evaluating, and advancing the state of the field. *Beilstein J. Nanotechnol.*, **6**, 1752–1762.

34. Lyklema, J., van Leeuwen, H. P., and Minor, M. (1999). DLVO-theory, a dynamic re-interpretation. *Adv. Colloid Interface Sci.*, **83**, 33–69.

35. Hill, J.-R., Maiti, A., and Subramanian, L. (2005). *Molecular Modeling Techniques in Material Sciences* (Taylor & Francis, Boca raton, FL).

36. Hopkins, J. C., Dryden, D. M., Ching, W.-Y., French, R. H., Parsegian, V. A., and Podgornik, R. (2014). Dielectric response variation and the strength of van der Waals interactions. *J. Colloid Interface Sci.*, **417**, 278–284.

37. Howard, P. H., and Muir, D. C. G. (2010). Identifying new persistent and bioaccumulative organics among chemicals in commerce. *Environ. Sci. Technol.*, **44**, 2277–2285.

38. Hunter, R. J. (2001). *Foundations of Colloid Science*, 2nd Ed. (Oxford University Press, New York).

39. Iler, R. K. (1979). *The Chemistry of Silica: Solubility, Polymerization, Colloid and Surface Properties, and Biochemistry* (Wiley, New York).

40. Ishida, N., Sakamoto, M., Miyahara, M., and Higashitani, K. (2002). Optical observation of gas bridging between hydrophobic surfaces in water. *J. Colloid Interface Sci.*, **253**, 112–116.

41. ISO (2015). *Nanotechnologies: Vocabulary. Part 2: Nano-Objects*. ISO/TS 80004-2.

42. Israelachvili, J. N. (2011). *Intermolecular and Surface Forces*, 3rd Ed. (Academic Press, Burlington, MA).

43. Israelachvili, J., and Wennerstrom, H. (1996). Role of hydration and water structure in biological and colloidal interactions. *Nature*, **379**, 219–225.

44. Iwahara, J., Esadze, A., and Zandarashvili, L. (2015). Physicochemical properties of ion pairs of biological macromolecules. *Biomolecules*, **5**, 2435–2463.

45. Jasinska-Stroschein, M., Kurczewska, U., and Orszulak-Michalak, D. (2016). Errors in reporting on dissolution research: methodological and statistical implications. *Pharm. Dev. Technol.*, 1–8.

46. Karickhoff, S. W., Brown, D. S., and Scott, T. A. (1979). Sorption of hydrophobic pollutants on natural sediments. *Water Res.*, **13**, 241–247.

47. Krug, H. F., and Wick, P. (2011). Nanotoxicology: an interdisciplinary challenge. *Angew. Chem. Int. Ed. Engl.*, **50**, 1260–1278.

48. Kühnel, D., Marquardt, C., Nau, K., Krug, H. F., Paul, F., and Steinbach, C. (2017). Environmental benefits and concerns on safety: communicating latest results on nanotechnology safety research—the project DaNa$^{2.0}$. *Environ. Sci. Pollut. Res.*, **24**(12), 11120–11125.

49. Leng, Y. (2012). Hydration force between mica surfaces in aqueous KCl electrolyte solution. *Langmuir*, **28**, 5339–5349.

50. Liden, G. (2006). Dustiness testing of materials handled at workplaces. *Ann. Occup. Hyg.*, **50**, 437–439.

51. Lyklema, J. (1991). *Fundamentals of Interface and Colloid Science* (Academic Press, San Diego).

52. Lyman, W. J., Reehl, W. F., and Rosenblatt, D. H. (1990). *Handbook of Chemical Property Estimation Methods : Environmental Behavior of Organic Compounds* (American Chemical Society, Washington, DC).

53. Mackay, D., and Shiu, W. Y. (1981). A critical review of Henry's law constant for chemicals of environmental interest. *J. Phys. Chem. Ref. Data*, **10**, 1175–1199.

54. Matsusaka, S., Maruyama, H., Matsuyama, T., and Ghadiri, M. (2010). Triboelectric charging of powders: a review. *Chem. Eng. Sci.*, **65**, 5781–5807.

55. Middlebrook, J. L., and Aronow, L. (1977). Physicochemical properties of glucocorticoid receptors from mouse fibroblasts. *Endocrinology*, **100**, 271–282.

56. Milas, M., Shi, X., and Rinaudo, M. (1990). On the physicochemical properties of gellan gum. *Biopolymers*, **30**, 451–464.

57. Misra, S. K., Dybowska, A., Berhanu, D., Luoma, S. N., and Valsami-Jones, E. (2012). The complexity of nanoparticle dissolution and its importance in nanotoxicological studies. *Sci. Total Environ.*, **438**, 225–232.

58. Moncho-Jorda, A., Louis, A. A., and Padding, J. T. (2012). How Peclet number affects microstructure and transient cluster aggregation in sedimenting colloidal suspensions. *J. Chem. Phys.*, **136**, 064517.

59. Mughal, A., El Demellawi, J. K., and Chaieb, S. (2014). Band-gap engineering by molecular mechanical strain-induced giant tuning of the luminescence in colloidal amorphous porous silicon nanostructures. *Phys. Chem. Chem. Phys.*, **16**, 25273–25279.

60. Namvar, A., Bolhassani, A., Khairkhah, N., and Motevalli, F. (2015). Physicochemical properties of polymers: an important system to

overcome the cell barriers in gene transfection. *Biopolymers*, **103**, 363–375.

61. National Research Council (2014). *A Framework to Guide Selection of Chemical Alternatives* (The National Academies Press, Washington, DC).

62. Neumann, A. W., David, R., and Zuo, Y. (2011). *Applied Surface Thermodynamics*, 2nd Ed. (Taylor & Francis, Boca Raton).

63. OECD (1981). Particle size distribution/fibre length and diameter distributions. In: *OECD Guidelines for Testing of Chemicals*, Vol. 110, pp. 1–13. Paris, France.

64. Parsegian, V. A. (2006). *Van der Waals Forces: A Handbook for Biologists, Chemists, Engineers, and Physicists* (Cambridge University Press, New York).

65. Pavan, M., and Worth, A. P. (2008). Review of estimation models for biodegradation. *QSAR Comb. Sci.*, **27**, 32–40.

66. Pensis, I., Mareels, J., Dahmann, D., and Mark, D. (2010). Comparative evaluation of the dustiness of industrial minerals according to European standard EN 15051, 2006. *Ann. Occup. Hyg.*, **54**, 204–216.

67. Persson, P. K., and Bergenstahl, B. A. (1985). Repulsive forces in lecithin glycol lamellar phases. *Biophys. J.*, **47**, 743–746.

68. Powers, K., Brown, S., Krishna, V., Wasdo, S., Moudgil, B., and Roberts, S. (2006). Research strategies for safety evaluation of nanomaterials. Part VI. Characterization of nanoscale particles for toxicological evaluation. *Toxicol. Sci.*, 296–303.

69. Prochaska, K., Konowal, E., Sulej-Chojnacka, J., and Lewandowicz, G. (2009). Physicochemical properties of cross-linked and acetylated starches and products of their hydrolysis in continuous recycle membrane reactor. *Colloids Surf. B*, **74**, 238–243.

70. Rabinovich, Y. I., Vakarelski, I. U., Brown, S. C., Singh, P. K., and Moudgil, B. M. (2004). Mechanical and thermodynamic properties of surfactant aggregates at the solid-liquid interface. *J. Colloid Interface Sci.*, **270**, 29–36.

71. Riebeling, C., Wiemann, M., Schnekenburger, J., Kuhlbusch, T. A., Wohlleben, W., Luch, A., and Haase, A. (2016). A redox proteomics approach to investigate the mode of action of nanomaterials. *Toxicol. Appl. Pharmacol.*, **299**, 24–29.

72. Rosen, M. J., and Kunjappu, J. T. (2012). *Surfactants and Interfacial Phenomena*, 4th Ed. (Wiley, Hoboken).

73. Sakthivel, T., Toth, I., and Florence, A. T. (1998). Synthesis and physicochemical properties of lipophilic polyamide dendrimers. *Pharm. Res.*, **15**, 776–782.

74. Schrader, M. E., and Loeb, G. I. (1992). *Modern Approaches to Wettability: Theory and Applications* (Plenum Press, New York).

75. Singh, S., Munjal, S., and Khare, N. (2015). Strain/defect induced enhanced coercivity in single domain $CoFe_2O_4$ nanoparticles. *J. Magn. Magn. Mater.*, **386**, 69–73.

76. Stefaniak, A. B., Hackley, V. A., Roebben, G., Ehara, K., Hankin, S., Postek, M. T., Lynch, I., Fu, W. E., Linsinger, T. P., and Thunemann, A. F. (2013). Nanoscale reference materials for environmental, health and safety measurements: needs, gaps and opportunities. *Nanotoxicology*, **7**, 1325–1337.

77. Tan, G. L., and French, R. H. (2006). Optical properties, electronic structure and London dispersion interactions for nanostructured interfacial and surficial films. *Mater. Sci. Eng. A*, **422**, 136–146.

78. Tang, R., Orme, C. A., and Nancollas, G. H. (2004). Dissolution of crystallites: surface energetic control and size effects. *ChemPhysChem*, **5**, 688–696.

79. USEPA (1985). *Toxic Substances Control Act Test Guidelines* (Office of Toxic Sustances).

80. USEPA (1997). *Chemical Assistance Manual for Premanufacture Notification Submitters* (O. o. P. P. a. T. United States Environmental Protection Agency, ed.), EPA 744-R-97-003, pp. 1–138.

81. Vakarelski, I. U., Brown, S. C., Basim, G. B., Rabinovich, Y. I., and Moudgil, B. M. (2010). Tailoring silica nanotribology for CMP slurry optimization: Ca(2+) cation competition in C(12)TAB mediated lubrication. *ACS Appl. Mater. Interfaces*, **2**, 1228–1235.

82. Vakarelski, I. U., Brown, S. C., Rabinovich, Y. I., and Moudgil, B. M. (2004). Lateral force microscopy investigation of surfactant-mediated lubrication from aqueous solution. *Langmuir*, **20**, 1724–1731.

83. Van de Waterbeemd, H. (2000). Intestinal permeability: prediction from theory, In: Dressman, J. (ed.), *Methods for Accessing Oral Drug Absorption* (Marcel Dekker, New York), pp. 31–49.

84. Voutchkova, A. M., Kostal, J., Steinfeld, J. B., Emerson, J. W., Brooks, B. W., Anastas, P., and Zimmerman, J. B. (2011). Towards rational molecular design: derivation of property guidelines for reduced acute aquatic toxicity. *Green Chem.*, **13**, 2373–2379.

85. Voutchkova, A., Kostal, J., and Anastas, P. (2010). Property-based approaches to design rules for reduced toxicity, In: Anastas, P. (ed.), *Handbook of Green Chemistry* (Wiley, New York).

86. Voutchkova-Kostal, A. M., Kostal, J., Connors, K. A., Brooks, B. W., Anastas, P. T., and Zimmerman, J. B. (2012). Towards rational molecular design for reduced chronic aquatic toxicity. *Green Chem.*, **14**, 1001–1008.

87. Wang, H., Kelley, S. P., Brantley, J. W., 3rd, Chatel, G., Shamshina, J., Pereira, J. F., Debbeti, V., Myerson, A. S., and Rogers, R. D. (2015). Ionic fluids containing both strongly and weakly interacting ions of the same charge have unique ionic and chemical environments as a function of ion concentration. *ChemPhysChem*, **16**, 993–1002.

88. Woodburn, K. B., Doucette, W. J., and Andren, A. W. (1984). Generator column determination of octanol/water partition coefficients for selected polychlorinated biphenyl congeners. *Environ. Sci. Technol.*, **18**, 457–459.

89. Yalkowsky, S. H. (1999). *Solubility and Solubilization in Aqueous Media* (American Chemical Society, Washington, DC; Oxford University Press, New York).

90. Yalkowsky, S. H., and Banerjee, S. (1992). *Aqueous Solubility: Methods of Estimation for Organic Compounds* (Marcel Dekker, New York).

91. Yalkowsky, S. H., He, Y., and Jain, P. (2010). *Handbook of Aqueous Solubility Data*, 2nd Ed. (CRC Press, Boca Raton, FL).

92. Luryi, S., Xu, J., and Zaslavsky, A. (2007). *Future Trends in Microelectronics: Up the Nano Creek* (Wiley, Hoboken), xiv, 459 p.

93. Zhang, H., Ji, Z., Xia, T., Meng, H., Low-Kam, C., Liu, R., Pokhrel, S., Lin, S., Wang, X., Liao, Y. P., Wang, M., Li, L., Rallo, R., Damoiseaux, R., Telesca, D., Madler, L., Cohen, Y., Zink, J. I., and Nel, A. E. (2012). Use of metal oxide nanoparticle band gap to develop a predictive paradigm for oxidative stress and acute pulmonary inflammation. *ACS Nano*, **6**, 4349–4368.

94. Zhu, X. D., Wang, Y. J., Sun, R. J., and Zhou, D. M. (2013). Photocatalytic degradation of tetracycline in aqueous solution by nanosized TiO_2. *Chemosphere*, **92**, 925–932.

Chapter 4

Common Physicochemical Properties

Paul Carpinone and Stephen Roberts

Particle Engineering Research Center, 1180 Center Drive, 2187 Mowry Road, Gainesville, FL 32611, USA

Center for Environmental & Human Toxicology, 2187 Mowry Road, Gainesville, FL 32611, USA

pcarpinoneuf@gmail.com

4.1 Introduction

As interest in nanotechnology blossomed in the late twentieth century, it became clear that proper characterization of nanomaterials was going to be a significant issue. The existence of novel and potentially beneficial properties of materials at the nanoscale compared to properties of the same materials at larger scales was the central premise that lead to nanotechnology research in a variety of areas. With this focus on exploiting nanomaterial properties, the question "Which properties need to be characterized?" naturally arose, not only in terms of communicating scientific findings, but also in terms of setting the stage for regulation of nanomaterials. What followed is nearly two decades of struggle to answer this simple question in an unambiguous manner.

Physicochemical Properties of Nanomaterials
Edited by Richard C. Pleus and Vladimir Murashov

ISBN 978-981-4774-80-2 (Hardcover), 978-1-351-16860-1 (eBook)
www.panstanford.com

Arguably, context matters, and the nanomaterial characterization needed for one purpose, for example, to determine whether a material fits the definition of a nanomaterial and is therefore subject to some regulation, might be different from characterization for another purpose, such as a safety assessment. In an attempt to identify a common minimum set of characteristics that should be identified, a 2008 workshop with broad industry, academic, and government participation offered a recommendation that a simple set of questions be answered [1]:

- What does the material look like (particle size, size distribution, agglomeration state/aggregation, shape)?
- What is the material made of (overall composition, surface composition, purity)?
- What factors affect how the material interacts with its surrounding (surface area; surface chemistry, including reactivity and hydrophobicity; surface charge)?

However, the temptation to develop lists of specific characteristic requirements has proven irresistible, and there are many such lists. Some have been produced by regulatory agencies (see later), some by standards-setting organizations (e.g., Organisation for Economic Co-operation and Development [OECD], ASTM International; see later), and others recommended by individual scientists and research groups [2–6]. The objective of this chapter is to show and contrast examples of physicochemical parameter lists for nanomaterials from various sources and to provide descriptions of what is meant by the most common parameters. The chapter is not intended to be an exhaustive compendium of physicochemical parameter lists, but rather it gives the reader a sense of the extent to which there are similarities and differences among current recommendations and requirements.

4.2 Promulgated Lists

Increasing interest in nanomaterials during the 1990s led to the establishment of the US National Nanotechnology Initiative (NNI) (1999) to create a central hub for nanotechnology activities among 20 participating departments and agencies of the US federal government [7]. The early 2000s saw major drives worldwide to establish standards related to nanotechnology. Beginning in 2003 with China's establishment of the national-level United Working Group for Nanomaterials Standardization, followed by the United States, United Kingdom, and Japan in 2004, national-level nanomaterial standardization efforts were initiated. International efforts at nanotechnology standardization followed in 2005, including activities by the International Organization for Standardization (ISO), ASTM International, and the OECD. Early deficiencies in characterization and terminology were well recognized, leading the aforementioned organizations to place specific emphasis on these issues. The wide diversity of nanomaterial geometries, compositions, and unique properties generated substantial interest in the development of guidance on the selection of physicochemical properties for characterization. The scientific community responded to this demand by developing characterization guidance and lists of important physicochemical properties for toxicological and risk assessment studies of nanomaterials. These lists are numerous and vary considerably in scope and detail (Table 4.1). At least 28 lists of important physicochemical properties, identifying over 60 properties deemed important for risk assessment, have been identified in the literature [8]. The lists outlined in Table 4.1, focusing primarily on lists from larger efforts, include over 100 different important properties of nanomaterials. A discussion of some of these lists from major organizations is provided in later sections.

4.2.1 The United States/Canada

In 2006, the US Food and Drug Administration (FDA) formed the Nanotechnology Task Force to investigate regulatory approaches for nanomaterials. The product report of this task force [36], issued in 2007, recognized that nanomaterials have unique properties and recommended that nanomaterial-specific guidance be provided. Nonbinding guidance specific to nanomaterials in cosmetics (including a list of important properties) [27], food ingredients (no list of properties) [37], and animal food (no list of properties) [38] has been published by the FDA. Beyond the list related to nanomaterials in cosmetics, the FDA has not published additional lists of nanomaterial characteristics. Although the FDA regulates

Table 4.1 Lists of important physicochemical properties for toxicological and risk assessment studies of nanomaterials

		SCCS (EU, 2012)[9]	Health Canada (2011)[18]	Oberdorster et. al. (2005)[3]	Council of Canadian Academies (2008)[11]	RIP-oN 2 (EU, 2011)[80]	NICNAS (Australia, 2013)[13]	ISO TC229 (2008)[14]	SCENIHR (EU, 2009)[15]	OECD (2010)[16]	Co-Nanomet (EC, 2010)[17]	OECD (2016)[18]	Powers et. al. (2006)[8]	OECD (2009)[19]	OECD Annex II (2009)[19]	NCL[120]	MINChar Initiative (2008)[21]	NANO Risk Framework (DuPont/Environmental Defense, 2007)[22]	NIST (2007)[23]	SCENIHR §3.2 (EU, 2007)[24]	SCENIHR §3.6 (EU, 2007)[24]	EPA (US, 2012)[25]	EPA (US, 2017)[4]	ISO TC 229 (2011)[26]	FDA (US, 2014)[27]	Montaño et. al. (Prepared for and reviewed by US EPA, 2014)[28]	DF4NanoGrouping (2015)[29]	ECHA (EU, 2012[87], 2015[30])	EFSA (EU, 2009)[31]	EFSA (EU, 2011)[32]	ISO TC229 Focused List (2008)[33]	SCENIHR (EU, 2015)[34]	ICCR (EU, 2011)[35]
External Dimensional Characteristics	Size/Distribution	•/⊕	•/•	prim.	•	○/○	•/•	•/•	•/•	○/○	○/-	•/•	•/•	⊕/•	•/•	•/•	•/•	•/•	•/○	•/•	•/•	•/-	•/•	⊕/•	•/•	•/-	prim./-	⊕/⊕	•/•	•/⊕	•/•	•/⊕	•/•
	Agglomeration, Aggregation	⊕	•	•	•	•	•	•		•	•		•	•	•	•	•	•	•	•	•	○	•	•	•					⊕	•	⊕	•
	Shape/Morphology/Aspect Ratio	⊕/•/⊕	•/•/-	•/-/-	•/•/-	•/-/-	•/-/-	•/-/-	•/•/•	-/•/-	•/•/-	•/-/•	•/-/-	○/•/-	•/•/•		•/-/-		-/•/•	-/•/-	•/•/•	•/•/-	•/⊕/•	•/-/-	•/•/-		•/•/•	•/⊕/⊕	•/•/•	⊕/•/-	•/-/-	⊕/•/⊕	•/-/-
	Surface Topography, Topology	⊕							•							•					•				•								
	Fractal Dimension										•								agglom.									⊕					
	Granulometry					•																						•					
Internal Dimensional Characteristics	Surface Area, SSA (mass)	BET	•	•	•	•	•	•	•	•	•	•	•	•	•		•	•	•	•	•	•	•	•	•		•	•	•	•	•	•	•
	Porosity	⊕		•		•				•		•	•	•	•			•		•			•		•							⊕	
	Pore Density														•																	•	
	Volume SSA	⊕	•																				○	•				⊕					
Identity	Identity/Purity	•/⊕	•/•				-/•	-/•	•/•	○/•				•/⊕	•/•	-/•	-/•						•/•	⊕/⊕	-/•		-/•		-/•	•/⊕	-/•	•/⊕	
	Composition	•	•	•	•		•	•	•		•	○	⊕	⊕/•	•	•	•	•	•	•	•	•		•	•	•	•		•		•	•	•
	Form, Appearance, Phase	⊕													•			•					•							•		⊕	
	Crystallography/Crystallinity	⊕/⊕		•/-	○/-		•/-		○/•	•/-	•/•	•/-	⊕/○	•/○	•/-		•/-	•/-	○/•	•/-	•/-	•/-	•/-	⊕/⊕	-/•		-/•			⊕/⊕		⊕/⊕	
	Crystallite Size									•				•	•																		
	Density	•				•							⊕		•			•		•			•		•			•		•		•	
	Dopants/Additives	⊕/⊕							-/•	-/•				-/⊕	-/•										-/•					-/⊕			
	Oxidation State	⊕																															
	Molecular Weight															•							•										
	Defect Structures								•																								
	Encapsulating Materials	⊕																					⊕							⊕		⊕	
	Formulants, Stabilizers	⊕					•								•															⊕		⊕	
	Chemical Name, Common Name, Identifiers, CAS, etc.	⊕								•				•	•			•					•		•								
	Molecular, Structural, and Chemical Formula	⊕						•	•	•				•	•			•					•		•							⊕	
	Medium Identity/Composition						•/•																					⊕/○					
Chemistry	Solubility	•	aq.		•	aq.		•	•	aq.	•	aq.	⊕	aq.	•	•		•	•	•	aq.	•	aq.	•	•		aq.	aq.	•	•	•	•	
	Dissolution Rate, Kinetics	⊕			⊕						•	•					⊕			•							•						
	Dissociation Constant	⊕				•							○		•								•					•					
	pH	•													•								•					⊕		•		•	
	Boiling Point/Melting Point/Freezing Point												-/•/-		-/•/-					-/•/-	•/-/-		•/•/-					•/•/•					
	Vapor Pressure																				•		•					•					
	Hygroscopicity	powd.																															
	Viscosity	•																										•		•		•	
Surface Chemistry	Surface Chemistry	○	•	•		•	•	•	•	•		•	•	•	•	○	•				•	•	adsorp.	•	•		•	adsorp.	properties	•	•	•	•
	Zeta Potential/Charge, Surface Charge	⊕/-	-/•	-/•	-/•	-/•	-/•	•/-	•/•	•/-	•/•	•/•	⊕/•	•/-	•/-	•/-	-/•	-/•	•/-	-/•	-/•		•/-	-/•	•/•		-/•		-/•	⊕/•	-/•	⊕/•	-/•
	Hydrophobicity/Partition Coefficient/Wettability	⊕/⊕/-				-/•/-		•/-/-	•/-/-	-/•/-	-/-/•		-/-/⊕	-/•/-	○/•/-		•/-/-		•/•/-		-/•/-		-/•/-				•/-/-	-/•/-	•/-/-	-/•/-	⊕/-/-	-/•/-	
	Henry's Law Constant																						•										
	Coating, Functionalization/Modifications	⊕/⊕			•/-		•/•			•/•			⊕/-	-/⊕	•/-	•/-			•/-						•/-		⊕/⊕		biomol. ads./-	⊕/⊕		⊕/⊕	
	PZC/IEP										•/•		-/⊕																				
	Zeta Potential Titrations (pH, etc.)												⊕																				
	Charge Density/Distribution												⊕/-						•/•														
	Surface Acidity					•							pKa																				
	Surface Contamination			•															•														
	Surface Energy					•							⊕																				
	Surface Composition, Moieties				⊕				•			•	⊕					•		•			•	⊕		•	•		•			⊕	
	Surface Structure		•										⊕																				
	Surface Tension					•			•																			•					
	Interfacial Tension	⊕																															
Reactivity	Catalytic Activity/Photocatalytic Activity	•/⊕	•/•						-/•	•/•		-/•	⊕/-	•/•	•/•										•/-					•/•		•/•	
	Reactivity	⊕	•		•												•		•	•		•								•		•	
	Radical/ROS Formation	⊕/-				-/•				•/-	-/○			•/-	•/-				-/•														
	Oxidizing Properties							•							•													•					
	Stability	•						•							•	•	•			○	•				•			•			•		
	Redox Potential, Activity	•				•				•				•	•				•											•		•	
	Reactive Sites	⊕							•																								
	Explosive Properties					•									•								•					•					
	Flammability					•									•								•					•					
	Surface Reactivity												•					•									•						
	Flash Point																											•					
	Autoignition Temperature																											•					
Suspension Properties	Dispersability		aq.							aq.		aq.		aq.	•			•						•			•						
	State of Dispersion					•																											
	Dispersants, Surface-Active Compounds	⊕																												⊕		⊕	
	Ionic Strength						•																										
	Diffusion Coefficient										•																						
	Hydrodynamic Radius, Diameter										•																						
	Settling Velocity										•								agglom.									⊕					
	Stokes Diameter										•																	•					
	Aerodynamic Diameter										•												•										
	Acoustophoretic Mobility										•																						
Composite Systems	Concentration, Particle Concentration	•		•	•			•/-			•						•									•		⊕	•	•		•/•	
	Structural Integrity		•																														
Bulk Powder Properties	Bulk Density/Tapped Density																	•/-															
	Pour Density	•								•				•	•															•			
	Dustiness	•								•		•		○	•													○		•		•	
Other and Advanced Properties	Protein Corona																										•						
	Electrical/Magnetic/Optical/Mechanical Properties		•/-/•/•										-/-/•/-							-/•/•/-		-/•/•/-											
	In situ Changes												•		•		•		•	•							size						
	Heterogeneity			•									⊕		○																		
	Degradation Products/By-products																						○/•					•/-					
	Particle Adhesion																																
	Surface Conductivity										•																						
	Scattering, Extinction Cross Section										•																						
	Absorption	UV													•																		
	Reflectivity	⊕																															
	NMR														•																		
	Mass Spectrum														•																		
	Chromatogram (GC,LC)														•																		
	Commercial Use									•				•	•								•										
	Method of Production, Preparation			•			•	•		•				•	•								•										
	Processing Chemicals/Precursors, Monomers, etc.																						-/•							⊕/-			
	Storage History, Stability			•											•																		
	Representative TEM Images									•				•														ns					
	Conductivity												⊕							•		•						•					
	Hardness												⊕							•							○						
	Areas in 2D Projections										•																						
	Spectra																						ns										
	Novel or Unique Properties																						•										
	Volatilization from Water and Soil																						•/•										
	Average Particle Mass/Surface Area																						•/•										
	Particle Physicochemical Structure			•																													

○ implied
⊕ defined explicitly in details/definitions of each list item
ns not specific
aq. aqueous/water
• identified
\- not identified

several products of specific concern, it can only require safety testing on products requiring premarket authorization (medicines/medical devices, food, cosmetics, and coloring additives). For many other consumer products, postmarket safety is regulated by the Consumer Product Safety Commission (CPSC). The CPSC joined the NNI in 2011 and received funding to collect data on the use of nanomaterials in consumer products the same year. Like the FDA, the CPSC indicated that safety regulation of nanomaterials can be achieved using existing mechanisms, but the CPSC does not provide a list of important physicochemical properties. In its 2016 budget request [39], the CPSC requested an additional $5 million to establish the Center for Consumer Product Applications and Safety Implications of Nanotechnology (CPASION), which will develop methods of identifying and characterizing nanomaterials in consumer products and their effects on human exposure.

Occupational and environmental exposures to nanomaterials are regulated and studied in the United States by the National Institute for Occupational Safety and Health (NIOSH), the Environmental Protection Agency (EPA), and the Occupational Safety and Health Administration (OSHA). Although NIOSH has published several guidance documents on nanomaterials in the workplace [40], no specific lists of important nanomaterial physicochemical properties are included. The EPA has provided brief lists of important properties as well as a detailed 2014 report [28] on characterization of engineered nanomaterials in the environment. In 2015, the EPA proposed recordkeeping and recording requirements for certain nanomaterials [41, 42] (the final rule was expected in October 2016 [42]), which would require unspecified physicochemical characterization data [43]. The final EPA rule [44] on nanomaterial reporting was published in January 2017 (effective date extended to August 2017) and required one-time reporting and three-year recordkeeping on certain specified nanomaterial classes. Materials that fall under the purview of this regulation include insoluble materials that are solid at standard temperature and pressure (STP) and are of a size between 1 and 100 nm, exhibit unique or novel properties, or contain particulate nanomaterials in concentrations over 1 wt%. Substantial focus is placed on certain listed physicochemical properties (size, zeta potential, specific surface area, dispersion stability, and surface reactivity) in identifying nanomaterials as discreet forms. Although the rule itself does not specify which physicochemical characterization data will be required, the EPA registration form for nanomaterials contains a worksheet with a detailed list of important physicochemical properties [45].

Finally, the US National Institute of Standards and Technology (NIST) has provided extensive guidance on nanomaterial characterization [46] through both characterization methods standards as well as work by the Nanotechnology Characterization Lab (NCL) [47]. One of the NCL's principal objectives is to "establish and standardize an analytical cascade for nanomaterial characterization" [48].

Canadian policies are similar to those in the United States in that existing regulatory approaches are used for nanomaterials. In 2007, Health Canada and Environment Canada proposed a regulatory framework for nanomaterials under the New Substances Notification Regulations (NSNR) as opposed to creating separate legislation [49]. A "New Substances Program Advisory Note" published in 2014 [50] detailed the required notification of new nanoscale materials via the NSNR. This advisory note also indicates that particle size data generally will be requested for certain enumerated materials and may be requested for others. Additional information, including characterization, fate, and toxicological information (not specified), may also be requested as part of the new material registration process. At the request of the Minister of Health, the Council of Canadian Academies prepared a detailed 2008 report on the regulatory challenges of nanomaterials [11]. This report contains lists of important properties as well as references to lists from the literature and other organizations. Health Canada has since released a policy statement in 2011 regarding the definition of nanomaterials [10], the current version of which contains guidance information including a list of important physicochemical properties. In July 2016, Environment Canada and Health Canada solicited comments on a proposed prioritization plan for nanomaterials [51]. This proposed plan, modeled after the DF4nanogrouping approach (European Centre for Ecotoxicology and Toxicology of Chemicals [ECETOC]) [29], prioritizes nanomaterials largely on the basis of their physicochemical properties, many of which are listed.

4.2.2 Europe

In general, like the United States and Canada, Europe evaluates nanomaterials on a case-by-case basis [52]. In 2007, the Registration, Evaluation and Authorization of Chemicals (REACH) legislation went into effect [53]. This overarching regulation establishes a system of registration and evaluation of chemical substances, including (but not specifically naming) nanomaterials. Later guidelines issued in 2008 [54] and 2010 [55] clarify that nanoscale forms of a substance are distinct and must be treated separately in REACH. The physicochemical data required by REACH is not specific to nanomaterials; however, detailed guidance has been provided for nanomaterials, including a list of physicochemical properties in 2011 [56] and measurement methods in 2012 [57]. The REACH Implementation Project on Nanomaterials (RIPoN) was formed by the European Commission in 2009 to provide guidance on implementation of REACH regulations for nanomaterials [58]. In 2011, RIPoN published a report that included a list of important physicochemical properties [12]. The OECD Working Party on Manufactured Nanomaterials has been referenced by the European Union (EU) for recommendations regarding additional physicochemical characterization endpoints beyond the REACH requirements [55, 57].

In 2009, the regulatory process for cosmetics was changed in the EU to include reporting requirements specific to products containing nanomaterials [59]. As of 2013, notification of all cosmetic products containing nanomaterials must be made six months prior to release for new products or immediately for existing products (a requirement more stringent than those for products without nanomaterials). Information such as the identity, size and physicochemical properties (not specifically identified), rate of use, and safety and toxicological information must be included in the notification.

The European Medicines Agency (EMA) and the European Food Safety Authority (EFSA) consider existing regulations and processes sufficient for nanomaterial-containing products but acknowledge that special expertise may be required to evaluate these products [31, 60]. The EMA provides limited guidance for specific nanomaterials (including lists of important properties) [61, 62]. The EFSA published a scientific opinion document in 2009 [31] that includes a list of important characteristics of nanomaterials and references several other lists (such as OECD lists and lists from open literature sources). On a larger scale, the European Commission's Scientific Committee on Consumer Safety (in conjunction with the EMA and the EFSA, among other organizations) has provided characterization guidance on nanomaterials in cosmetics [9], including a list of important properties. The EU Scientific Committee on Emerging and Newly Identified Health Risks (SCENIHR) has published several opinions on the determination of potential health effects of nanomaterials, including lists of important physicochemical properties [15, 24, 34].

4.2.3 Australia

Australia employs a regulatory approach consistent with OECD recommendations [63, 64]. Industrial nanomaterials, including formulations containing nanomaterials, are regulated through the National Industrial Chemicals Notification and Assessment Scheme (NICNAS) as of 2011. This approach is similar to that of Canada, where nanomaterials must be reported to the government, self-assessment of safety is not permitted, and additional physicochemical characterization is required [65]. Particle size data (primary particle size and number distribution) is required at a minimum for declared nanomaterials, materials where uncertainty exists over the presence of nanomaterials, and insoluble dispersions and powders [13]. Additional physicochemical characterization data may be required, and a list of important parameters is provided [13]. The Australian Pesticides and Veterinary Medicines Authority (APVMA) recently updated regulations involving risk assessment of products under their purview in 2014 and issued a report on nanotechnology regulation in 2015 [14]. This report references several lists of important physicochemical properties from ISO TC 229, OECD [66], and scientific literature [17].

4.2.4 Other Countries

In addition to the major national-level efforts discussed in Sections 4.2.1–4.2.3, national-level efforts at nanotechnology standardization exist in several other countries [67]. Many of these countries participate in or interface with the international standardization efforts discussed in Section 4.2.5.

4.2.5 International Organizations

International efforts on defining nanomaterial physicochemical characterization requirements and properties of importance have largely occurred through work by the OECD, the ISO/International Electrotechnical Commission (IEC), and ASTM International. Perhaps the most significant international effort is that of the OECD, whose nanotechnology working parties include the EU and over 30 member and nonmember countries, as well as several international organizations (ISO, World Health Organization [WHO], United Nations Environment Programme [UNEP], etc.) [68]. Two OECD working parties related to nanotechnology were founded in 2006 [69] and 2007 [70]: the Working Party on Manufactured Nanomaterials and the Working Party on Nanotechnology, respectively. The OECD has published, and continues to publish, numerous documents on the characterization of nanomaterials, including a list of physicochemical characteristics of importance [19]. The OECD list of characteristics is often cited by represented organizations [9, 10, 14, 31].

ISO efforts on nanotechnology standardization began with the founding of "TC 229: Nanotechnologies" in 2005 [71] to address standardization and characterization of nanomaterials. ISO TC 229 membership currently includes 50 participating and observing countries and 10 liaison organizations [71]. ISO TC 229 published a list of important physicochemical properties of nanomaterials in 2012 [72]. ISO TC 229 interfaces closely [72] with IEC TC 113, founded in 2006, on matters related to nanotechnology standardization. The IEC and the ISO share two working groups on nanotechnology, with IEC standards principally focused on electrical and electronic systems containing nanomaterials.

ASTM International founded a technical committee on nanotechnology (E56) with a subcommittee on Characterization: Physical, Chemical, and Toxicological Properties in 2005 [73]. Although it has authored several standards on nanomaterial and toxicological characterization [74], it does not provide a list of important properties.

4.3 Specific Physicochemical Parameters

Broadly speaking, nanomaterials may exist in a wide range of possible forms, including free forms (such as free particles), fixed forms (such as semiconductor devices), and intermediate forms (such as composites and solid formulations). This diversity of nanomaterial forms leads to an equally diverse set of potentially important physical and chemical characteristics, as outlined in the previous section (Table 4.1) and discussed in Chapter 3. These properties may also change when a nanomaterial is exposed to different conditions for different amounts of time, requiring characterization to be considered at multiple points. From a safety and regulatory perspective, the nanomaterial properties of most concern are those related to free forms, such as particulate materials. These nanomaterials represent the greatest potential for release, mobility, and biological interaction. While it may be impossible to exhaustively list all potentially important physicochemical properties for all nanomaterials under all conditions, the characteristics discussed in this section include the properties of highest concern. These properties of importance can be broadly classified into the following categories:

- **General/Descriptive characteristics**:
  - Dimensional characteristics: Characteristic dimensions, structure, and properties related to the physical dimensions of the material
  - Identity: Chemical and physical identify of the material
  - Surface chemistry: Surface-specific chemical and physical properties
- **Advanced and application-specific characteristics**:
  - Reactivity: The reactivity of the material toward light, heat, other materials, etc.
  - Suspension properties: Properties that influence the state of dispersion or dispersibility in suspended nanomaterials
  - Bulk powder properties: Properties specific to the behavior of nanomaterials in bulk powder form
  - Other advanced characteristics

4.3.1 Size, Shape, and Dimensional Characteristics

The definition of "nanomaterial" typically encompasses one or both of the following features: nanoscale phenomena and nanoscale size. Regardless of complexity, most definitions include, at a minimum, the criteria that some dimension of a nanomaterial exists at a size below 100 nm. Determination of the critical dimensions of a nanomaterial is the typical first stage in identifying and characterizing the nanomaterial. Defining size can encompass a wide range of possible dimensions in a nanomaterial: primary particle size, agglomerate size, internal dimensions, roughness, etc. Not all possible dimensions are applicable to all nanomaterial systems; the characteristic dimensions of a macroscopic porous body with nanoscale internal features, for example, differ considerably from those of a solid spherical nanoparticle. Careful study is required to define the dimensions of importance for a given system. Dimensional characteristics encompass the size, shape, and orientation (structure) of a nanomaterial and may be subdivided into internal dimensions (such as pore size) and external dimensions (such as particle size). These subdivisions will be discussed individually in the following sections.

4.3.1.1 External dimensional characteristics

The external dimensional characteristics of principal importance in nanoscale materials are shown in Table 4.2. For particulate nanomaterials, the principal dimensional characteristics are particle size and size distribution. In countries with enhanced reporting and testing requirements for nanomaterials, such as the EU [75, 76], Canada [10], the United States [44], and Australia [77], particle size is one of the criteria used in the decision to treat a material as "new" or "nanoscale," thereby triggering additional regulatory requirements. Particle size [78–84], shape [85–87], and topography [88, 89] are also well known to influence the behavior, fate, and toxicity of nanomaterials. Defining the size of particulate nanomaterials can be a complex process, particularly for anisotropic and irregularly shaped materials. Anisotropic particles may require several metrics for adequate characterization. Rod- and plate-shaped particles, at a minimum, would have two characteristic dimensions and one aspect ratio showing how these dimensions are related (Figs. 4.1

Table 4.2 External dimensional characteristics of nanomaterials and associated properties

	Definition/Notes	Common metrics	Common characterization methods
Particle size	External dimension of the dispersed phase, including agglomerates, emulsions, and suspensions in nonfluid media	Feret's diameter, Martin's diameter, equivalent sphere, min./max. dimension, etc.	Microscopy/image analysis, SPM, DLS, laser diffraction, sedimentation methods, BET, scattering techniques (XRD, SAXS, SANS, etc.), DMA, etc.
Primary particle size	External dimension of the smallest identifiable and physically continuous particles or dispersed phase	Feret's diameter, Martin's diameter, equivalent sphere, min./max. dimension, etc.	Microscopy/image analysis, SPM, DLS, laser diffraction, sedimentation methods, BET, scattering techniques (XRD, SAXS, SANS, etc.), DMA, etc.
Size distribution	Distribution of particle sizes using one of the previously listed particle size metrics	Number, surface, and volume distributions, summary statistics of these, PDI, etc.	Microscopy/image analysis, SPM, DLS, laser diffraction, sedimentation methods, BET, scattering techniques (XRD, SAXS, SANS, etc.), DMA, etc.

	Definition/Notes	Common metrics	Common characterization methods
Shape/ aspect ratio	Characteristic dimensions of anisotropic particles or ratios thereof; metrics describing particle shape	Sizes (as above), aspect ratio, circularity, shape descriptors, etc.	Microscopy/ image analysis, SPM
Roughness	Roughness, dimensional characteristics of surface features	Roughness metrics, lateral correlation length, other characteristic dimensions	Microscopy/ image analysis, SPM, diffraction/ scattering techniques, profilometry
Surface topography	Description of the positioning, dimensions, and orientation of surface features; often referring to length scales larger than roughness but may be inclusive of roughness	Dimensions, shape, symmetry and orientation descriptors, spacing and ordering of features, RDF	Microscopy/ image analysis, SPM, diffraction/ scattering techniques, profilometry
Fractal dimension	Ratio indicating how surface features change with scale	Fractal dimension	Microscopy/ image analysis, SPM, diffraction/ scattering techniques, profilometry

DLS, dynamic light scattering; BET, Brunauer–Emmett–Teller; XRD, X-ray diffraction; SAXS, small-angle X-ray scattering; SANS, small-angle neutron scattering; DMA, differential mobility analyzer; PDI, polydispersity index; SPM, scanning probe microscopy; RDF, radial distribution function.

and 4.2). Figure 4.1 illustrates the complexities in defining particle size. Numerous metrics for defining particle size exist but are infrequently specified and/or only applicable to imaging techniques. Additionally, the majority of common ensemble particle-sizing methods operate under the assumption that analyzed particles are spherical (or substantially close to spherical), which is often not the case. Imaging-based particle-sizing methods are powerful tools in characterizing nanomaterials, particularly those with complex or anisotropic structures. However, these methods typically employ 2D imaging techniques, which may bias image analysis toward one specific particle orientation (e.g., the thickness of plate-shaped particles may be poorly represented due to preferential orientation, or the dimensions of the 2D projection of a particle may vary based on the orientation of the particle with respect to the imaging apparatus). Three-dimensional imaging techniques are infrequently used but have the potential to generate a rich data set for complex particle systems.

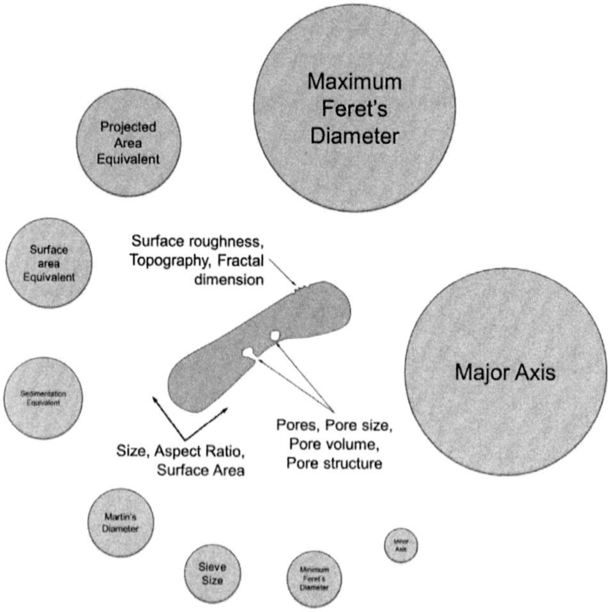

Figure 4.1 Dimensional characteristics of nanomaterials. Examples of several particle size metrics for the central particle are illustrated.

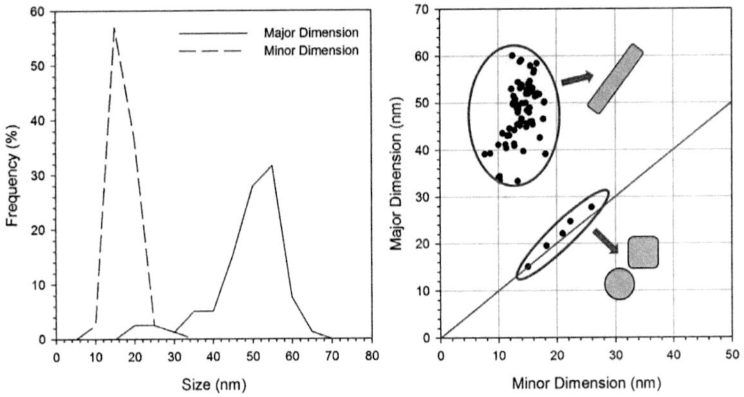

Figure 4.2 Major and minor dimensions and aspect ratio distributions of gold nanorods.

The characteristic dimensions of nanomaterials are rarely perfectly monodisperse, making the distribution of dimensions a key piece of data in characterizing nanomaterials. Data derived from these distributions, such as mean, median, mode, d90, and d10, are used for specifying nominal particle sizes and in providing summary statistics. Size distributions and summary statistics may be given in terms of particle number, surface area, or volume to highlight specific features of the size distribution. Consideration of both number and volume distributions provides a clearer picture of broad or polydisperse size distributions and helps to address the issue of fines (Fig. 4.3). The production and handling of particulate materials will often result in the generation of incidental fines, which may be nanoscale. By mass, these particles represent an insignificant percentage of the total material, but by number they are much more significant. Some regulatory agencies [10, 75] include both incidental and deliberately manufactured nanomaterials within the scope of their nanomaterial regulations and have introduced regulatory definitions based on specific particle size distributions. Most often, the number distribution is used, which tends to heavily weight smaller, more numerous particles. The EU defines [75, 76] a nanomaterial as a material containing particles with at least one external dimension between 1 and 100 nm where these particles comprise at least 50% of particles by number. This percentage threshold may be decreased to as low as 1% when ". . . warranted by concerns for the environment, health, safety or competitiveness . . .," and the definition provides that fullerenes, graphene flakes, and single-walled carbon nanotubes with dimensions below 1 nm will also be included. Australia's NICNAS defines a nanomaterial as a manufactured material with unique properties, typically ranging between 1 and 100 nm, which either has nanoscale structures or has a dimension at the nanoscale. NICNAS and the Australian Pesticides and Veterinary Medicines Authority (AVPMA) 2014 definitions include materials containing particles where 10% or more of the particles fit the definition of a nanomaterial [77]. The US EPA recently clarified its 2017 reporting rule to exempt materials where 1% or less of particles by mass is below a size of 100 nm [44].

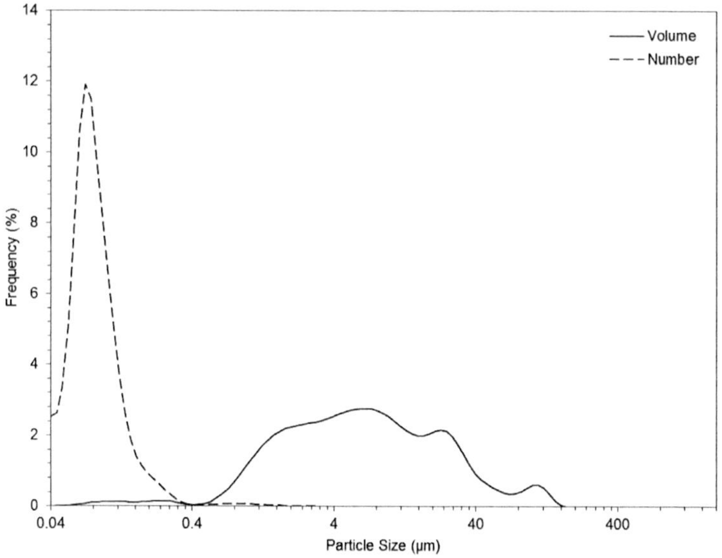

Figure 4.3 Number and volume particle size distributions of a nanoscale powder dispersed in water.

An additional degree of complexity arises from the fact that for various reasons, collections of dispersed particles can assemble into larger agglomerate particles. While the primary particles retain their size-related properties, such as reactivity and high surface area, the collective particle itself exhibits different properties than either a solid particle of the same size or the individual primary particles.

Agglomeration, coagulation, and flocculation are frequently cited issues with suspensions and are characterized, in part, using size distributions. For a given material, these behaviors vary with the dispersion medium, dispersion method, and time, among other factors. A dry powder, for example, will likely exhibit distinctly different particles sizes when aerosolized versus when dispersed in a liquid medium. Characterization of the particle size under a relevant set of conditions and time points is particularly important for determining toxicological parameters such as dose and exposure.

Materials may also exhibit nanoscale external surface features, such as surface roughness or topography. Many common macroscopic objects not generally considered to be nanomaterials exhibit nanoscale surface topography. Perhaps of more concern are materials with deliberately created nanoscale surface features, such as nanowires or nanotubes grown on a substrate. Materials with nanoscale surface features can be characterized using roughness metrics, fractal dimension, and other relevant dimensional characteristics for pattered features or adhered particles.

4.3.1.2 Surface area and internal dimensions

Although considerable interest has been given to particulate nanomaterials, by many definitions, a range of other materials may be classified as nanoscale due to their internal (rather than external) dimensions. A major class of nanomaterials includes porous bodies with nanoscale pore structures. Biological effects have been attributed to the porosity and pore structure for some materials [90, 91]. Porous materials with nanoscale internal dimensions do not necessarily have to also possess external dimensions on the nanometer scale. Materials such as porous ceramics and carbons fall into this category. Other materials, such as mesoporous silica particles, possess both nanoscale external and internal features (Fig. 4.4). Macroscopic porous bodies often receive less attention than other nanomaterials due to the fact that macroscopic bodies are less likely to biologically interact than a particle and that many materials (such as activated carbon and porous ceramics) have been in the marketplace for decades. The principal internal dimensional characteristics of nanomaterials are outlined in Table 4.3.

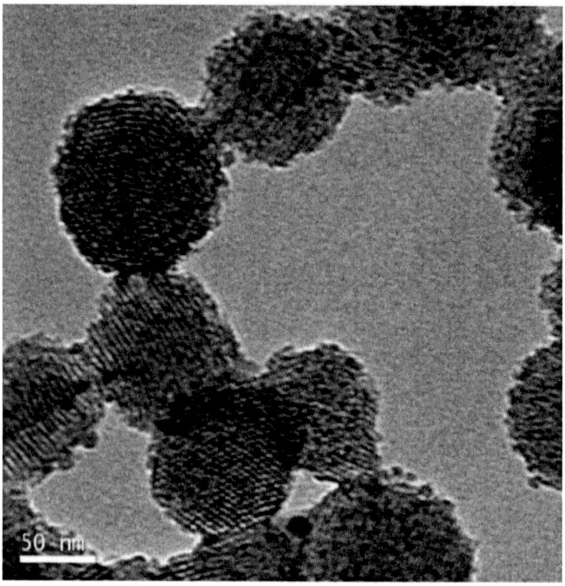

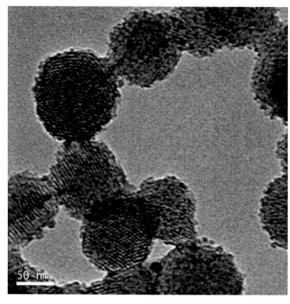

Figure 4.4 Internal dimensional characteristics of nanomaterials: mesoporous silica particles exhibiting both nanoscale internal and external dimensions.

Table 4.3 Internal dimensional characteristics of nanomaterials and associated properties

	Definition/Notes	Common metrics	Common characterization methods
Surface area	Typically, the accessible surface area of a material	Surface area, specific surface area (by mass and volume)	Gas and vapor sorption
Density	Material density (including closed porosity)	Volumetric mass density	Gas pycnometry
Bulk/ Apparent/ Pour density	Density of a material or bulk powder, including all porosity and interparticle voids	Volumetric mass density	Volume measurements

	Definition/Notes	Common metrics	Common characterization methods
Pore volume and/or number	Total volume occupied by pores within a material (and/or total number of pores)	Volume/specific volume, number/pore density	Gas and vapor sorption, Hg porosimetry, pycnometry
Pore size	Dimension(s) of pores within the material structure	Pore radius	Microscopy/image analysis, CT, Hg porosimetry, porometry, gas/vapor sorption, scattering methods
Pore size distribution	Distribution of pore sizes within the material	Volume and number distributions	Microscopy/image analysis, CT, Hg porosimetry, porometry, gas/vapor sorption, scattering methods
Pore shape and structure	Shape, structure, tortuosity, and connectivity of pores	Shape and structure descriptors	Microscopy/image analysis, CT, Hg porosimetry, gas/vapor sorption, scattering methods
Fractal dimension	Ratio indicating how pore structures change with scale	Fractal dimension	Microscopy/image analysis, CT, Hg porosimetry, gas/vapor sorption, scattering methods

CT, computed tomography.

One of the most widely listed properties of importance for nanomaterials is surface area. Characteristics often associated with nanomaterials, such as reactivity, adsorbency, and dissolution, are strongly surface mediated. The surface area of nanomaterials is also a factor known to influence toxicity [92, 93]. Fine particle size, porosity, and surface topography are the principal contributing factors to the high specific surface areas often found in nanomaterials. For materials where internal dimensions contribute to the structure or surface area, metrics such as porosity, pore type, structure, and critical dimensions are most important. As with internal dimensions, careful study must be conducted to determine the characteristic external dimensions applicable to a particular system.

Characterization of surface area and pore structure is strongly dependent on the type of porosity found in a material. Pores may be closed or open, may or may not extend through a material, may vary in tortuosity, and/or be linked or branched (Fig. 4.5). The definition of a pore itself is also subjective—the nanoscale void spaces between primary particles in contact with one another may be variably interpreted as porosity. Pore dimensions and structures may also change throughout a material (Fig. 4.6). Analogous to the particle size, the pore size and size distributions are the principal metrics used to characterize the internal dimensions of porous materials. Accessible (open) porosity and surface area may be probed by a wide range of techniques, including intrusion porosimetry methods and sorption methods, while closed porosity is generally restricted to imaging and scattering methods.

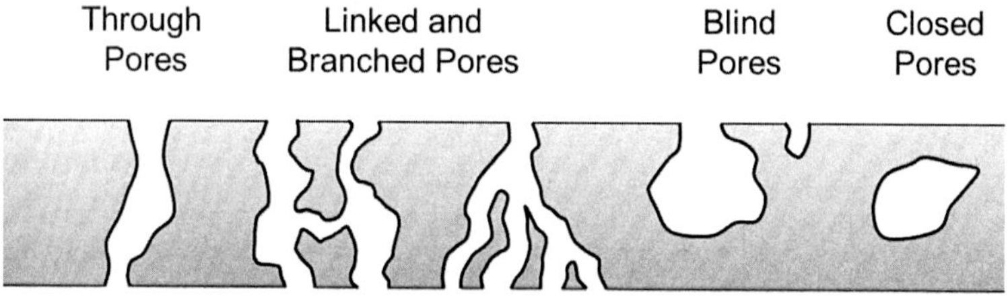

Figure 4.5 Internal dimensional characteristics of nanomaterials: illustration of common pore structures.

In addition to the dimensions and structures of porous materials, the total pore volume (and/or number) is another important characteristic. Pore volume may be obtained using many of the same methods used for pore size analysis as well as density measurements in certain circumstances. The gas pycnometer density of a material can provide insight into pore structures of solid materials. The volume of closed pores contribute to the volume measured by gas pycnometry, while open pores will not, and if the nonvoid material density is known, the closed pore volume may be estimated. For macroscopic porous bodies, the volume occupied by the body itself can be used to determine the open pore volume in conjunction with gas pycnometer data.

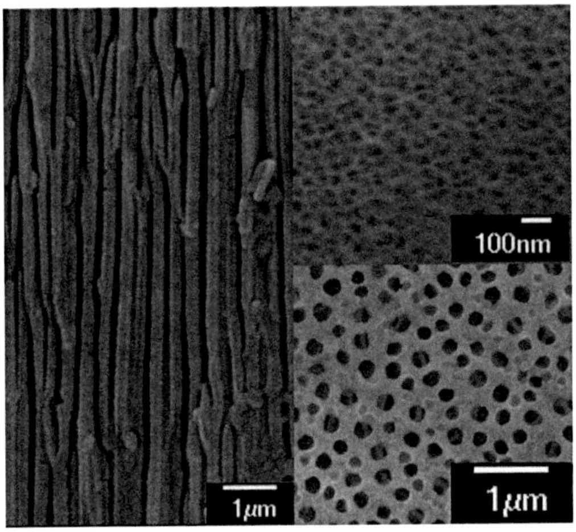

Figure 4.6 Internal dimensional characteristics of nanomaterials: anodic alumina membrane showing pore structure changes through the material thickness. The cross section (left), top surface (top right), and bottom surface (bottom right) are shown.

4.3.2 Chemical Identity and Properties

The chemical and physical identities of a nanomaterial are determining factors for a variety of toxicologically relevant properties, such as reactivity and dissolution. Additionally, as with all substances, the atomic, chemical, and physical purities of a nanomaterial are important. The principal metrics of identity and purity are listed in Table 4.4.

Verifying the elemental composition and purity is an important initial step in the characterization of a nanomaterial. Dopants are often used in nanomaterials to alter optical or physical properties, and impurities from manufacture are well known to exist in many nanomaterials. Carbon nanotubes, for example, often contain significant quantities of inorganic impurity particles left over from manufacture, which are known to affect biological response [94, 95]. Chemical identity and purity are the next concerns. For inorganic nanomaterials, the valence state and bonding properties are perhaps the most important chemical identity factors, while for organic materials, structure and isomerism are key properties.

Table 4.4 Properties related to the chemical and physical identity of a nanomaterial

	Definition/Notes	Common metrics	Common characterization methods
Elemental composition and purity	Elemental composition	Atomic and mass composition, stoichiometry	Wide range of techniques: ICP/AA, CHNO/S, EDS/WDS/XRF, etc.
Phase/ Crystallography	Phase composition and structure, defects and defect structure, amorphous content and structure	Crystal structure, phase composition, amorphous content, RDF	Scattering techniques (XRD, neutron diffraction, etc.), TEM
Crystallite size	Size of crystalline domains	Crystallite size, size distribution	Scattering techniques (XRD, neutron diffraction, electron diffraction, etc.), TEM
Chemical identity and purity	Valence, bonding state, chemical structure	Chemical structure, composition	Wide range of techniques: XPS, XAS, IR/Raman, NMR, MS tech, EELS, etc.
Density	Material density (including closed porosity)	Volumetric mass density	Pycnometry

	Definition/Notes	Common metrics	Common characterization methods
Solubility	Solubility of a nanomaterial, leaching of soluble species, and kinetics of these	Solubility, K_{sp}, dissolution kinetics, identity of solubilized species	Wide range of techniques: gravimetry, LC, GC, ICP/AA, etc.
Hydration	Quantity and mechanism of moisture incorporation into a material	Hydration, stoichiometry	TGA/DSC, TPR/TPD, gravimetry, titrimetry, vapor sorption
Effect on pH	Effect on pH when dispersed (if relevant)	pH, K_a, buffer capacity	pH/titrimetry
Form and appearance	Form and appearance of a nanomaterial	Appearance	Visual inspection

ICP, inductively coupled plasma; AA, atomic absorption; CHNO/S, carbon hydrogen nitrogen oxygen sulfur elemental analysis; EDS, energy-dispersive X-ray spectroscopy; WDS, wavelength-dispersive spectroscopy; XRF, X-ray fluorescence spectroscopy; XRD, X-ray diffraction; RDF, radial distribution function; TEM, transmission electron microscopy; XPS, X-ray photoelectron spectroscopy; XAS, X-ray absorption spectroscopy; IR, infrared; NMR, nuclear magnetic resonance; MS, mass spectrometry; EELS, electron energy loss spectroscopy; LC, liquid chromatography; GC, gas chromatography; TGA, thermogravimetric analysis; DSC, differential scanning calorimetry; TPR, temperature-programmed reaction; TPD, temperature-programmed desorption.

The solubility of a nanomaterial in a relevant system is important particularly when leaching is a concern. In some regulatory systems (such as Australia's NICNAS [13]) or the US EPA [44], solubility is also a property used to determine whether or not a material is considered a nanomaterial and may be subject to additional testing and reporting requirements. The solubility and subsequent effects of solubilized species have been shown to influence toxicity [96–98]. Some nanomaterials may cause a pH change when exposed to an aqueous medium due to dissolution, reaction, or protonation/deprotonation of surface groups. The high specific surface area of many nanomaterials may permit sufficient numbers of pH-active sites to be available. Materials exhibiting this behavior may be characterized using the dissociation constant, buffer capacity, or pH change.

Since nanomaterials may exist in multiple crystallographic forms, identification of the phase composition, crystallography, and amorphous content are important. The chemical, physical, and toxicological [99, 100] properties of a material may differ significantly between different crystalline and amorphous phases of the same compound. For example, solubility of many amorphous or disordered materials is significantly higher than their corresponding crystalline analogs [101]. Photocatalytic activity and radical generation are also strongly related to phase composition [100, 102, 103]. Finally, for crystalline materials, the size and quality of the crystalline domains within a material can significantly affect the chemical and physical properties of that material [104].

4.3.3 Surface Chemistry

Surface chemistry is often the dominant source of interactions in many nanomaterial systems and contributes directly to colloidal stability, adsorptivity, reactivity, and many nanoscale phenomena. Surface chemistry is dynamic and varies with the media in contact with the nanomaterial and the nanomaterial composition, among other factors. Nanomaterial surfaces are frequently modified to alter their physical and chemical properties or enhance stability, potentially adding an additional layer of complexity. Surface-mediated factors such as charge [105–107], chemistry [105, 108, 109], and hydrophobicity [110–112] are well known to influence toxicity and biological effects. Characterization of the surface chemistry of nanomaterials is therefore critical. The principal surface chemical properties for nanomaterials are outlined in Table 4.5.

Table 4.5 Properties related to nanomaterial surface chemistry

	Definition/Notes	Common metrics	Common characterization methods
Surface composition	Elemental composition of nanomaterial surface	Atomic and mass composition, stoichiometry	XPS, SIMS, Auger spectroscopy
Surface structure	Crystallographic structure and orientation of the surface	Crystal structure and orientation	Scattering techniques (XRD, LEED, etc.), TEM, SPM
Surface chemistry	Valence, bonding state, chemical structure, adsorbate composition	Chemical structure, composition	XPS, IR/Raman, SIMS, TEM, gas and vapor sorption methods, etc.
Surface potential and zeta potential	Charge at surface (surface potential) or boundary layer (zeta potential) in medium of interest	Charge, IEP/PZC, titration data (charge vs. pH/concentration)	DLS, streaming potential, electroacoustic methods, optical methods
Wettability and hydrophobicity	Hydrophobicity or hydrophilicity of a material, wettability	Partition coefficient, surface energy, contact angle	Intrusion porosimetry, octanol–water partition coefficient, contact angle
Adsorbate structure	Structure and density of adsorbates on a material surface	Adsorbate surface density and structure, adsorption isotherm	Various techniques: SPM, scattering techniques, IR and fluorescence spectroscopy, chemical analysis methods, etc.

XPS, X-ray photoelectron spectroscopy; SIMS, secondary ion mass spectroscopy; XRD, X-ray diffraction; LEED, low-energy electron diffraction; TEM, transmission electron microscopy; SPM, scanning probe microscopy (includes atomic force microscopy and scanning tunneling microscopy); IR, infrared; IEP, isoelectric point; PZC, point of zero charge; DLS, dynamic light scattering; AFM, atomic force microscopy; STM, scanning tunneling microscopy.

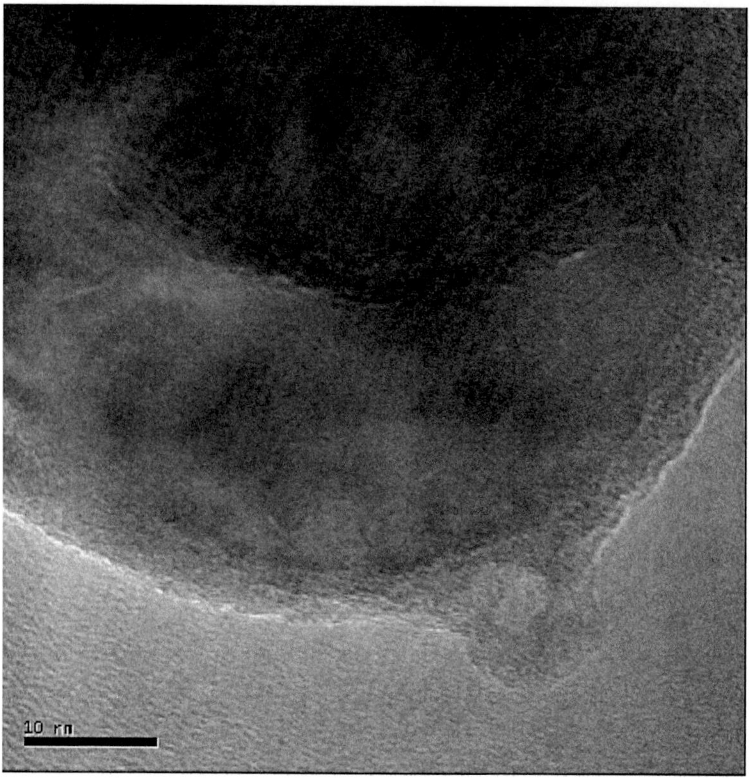

Figure 4.7 Surface chemistry of nanoscale aluminum particles: TEM image of nanoscale aluminum particles showing a crystalline aluminum core and an amorphous hydrated oxide surface layer.

The surface composition of a nanomaterial may vary significantly from its bulk composition in terms of its elemental, chemical, and structural characteristics. The method of preparation, environmental exposure, intentional modifications, etc., all may contribute to differences in the elemental composition of the surface. In the example shown in Fig. 4.7, crystalline aluminum nanoparticles, due to reactivity with moisture and oxygen, will form a thin, hydrated amorphous oxide layer on the surface. This layer will largely determine the charge behavior of these particles when dispersed in water (Fig. 4.8). The surface composition of suspended nanomaterials is typically not measured in situ due to the limitations of the relevant characterization techniques. In situ surface composition of suspended nanomaterials therefore must be inferred from other metrics or related to ex situ measurements (when possible). In addition to composition, crystallographic orientation and crystallinity are important characteristics of the surface of nanomaterials. Surface structure and orientation affect properties such as reactivity, adsorbate type and density, charge, and adsorbate structure. Crystalline nanomaterials may exist in the form of random polycrystals, oriented polycrystals, or single crystals. In each case, the type and extent of crystallographic orientations exposed on the surface will vary. This is particularly important in anisotropic materials, where different geometric orientations of the material will often exhibit different crystallographic orientations. Anisotropic materials, for example, may exhibit significant differences in surface charge on the basis of crystallographic orientation (Fig. 4.9).

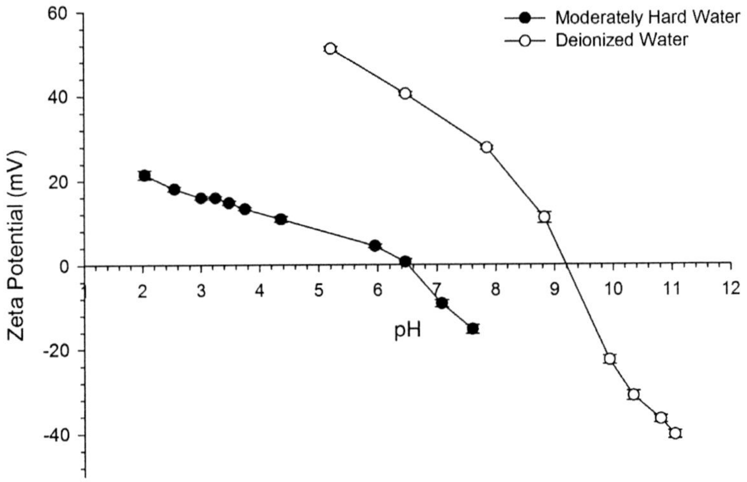

Figure 4.8 Surface chemistry of nanoscale aluminum particles: zeta potential titration of nanoscale aluminum particles in deionized water and moderately hard tap water. Zeta potential titration in deionized water is consistent with pure aluminum oxide. The presence and type of ions in moderately hard water result in a shift in the isoelectric point and a depression in the magnitude of the zeta potential compared to deionized water.

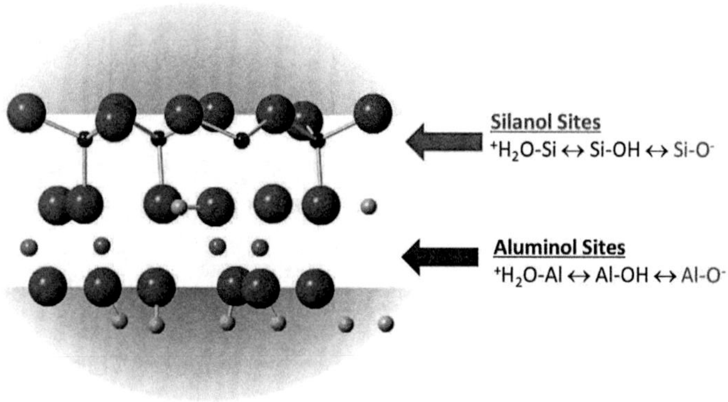

Figure 4.9 Surface chemistry of anisotropic materials: Illustration of the effects of crystallographic orientation on the surface potential of kaolin clay [132]. The faces and edges have sites that differ in the point of zero charge, resulting in pH-dependent charge differences between locations.

In addition to surface compositional and structural differences, chemical changes in the surface are also possible. Chemistry differences from the bulk, such as valence, hydration, and bonding, are important in most surface-mediated processes. The chemistry of a surface may vary with the medium in contact with the surface and can directly determine charge, colloidal stability, and adsorbate type/structure. The surface chemistry of nanomaterials is often modified for the purposes of enhancing stability and mediating the interactions of the materials with their environment. Common methods of surface modification involve the adsorption of a desired compound, chemical modification of the existing surface, or a combination thereof. Adsorption and desorption isotherms provide several pieces of important information about surface modification via adsorbates, including strength of interaction, adsorbate density, and adsorbate structure. Adsorbate structure, which may be inferred from simultaneous measurements of the adsorption isotherm and layer thickness, may also be probed directly using methods such as scanning probe microscopy (SPM), Fourier transform infrared spectroscopy (FTIR), and scattering techniques. For systems involving the chemical modification of an existing surface, determination of the number of active sites or the extent of conversion may be measured.

The surface composition and chemistry are critical determiners of dispersion stability in particulate materials. The mechanisms of dispersion stability and consequences of surface chemistry will be discussed in more detail in Section 4.3.4.2; however an introduction will be presented here. Charge-related properties are among the most commonly listed physicochemical properties of nanomaterials. Charge-related properties govern the efficacy of electrostatic stabilization, one of the most common mechanisms of dispersion in particulate systems. Particles stabilized by this mechanism will resist agglomeration due to repulsive interparticle forces if they exhibit a sufficient charge. The medium in which the particles are suspended plays a major role in determining the length scales at which the surface charge is propagated, which, in turn, determines charge effectiveness. A medium containing a sufficient concentration of ions, for example, may screen the surface charge to the extent that the dispersion is no longer stable. The zeta potential, which is often conflated with surface potential, is the potential measured at the shear plane rather than the surface, and provides a practical indication of dispersion stability. The zeta potential is also significantly easier to directly measure than the surface potential. Determining both the surface potential and the zeta potential can provide a clearer picture of the dispersion system. The surface potential can reveal information about the surface chemistry, active sites, and potential interactions with other species, while the zeta potential will show the effective charge in a medium and provide an indication of dispersion stability. The zeta potential may also be used in the characterization of adsorbates, as adsorbates will often change the zeta potential in a manner dependent on the adsorbate density, structure, and/or environment. Finally, charge-related properties of nanomaterials will mediate the interaction of nanomaterials with external surfaces, which also often exhibit a charge. From the standpoint of nanomaterial safety, adhesion of nanomaterials to and interaction with biologically relevant surfaces (such as cell membrane and tissue surfaces) are cases where charge-related properties may strongly determine biologic activity. For macroscopic and planar materials, analogous streaming potential measurements may be employed to characterize these systems.

Wettability and hydrophobicity are important and often-cited physicochemical characteristics of nanomaterials. The hydrophobicity of a material can determine dispersion stability in a medium as well as the type and structure of an adsorbate, among other factors. The combined effects of nanoscale surface features and material hydrophobicity can also dramatically alter the wettability relative to a nontextured material [113, 114]. There is no specific and universally accepted scale of hydrophobicity. Metrics such as the octanol–water partition coefficient and contact angle are used to characterize materials on a method-dependent scale. For particulate materials, the octanol–water partition coefficient is an often-cited method, while for planar materials, the contact angle is commonly used.

4.3.4 Advanced and Application-Specific Characteristics

The previous sections focused on the descriptive physical and chemical properties of nanomaterials. This, however, represents only part of the potentially important physicochemical properties. Beyond descriptive information, consideration must be given to the behavior of nanomaterials in their intended application, the behavior of nanomaterials when exposed to relevant environments, and the properties unique to nanomaterials that are distinctly different from the bulk. The potential list of advanced properties of nanomaterials is evolving with the development of new materials and applications. Due to the increasing diversity in these applications, potential advanced properties can span over a wide range of disciplines. Since advanced properties are also typically tied to specific materials and/or applications, the list in this section is not intended to be exhaustive. Factors of particular importance are those recognized to have significant potential impacts on public or environmental health. The groups of advanced and application-specific characteristics include:

- Reactivity
    - Photocatalytic properties
    - Reactivity
    - Radical formation
    - Redox potential
    - ROS generation

- Suspension properties
- Protein corona
- Bulk powder properties
- Composite materials
- Mechanical, magnetic, optical, and electronic properties

4.3.4.1 Reactivity

Reactivity, catalysis, and other surface-mediated processes may be strongly augmented by the high specific surface areas found in many nanomaterials. An example of this is illustrated with aluminum particles in Fig. 4.10. Terms such as "catalytic activity," "surface reactivity," and "reactivity" are recognized to be broadly defined characteristics [18]. Reactivity in general is strongly dependent on the environment to which a nanomaterial may be exposed. Careful consideration must be given to the application of the nanomaterial in order to determine the relevant types of reactivity. Reactivity to common materials and conditions, such as water, air, light, and heat, should be considered, in addition to application-specific conditions. Toxicological outcomes for many nanomaterials have been attributed to various types of reactivity [99, 115].

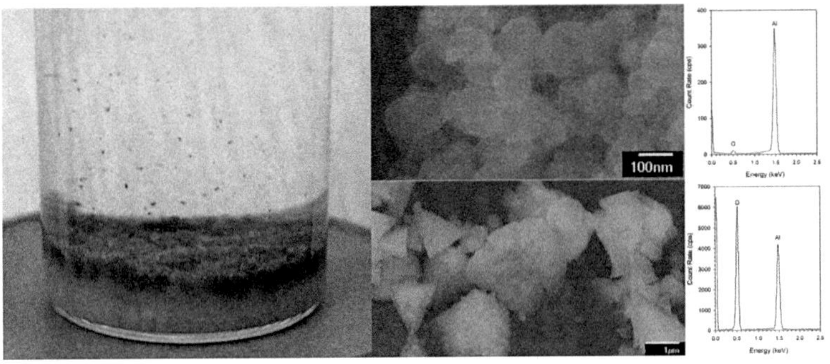

Figure 4.10 Image of nominally 50 nm aluminum particles (left image, gray layer) spontaneously reacting in water to form a hydrated aluminum oxide (left image, white layer) and hydrogen gas. The same behavior is not observed when larger particles are exposed to water under similar conditions. Scanning electron micrographs of as-received particles (center top) and particles after suspension in deionized water (center bottom). Corresponding EDS data (far right) shows a significant increase in oxygen content after suspension in water.

Three different aspects of reactivity are most often considered for nanomaterials: surface reactivity, chemical reactivity/catalytic activity, and photoreactivity/photocatalytic activity. Surface reactivity has been variably defined, ranging from a synonym for surface chemistry (OECD [14, 116]) to the impacts of surface charge (Australia [14]) on biological systems to chemical reactivity (OECD [18]). Surface reactivity and chemical reactivity are often conflated, as many chemical reactions involving solids propagate from the surface inward. Photocatalytic activity is perhaps the best-defined category of reactivity and has received significant attention due to the incorporation of nanoscale titanium oxide and zinc oxide particles in sunscreens. Materials exhibiting photocatalytic activity have the ability to generate reactive species, such as free radicals and reactive oxygen species, when exposed to certain wavelengths of light. These species subsequently can exhibit toxicity [92, 117]. Photoreactive materials, on the other hand, may undergo chemical reactions triggered by certain wavelengths of light but may not be catalytic in nature. These reactions can result in changes to particle morphology [118] as well as chemistry and toxicity [119]. There are many possible endpoints identified for the characterization of reactivity, and most lists are not considered to be comprehensive. At the most fundamental level, reactivity can be considered as any change in the physicochemical properties of a nanomaterial system. The enumerated endpoints related to reactivity most often focus on the generation of potentially damaging species, such as reactive oxygen species and radicals. Aside from these, endpoints such as redox potential, oxidizing properties, photocatalytic properties, reactive sites (number and type), and surface charge (or other surface chemical properties) are commonly listed. Other properties of importance may include the extent of reaction or equilibrium constant, thermochemistry of the reaction, rate and kinetics data, biological effect (e.g., hemolysis), etc.

4.3.4.2 Suspension stability

For particulate and suspended nanomaterials, dispersion stability and dispersibility are among the most frequently cited properties of importance. In terms of the potential biological effects of nanomaterials, dispersibility and dispersion stability are recognized as determining factors in the mechanism and extent of exposure as well as biological response. Dispersion stability is dependent on most of the aforementioned physicochemical characteristics of nanomaterials: the surface chemistry is the principal mediator of interparticle interactions, the dimensions of the nanomaterial play a role in determining the balance of interparticle forces that determine stability, and reactivity details how and if these properties change with time and condition. In addition to properties specific to the nanomaterials themselves, suspension stability and dispersibility are strongly dependent on the mechanism of dispersion and the medium. Additional characteristics, such as the mechanism and energetics of stability, conditions that promote or inhibit suspension stability, the kinetics of agglomeration, segregation, and partitioning provide a more complete picture of the suspension system.

The mechanisms determining suspension stability can be understood by examining the sources of interparticle forces and the distances over which they are applicable (Fig. 4.11). For a suspension to be stable, the net effect of the interparticle forces must result in sufficient repulsion between particles. The principal repulsive forces include electrostatic, steric, and solvation forces, while the principal attractive forces include hydrophobic, depletion, and van der Waals forces. Electrostatic and steric stabilization are perhaps the most common mechanisms of stability in particle systems. Factors that affect these stabilization mechanisms are outlined in Table 4.6. Electrostatic stabilization requires that the coulombic repulsion between particles be sufficient to overcome attractive forces, particularly van der Waals forces, as particles come in close proximity to one another. This mechanism is predicated on maintaining a zeta potential of sufficient magnitude. Properties that promote or inhibit this mechanism include the medium permittivity/polarizability and ionic strength, certain dispersion aids (such as surfactants), specifically adsorbing ions, the type and concentration of charged surface groups, potential determining ions, and other adsorbates that may alter the surface chemistry. By contrast, steric stabilization provides a strong entropically driven repulsive force that has fewer dependencies and is effective over a longer distance than electrostatic repulsion. Solvated polymer surfaces and polymer adsorbates provide this type of stabilization, which is somewhat dependent on the degree of solvation but not strongly dependent on salt type and concentration. Polymer adsorbates also introduce the potential for depletion stabilization and depletion flocculation. In addition to depletion flocculation, polymers permit flocculation by either bridging multiple particles (typically higher-molecular-weight polymers) or by providing charge neutralization (typically lower-molecular-weight polymers) (Fig. 4.12). The resultant agglomerate particles may vary in strength of adhesion and consequently the potential for redispersion. In addition to the properties outlined in the surface chemistry section, important characteristics/metrics related to dispersion stability and mechanism of stabilization include zeta potential titrations (pH, dilution, ionic strength, dispersant concentration, potential-determining ion concentration if not H^+/OH^-), adsorption isotherms, medium ion types and concentrations, surfactant concentration and structure, and stability diagrams. Attention must also be given to interactions between factors, such as the salting out of surfactants. Lastly, the temperature of a suspension may impact the performance of many dispersants (and hence stability), in addition to kinetics concerns in unstable suspension systems.

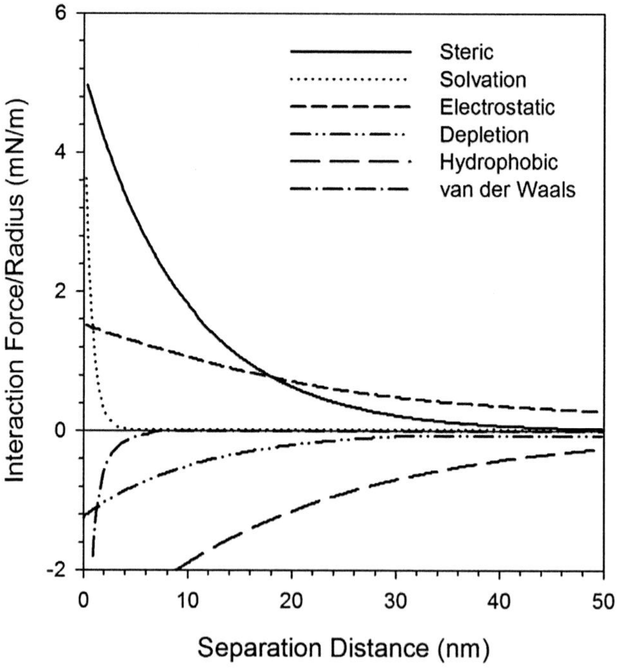

Figure 4.11 Plot of interparticle interaction forces and their associated length scales.

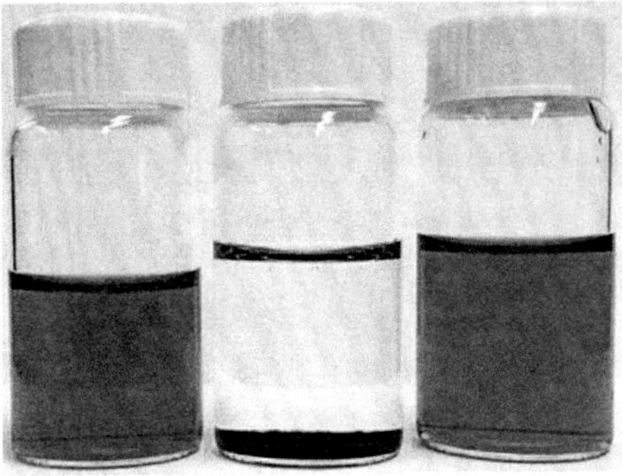

Figure 4.12 Gold nanoparticles, 4 nm, (left) before coating with chitosan (dispersed), (center) coated particles after settling (exhibiting bridging flocculation), and (right) coated particles after agitation (dispersed).

For particulate materials that are not already present in a stable dispersion, the ability of a material to be dispersed in a medium is an important consideration. Dry powders are often poorly dispersible due to close interparticle contact and associated strong attractive forces. Dependence on infinitely variable factors such as mixing method and kinetics generally leads to dispersibility being characterized in a qualitative manner. Particle size measurements taken at various time points after a dispersion process in addition to the stability characteristics discussed previously can be employed to characterize the degree of dispersibility of a material.

The dispersion stability itself can be evaluated by comparison of the particle size distribution to the primary or initial particle size distribution over time in a given medium and set of conditions. The dispersion stability is a kinetics problem—the frequency at which particles interact (e.g., due to concentration, thermal motion, and/or shear) and the strength of that interaction will determine the rate of agglomeration and particle size distribution at a given point in time. The structure of the agglomerate particle and the ability to redisperse these particles are dependent on the strength of interaction and type of agglomeration (e.g., coagulation and/or flocculation). Most often, the strength of interactions leading to coagulation (van der Waals forces) will result in smaller, denser, poorly redispersible agglomerate particles. Particles produced solely through flocculation may be redispersible by mechanical means dependent on the interaction of the flocculant with the particle surface.

Table 4.6 Factors affecting the stability of a suspension, their effects, and dependencies

	Mechanism	Effect	Dependencies
Medium polarizability and ionic strength	Alters the propagation of charge in the medium	Alters the effectiveness of charged surface groups (decreasing charge effectiveness diminishes electrostatic stabilization); increased ionic strength screens charges	Medium type and ionic strength
Medium hydrophobicity	Alters solvation	May increase or decrease stability on the basis of compatibility of medium with particle	Medium and particle type
Dispersion aids (surfactants)	Alters zeta potential and hydrophobicity	May promote or retard stability based on the surfactant structure and surface chemistry	Surfactant type and concentration, strength of interaction between particle and surfactant
Dispersion aids (polymers)	Alters zeta potential, hydrophobicity, steric effects, and/or solvation effects	May alter zeta potential and hydrophobicity, increases stability by steric repulsion, increases or decreases stability by depletion effects and/or hydrophobicity	Polymer type, strength of interaction with the surface, and concentration

	Mechanism	Effect	Dependencies
Specifically adsorbing ions	Alters zeta potential	Alters zeta potential and isoelectric point, typically reduces charge effectiveness	Ion valence, activity, and concentration
Potential-determining ions	Alters surface charge	Interacts with surface groups to determine charge, may increase or decrease stability by changing charge magnitude and polarity	Ion activity and concentration, surface chemistry
Other adsorbates	Variable	May promote or inhibit stability on the basis of interaction type	Concentration and type of adsorbate, mechanism and strength of interaction

4.3.4.3 Bulk powder properties

Several characteristics of bulk powder nanomaterials have been deemed important, particularly in regard to material handling and dispersibility. Dry powder nanomaterials may vary in degree of compaction, which may affect dispersibility and other properties. In addition to the pycnometer density of the material, the bulk density (volume occupied by a given mass of powder) is an important characteristic. The tapped density, the bulk density of a powder after mechanical agitation (tapping), and the Hausner ratio are simple metrics that may be used to describe the compressibility of powders. Powder cohesiveness and bulk powder flow properties (flowability, powder mechanics, segregation, angle of repose, etc.) are related to both the particle size distribution as well as interparticle forces. Finally, the potential for release of a dry powder nanomaterial by aerosolization represents a major route of exposure. Dustiness is an often-cited (but poorly defined) metric of the ability of a powder to be aerosolized.

4.3.4.4 Protein corona

Perhaps the most commonly cited advanced property is the adsorption of proteins when a nanomaterial enters a complex physiological environment (often referred to as the protein corona). Adsorbed proteins mediate the interaction of nanomaterials with their environment and can therefore alter the physiological response to these materials [120]. Adsorbed proteins may also influence other nonbiological properties, such as suspension stability, charge, and hydrophobicity, as shown in Fig. 4.13. A complex set of interactions between proteins and nanomaterial surfaces dictate which proteins adsorb and how protein-coated surfaces associate with other proteins in the surrounding environment [121]. Adsorption of proteins can result in changes to the protein conformation [122, 123], differential and competitive binding with other proteins in the environment [124–128], and can exhibit dependencies on time and temperature [129]. The protein corona is often divided into hard and soft coronas, defined as the proteins that strongly bind and weakly associate with the particle surface, respectively. It is generally difficult to probe the entire protein corona without alteration. The hard protein corona is considerably easier to probe than the soft corona, as the hard corona is less likely to be altered by separation processes than the soft corona. Consequently, the soft corona is not as well understood [121]. Characterization of the protein corona is a complex and developing subject but is recognized as a critical step in understanding the physiological behavior of nanomaterials [120, 121, 128]. The concepts discussed in this section on protein adsorption may also be extended to other functional biomolecules.

4.3.4.5 Composite materials

Nanomaterials are often incorporated into various composite materials, such as cosmetics, foods, and reinforced composites. For these materials, parameters such as the concentration of nanomaterials and state of dispersion of the nanomaterials within the composite are important. As discussed previously, the quantity of nanomaterials present in a composite material may dictate how that material is treated from a regulatory standpoint [75, 76]. Factors that affect the potential release of these materials are also important [130], such as the strength of adhesion between the matrix and

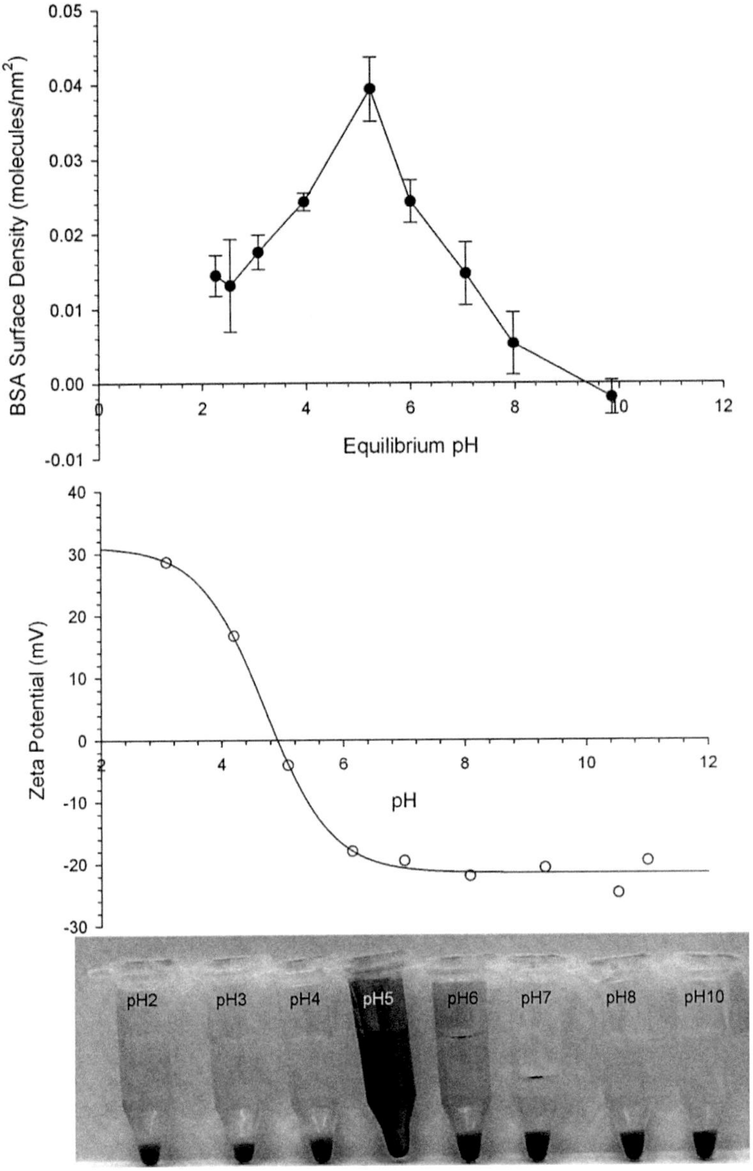

Figure 4.13 Effects of adsorption of bovine serum albumin (BSA) on adsorbate density (top) zeta potential (center) and hydrophobicity (bottom) as a function of pH on gold nanoparticles. The isoelectric point of BSA is 4.92, coincident with the point at which adsorption density is maximized, the zeta potential is neutral, and adhesion of coated particles to hydrophobic polypropylene centrifuge tubes is observed.

nanomaterial, the degree of exposure of the nanomaterials to the surface, the chemical and mechanical stability of the matrix, and the solubility of the matrix.

4.3.4.6 Other properties

Characteristics such as the magnetic, mechanical, optical, and electronic properties are infrequently cited in most lists of important physicochemical properties of nanomaterials. Some organizations, such as the ISO [131], have acknowledged a need for additional information on these advanced physicochemical properties. ISO TC 229 [131] has produced a draft roadmap that includes these broad properties as part of an advanced character set for most nanomaterial classes. These properties are occasionally found in lists of important physicochemical properties, such as the optical properties listed in the European Commission (EC) guidance on nanomaterials in cosmetics [9]. Material-specific guidelines (e.g., for carbon nanotubes) occasionally will list individual advanced properties related specifically to that material.

4.4 Summary and Conclusions

Physicochemical characterization of nanomaterials is critically important in establishing their identity, predicting potential uses and limitations, and, in some cases, determining how they will be regulated. The tremendous diversity in the types of nanomaterials and the different contexts in which physicochemical characterization information are used make it virtually impossible to derive a "one size fits all" list of parameters to measure. This is evident from the example lists provided in this chapter. Many of the parameters that the various lists have in common have been proposed as minimum characterization requirements. However, describing them as "minimum" implies "adequate." It can be argued that all of the parameters on these short lists are important to measure nearly all the time but that short lists are rarely sufficient for any given purpose and therefore may be counterproductive.

Lists of nanomaterial physicochemical parameters to characterize will certainly evolve in the future as more sophisticated instrumentation and approaches become available, and research provides clearer pictures of which characteristics are most important to consider. It is reasonable to expect that the characteristics regarded as most important will vary by material, application, and field of science or technology studying the material. As a consequence, we expect the lists of physicochemical parameters to characterize will proliferate rather than consolidate, reflecting the specialized needs of different fields and uses for the information. New approaches will also allow characterization to take place under more complex and realistic circumstances of nanomaterial use, rather than simply characterizing the material "as manufactured" or "as supplied."

References

1. The minimum information for nanomaterial characterization (MINChar) initiative. https://characterization matters.wordpress.com/2008/11/2.
2. Fadeel, B., Fornara, A., Toprak, M. S., and Bhattacharya, K. (2015). Keeping it real: the importance of material characterization in nanotoxicology. *Biochem. Biophys. Res. Commun.*, **468**(3), 498–503. doi: 10.1016/j.bbrc.2015.06.178.
3. Oberdörster, G., Maynard, A., Donaldson, K., Castranova, V., Fitzpatrick, J., Ausman, K., et al. (2005). Principles for characterizing the potential human health effects from exposure to nanomaterials: elements of a screening strategy. *Part. Fibre Toxicol.*, **2**(1), 1.
4. Powers, K. W., Palazuelos, M., Moudgil, B. M., and Roberts, S. M. (2007). Characterization of the size, shape, and state of dispersion of nanoparticles for toxicological studies. *Nanotoxicology*, **1**(1), 42–51.
5. Powers, K. W., Brown, S. C., Krishna, V. B., Wasdo, S. C., Moudgil, B. M., and Roberts, S. M. (2006). Research strategies for safety evaluation of nanomaterials. Part VI. Characterization of nanoscale particles for toxicological evaluation. *Toxicol. Sci.*, **90**(2), 296–303. doi: kfj099 [pii].
6. Warheit, D. B. (2008). How meaningful are the results of nanotoxicity studies in the absence of adequate material characterization? *Toxicol. Sci.*, **101**(2), 183–185.
7. The National Science and Technology Council. (2014). National nanotechnology initiative strategic plan.
8. Stefaniak, A. B., Hackley, V. A., Roebben, G., Ehara, K., Hankin, S., Postek, M. T., et al. (2013). Nanoscale reference materials for environmental,

health and safety measurements: needs, gaps and opportunities. *Nanotoxicology*, **7**(8), 1325–1337.

9. Scientific Committee on Consumer Safety. (2012). Guidance on the safety assessment of nanomaterials in cosmetics, No. SCCS/1484/12. European Commission.
10. Health Canada. (2011). Policy statement on health Canada's working definition for nanomaterial. http://www.hc-sc.gc.ca/sr-sr/pubs/nano/pol-eng.php.
11. Council of Canadian Academies. (2008). Small is different: a science perspective on the regulatory challenges of the nanoscale (full report), No. T174.7 620'.5 C2008-905348-6. Ottawa, Canada.
12. Hankin, S. M., Peters, S. A. K., Poland, C. A., Foss Hansen, S., Holmqvist, J., Ross, B. L., et al. (2011). Specific advice on fulfilling information requirements for nanomaterials under REACH (RIP-oN 2): final project report, No. RNC/RIP-oN2/FPR/1/FINAL.
13. Specified conditions for requesting additional data requirements - NICNAS (2016). https://www.nicnas.gov.au/regulation-and-compliance/nicnas-handbook/handbook-appendixes/guidance-and-requirements-for-notification-of-new-chemicals-that-are-industrial-nanomaterials/specified-conditions-for-requesting-additional-data-requirements.
14. Australian Pesticides and Veterinary Medicines Authority. (2015). Nanotechnologies for pesticides and veterinary medicines: regulatory considerations final report.
15. European Commission. (2009). Scientific committee on emerging and newly identified health risks: risk assessment of products of nanotechnologies.
16. Organisation for Economic Co-operation and Development (OECD). (2010). List of manufactured nanomaterials and list of endpoints for phase one of the sponsorship programme for the testing of manufactured nanomaterials: revision, No. ENV/JM/MONO(2010)46.
17. Stintz, M., Babick, F., and Roebben, G. (2010). Draft report for the co-nanomet workshop "instruments, standard methods and reference materials for traceable nanoparticles characterization". Nuremberg, Germany.
18. Organisation for Economic Co-operation and Development (OECD). (2016). Physical-chemical parameters: measurements and methods relevant for the regulation of nanomaterials, No. ENV/JM/MONO(2016)2.

19. Organisation for Economic Co-operation and Development (OECD). (2010). Guidance manual for the testing of manufactured nanomaterials: OECD's sponsorship programme; first revision, No. ENV/JM/MONO(2009)20/REV.
20. Working with the NCL - assay cascade protocols - nanotechnology characterization laboratory. http://ncl.cancer.gov/working_assay-cascade.asp.
21. MINChar Initiative. (2008). The parameters list | minimum information for nanomaterial characterization initiative. https://characterizationmatters.wordpress.com/parameters/.
22. DuPont - Environmental Defense Nano Partnership. (2007). NANO risk framework.
23. National Institute of Standards and Technology. (2007). Material standards for environmental health & safety for engineered nanoscale materials.
24. European Commission. (2007). Scientific committee on emerging and newly-identified health risks: opinion on the appropriateness of the risk assessment methodology in accordance with the technical guidance documents for new and existing substances for assessing the risks of nanomaterials.
25. U.S. Environmental Protection Agency. (2012). Nanomaterial case study: Nanoscale silver in disinfectant spray, No. EPA/600/R-10/081F.
26. Pleus, R. (2011). Guidance on physicochemical characterization for manufacture nano-objects submitted for toxicological testing. *11th IEEE International Conference on Nanotechnology*, Portland, OR, pp. 20-21. doi: 10.1109/NANO.2011.6144672.
27. U.S. Food and Drug Administration. (2014). Guidance for industry: safety of nanomaterials in cosmetic products.
28. Montaño, M., Ranville, J., Lowry, G., Blue, J., Hiremath, N., Koenig, S., et al. (2014). Detection and characterization of engineered nanomaterials in the environment: Current state-of-the-art and future directions report, Annotated Bibliography, and Image Library. U.S. Environmental Protection Agency, Washington, DC, EPA/600/R-14/244.
29. Arts, J. H., Hadi, M., Irfan, M. A., Keene, A. M., Kreiling, R., Lyon, D., et al. (2015). A decision-making framework for the grouping and testing of nanomaterials (DF4nanoGrouping). *Regul. Toxicol. Pharm.*, **71**(2 Suppl), S1–27. doi: 10.1016/j.yrtph.2015.03.007.
30. European Chemicals Agency. (2015). Guidance on information requirements and chemical safety assessment chapter R.7a: endpoint specific guidance, No. ECHA -15- G-04.1-EN.

31. European Food Safety Authority. (2009). Scientific opinion of the scientific committee on a request from the European commission on the potential risks arising from nanoscience and nanotechnologies on food and feed safety. *EFSA J.*, **7**(3), 1. doi: 10.2903/j.efsa.2009.958.

32. European Food Safety Authority. (2011). Guidance on the risk assessment of the application of nanoscience and nanotechnologies in the food and feed chain. *EFSA J.*, **9**(5), 2140. doi: 10.2903/j.efsa.2011.2140.

33. Hight Walker, A. R. (2009). Developing nano-measurements and standards: the NIST role.

34. European Commission. (2015). Scientific committee on emerging and newly identified health risks SCENIHR: opinion on the guidance on the determination of potential health effects of nanomaterials used in medical devices, No. ND-AS-14-001-EN-N.

35. Ansell, J., and Rauscher, H. (2011). Report for international cooperation on cosmetic regulation: report of the joint regulator - industry ad hoc working group: currently available methods for characterization of nanomaterials.

36. U.S. Food and Drug Administration. (2007). Nanotechnology task force report 2007.

37. U.S. Food and Drug Administration. (2014). Guidance for industry: assessing the effects of significant manufacturing process changes, including emerging technologies, on the safety and regulatory status of food ingredients and food contact substances, including food ingredients that are color additives.

38. U.S. Food and Drug Administration. (2015). Guidance for industry: use of nanomaterials in food for animals, No. 220.

39. U.S. Consumer Product Safety Commission. (2015). Fiscal year 2016 performance budget request.

40. CDC - nanotechnology - guidance and publications - NIOSH workplace safety and health topic. https://www.cdc.gov/niosh/topics/nanotech/pubs.html.

41. US Government Publishing Office. (2015). Proposed rules. *Fed. Regist.*, **80**(65), 18330.

42. Nanoscale materials; chemical substances when manufactured, imported, or processed as nanoscale materials; reporting and recordkeeping requirements - Reg DaRRT | Laws & regulations | US EPA (2015). https://yosemite.epa.gov/opei/RuleGate.nsf/byRIN/2070-AJ54.

43. Chemical substances when manufactured or processed as nanoscale materials: TSCA reporting and recordkeeping requirements. (2016). http://www.regulations.gov/document?D=EPA-HQ-OPPT-2010-0572-0001.
44. US Environmental Protection Agency. *Chemical Substances When Manufactured or Processed as Nanoscale Materials: TSCA Reporting and Recordkeeping Requirements*. www.regulations.gov/document?D=EPA-HQ-OPPT-2010-0572-0137.
45. US Environmental Protection Agency. TSCA §8(a) Reporting for Chemical Substances when Manufactured or Processed as Nanoscale Materials: Data Submission Form. 2017, 9600-07.
46. Nanotechnology portal. http://www.nist.gov/nanotechnology-portal.cfm.
47. Working with the NCL - assay cascade protocols - nanotechnology characterization laboratory. http://ncl.cancer.gov/working_assay-cascade.asp.
48. About the NCL - mission - nanotechnology characterization laboratory. http://ncl.cancer.gov/about_mission.asp.
49. Environment Canada & Health Canada. (2007). Proposed regulatory framework for nanomaterials under the Canadian environmental protection act, 1999, No. {0502.096/8/00020048.DOC}.
50. Environment Canada. (2014). New substances program advisory note 2014-02: assessment of nanomaterials under the new substances notification regulations (chemicals and polymers), No. 2014-02.
51. Environment and climate change Canada - consultation document - proposed prioritization approach for nanoscale forms of substances on the domestic substances list. (2016). https://www.ec.gc.ca/lcpe-cepa/default.asp?lang=En&n=FA3C8DBF-1.
52. European Commission. (2013). Nanomaterials - chemicals - environment - European commission. http://ec.europa.eu/environment/chemicals/nanotech/index_en.htm.
53. European Parliament & Council of the European Union. (2006). Regulation (EC) no 1907/2006 of the European Parliament and of the council. *Off. J. Eur. Union*, (L 396), 1.
54. European Commission. (2008). Nanomaterials in REACH, No. CA/59/2008 rev. 1.
55. European Commission. (2010). Nanomaterials in IUCLID 5.2, No. 1.0.
56. European Chemicals Agency. Guidance on information requirements and chemical safety assessment - ECHA. https://echa.europa.eu/web/

guest /guidance-documents/guidance-on-information-requirements-and-chemical-safety-assessment.

57. European Chemicals Agency. (2012). Guidance on information requirements and chemical safety assessment: Appendix R7-1 recommendations for nanomaterials applicable to chapter R7a endpoint specific guidance, No. ECHA-12-G-03-EN.
58. RIPON - nanomaterials - environment - European commission. (2016). http://ec.europa.eu/environment/chemicals/nanotech/reach-clp/ripon_en.htm.
59. European Parliament & Council of the European Union. (2009). Regulation (EC) no 1223/2009 of the European Parliament and of the council of 30 November 2009 on cosmetic products. *Off. J. Eur. Union*, (L 342), 59.
60. European Medicines Agency. (2006). Reflection paper on nanotechnology-based medicinal products for human use, No. EMEA/CHMP/79769/2006.
61. European Medicines Agency. (2013). Reflection paper on surface coatings: general issues for consideration regarding parenteral administration of coated nanomedicine products, No. EMA/325027/2013.
62. European Medicines Agency. (2015). Reflection paper on the data requirements for intravenous iron-based nano-colloidal products developed with reference to an innovator medicinal product, No. EMA/CHMP/SWP/620008/2012. London, United Kingdom.
63. Organisation for Economic Co-operation and Development (OECD). (2015). Developments on the safety of manufactured nanomaterials: 2013, No. ENV/ JM/MONO(2015)41.
64. Our approach to regulating industrial nanomaterials - NICNAS (2016). https://www.nicnas.gov.au/communications/issues/nanomaterials-nanotechnology/our-approach-to-regulating-industrial-nanomaterials.
65. Nanomaterials that are 'new chemicals' - NICNAS (2016). https://www.nicnas.gov.au/communications/issues/nanomaterials-nanotechnology/nicnas-regulatory-activities-in-nanomaterials.
66. Organisation for Economic Co-operation and Development (OECD). (2010). List of manufactured nanomaterials and list of endpoints for phase one of the sponsorship programme for the testing of manufactured nanomaterials, Revision No. NV/JM/MONO(2010)46.

67. Locascio, L. E., Reipa, V., Zook, J. M., and Pleus, R. C. (2011). Nanomaterial toxicity: emerging standards and efforts to support standards development. In: V. Murashov, and J. Howard (eds.), *Nanotechnology Standards* (Springer, New York), p. 179.

68. Organisation for Economic Co-operation and Development (OECD). (2011). OECD work on the safety of manufactured nanomaterials.

69. Organisation for Economic Co-operation and Development (OECD). (2011). Nanosafety at the OECD: the first five years 2006–2010.

70. OECD working party on nanotechnology (WPN): Vision statement - OECD. https://www.oecd.org/sti/nano/oecdworkingpartyonnano-technology wpnvisionstatement.htm.

71. ISO - technical committees - ISO/TC 229 - nanotechnologies. (2016). http://www. iso.org/iso/iso_technical_committee?commid=381983.

72. International Organization for Standardization. (2012). Nanotechnologies: guidance on physico-chemical characterization of engineered nanoscale materials for toxicologic assessment, No. ISO/TR 13014:2012.

73. ASTM International. (2009). ASTM International Technical Committee E56 on Nanotechnology.

74. Nanotechnology standards. https://www astm.org/Standards / nanotechnology-standards.html.

75. European Parliament & Council of the European Union. (2011). Commission recommendation of 18 October 2011 on the definition of nanomaterial. *Off. J. Eur. Union*, **54**(L 275), 38.

76. European Commission. (2016). Definition - nanomaterials - environment - European Commission. http://ec.europa.eu/environment/chemicals/nanotech/faq/definition_en.htm.

77. NICNAS working definition for 'industrial nanomaterial' - NICNAS (2016). https://www.nicnas.gov.au/communications/issues/nanomaterials-nano technology/our-approach-to-regulating-industrial-nanomaterials.

78. Noël, A., Maghni, K., Cloutier, Y., Dion, C., Wilkinson, K., Halle, S., et al. (2012). Effects of inhaled nano-TiO_2 aerosols showing two distinct agglomeration states on rat lungs. *Toxicol. Lett.*, **214**(2), 109–119.

79. Service, R. F. (2003). American chemical society meeting. Nanomaterials show signs of toxicity. *Science*, **300**(5617), 243. doi: 10.1126/science.300.5617.243a.

80. Kawano, T., Yamagata, M., Takahashi, H., Niidome, Y., Yamada, S., Katayama, Y., et al. (2006). Stabilizing of plasmid DNA in vivo by PEG-modified cationic gold nanoparticles and the gene expression assisted with electrical pulses. *J. Control. Release*, **111**(3), 382–389. doi: 10.1016/j.jconrel.2005.12.022.

81. Cho, W. S., Cho, M., Jeong, J., Choi, M., Han, B. S., Shin, H. S., et al. (2010). Size-dependent tissue kinetics of PEG-coated gold nanoparticles. *Toxicol. Appl. Pharmacol.*, **245**(1), 116–123. doi: 10.1016/j.taap.2010.02.013.

82. Balasubramanian, S. K., Poh, K., Ong, C., Kreyling, W. G., Ong, W., and Liya, E. Y. (2013). The effect of primary particle size on biodistribution of inhaled gold nano-agglomerates. *Biomaterials*, **34**(22), 5439–5452.

83. Horie, M., Fukui, H., Endoh, S., Maru, J., Miyauchi, A., Shichiri, M., et al. (2012). Comparison of acute oxidative stress on rat lung induced by nano and fine-scale, soluble and insoluble metal oxide particles: NiO and TiO_2. *Inhalation Toxicol.*, **24**(7), 391–400.

84. Hillyer, J. F., and Albrecht, R. M. (2001). Gastrointestinal persorption and tissue distribution of differently sized colloidal gold nanoparticles. *J. Pharm. Sci.*, **90**(12), 1927–1936.

85. Porter, D. W., Wu, N., Hubbs, A. F., Mercer, R. R., Funk, K., Meng, F., et al. (2013). Differential mouse pulmonary dose and time course responses to titanium dioxide nanospheres and nanobelts. *Toxicol. Sci.*, **131**(1), 179–193. doi: 10.1093/toxsci/kfs261.

86. Schinwald, A., Chernova, T., and Donaldson, K. (2012). Use of silver nanowires to determine thresholds for fibre length-dependent pulmonary inflammation and inhibition of macrophage migration in vitro. *Part. Fibre Toxicol.*, **9**(1), 1.

87. Pal, S., Tak, Y. K., and Song, J. M. (2007). Does the antibacterial activity of silver nanoparticles depend on the shape of the nanoparticle? A study of the gram-negative bacterium Escherichia coli. *Appl. Environ. Microbiol.*, **73**(6), 1712–1720. doi: AEM.02218-06 [pii].

88. Lee, J., Kang, B., Hicks, B., Chancellor, T. F., Chu, B. H., Wang, H., et al. (2008). The control of cell adhesion and viability by zinc oxide nanorods. *Biomaterials*, **29**(27), 3743–3749.

89. Rabolli, V., Thomassen, L. C., Princen, C., Napierska, D., Gonzalez, L., Kirsch-Volders, M., et al. (2010). Influence of size, surface area and microporosity on the in vitro cytotoxic activity of amorphous silica nanoparticles in different cell types. *Nanotoxicology*, **4**(3), 307–318.

90. Yu, T., Greish, K., McGill, L. D., Ray, A., and Ghandehari, H. (2012). Influence of geometry, porosity, and surface characteristics of silica

nanoparticles on acute toxicity: their vasculature effect and tolerance threshold. *ACS Nano*, **6**(3), 2289–2301.

91. Lin, Y., and Haynes, C. L. (2010). Impacts of mesoporous silica nanoparticle size, pore ordering, and pore integrity on hemolytic activity. *J. Am. Chem. Soc.*, **132**(13), 4834–4842.

92. Xiong, S., Tang, Y., Ng, H. S., Zhao, X., Jiang, Z., Chen, Z., et al. (2013). Specific surface area of titanium dioxide (TiO_2) particles influences cyto-and photo-toxicity. *Toxicology*, **304**, 132–140.

93. Duffin, R., Tran, L., Brown, D., Stone, V., and Donaldson, K. (2007). Proinflammogenic effects of low-toxicity and metal nanoparticles in vivo and in vitro: highlighting the role of particle surface area and surface reactivity. *Inhalation Toxicol.*, **19**(10), 849–856.

94. Pulskamp, K., Diabaté, S., and Krug, H. F. (2007). Carbon nanotubes show no sign of acute toxicity but induce intracellular reactive oxygen species in dependence on contaminants. *Toxicol. Lett.*, **168**(1), 58–74.

95. Hull, M. S., Kennedy, A. J., Steevens, J. A., Bednar, A. J., Weiss, J., Charles A., and Vikesland, P. J. (2009). Release of metal impurities from carbon nanomaterials influences aquatic toxicity. *Environ. Sci. Technol.*, **43**(11), 4169–4174.

96. Franklin, N. M., Rogers, N. J., Apte, S. C., Batley, G. E., Gadd, G. E., and Casey, P. S. (2007). Comparative toxicity of nanoparticulate ZnO, bulk ZnO, and $ZnCl_2$ to a freshwater microalga (pseudokirchneriella subcapitata): the importance of particle solubility. *Environ. Sci. Technol.*, **41**(24), 8484–8490.

97. Li, H., Li, M., Shih, W. Y., Lelkes, P. I., and Shih, W. (2011). Cytotoxicity tests of water soluble ZnS and CdS quantum dots. *J. Nanosci. Nanotechnol.*, **11**(4), 3543–3551.

98. Xia, T., Zhao, Y., Sager, T., George, S., Pokhrel, S., Li, N., et al. (2011). Decreased dissolution of ZnO by iron doping yields nanoparticles with reduced toxicity in the rodent lung and zebrafish embryos. *ACS Nano*, **5**(2), 1223–1235.

99. Warheit, D. B., Webb, T. R., Reed, K. L., Frerichs, S., and Sayes, C. M. (2007). Pulmonary toxicity study in rats with three forms of ultrafine-TiO_2 particles: differential responses related to surface properties. *Toxicology*, **230**(1), 90–104.

100. Sayes, C. M., Wahi, R., Kurian, P. A., Liu, Y., West, J. L., Ausman, K. D., et al. (2006). Correlating nanoscale titania structure with toxicity: a cytotoxicity and inflammatory response study with human dermal fibroblasts and human lung epithelial cells. *Toxicol. Sci.*, **92**(1), 174–185. doi: kfj197 [pii].

101. Murdande, S. B., Pikal, M. J., Shanker, R. M., and Bogner, R. H. (2010). Solubility advantage of amorphous pharmaceuticals. I. A thermodynamic analysis. *J. Pharm. Sci.*, **99**(3), 1254–1264.

102. Ding, Z., Lu, G., and Greenfield, P. (2000). Role of the crystallite phase of TiO_2 in heterogeneous photocatalysis for phenol oxidation in water. *J. Phys. Chem. B*, **104**(19), 4815–4820.

103. Hurum, D. C., Agrios, A. G., Gray, K. A., Rajh, T., and Thurnauer, M. C. (2003). Explaining the enhanced photocatalytic activity of degussa P25 mixed-phase TiO_2 using EPR. *J. Phys. Chem. B*, **107**(19), 4545–4549.

104. Strauss, M., Pastorello, M., Sigoli, F. A., e Silva, J. M. de Souza, and Mazali, I. O. (2014). Singular effect of crystallite size on the charge carrier generation and photocatalytic activity of nano-TiO_2. *Appl. Surf. Sci.*, **319**, 151–157.

105. Choi, H. S., Ashitate, Y., Lee, J. H., Kim, S. H., Matsui, A., Insin, N., et al. (2010). Rapid translocation of nanoparticles from the lung airspaces to the body. *Nat. Biotechnol.*, **28**(12), 1300–1303.

106. Feswick, A., Griffitt, R. J., Siebein, K., and Barber, D. (2013). Uptake, retention and internalization of quantum dots in daphnia is influenced by particle surface functionalization. *Aquat. Toxicol.*, **130**, 210–218.

107. Heiden, T. C. K., Dengler, E., Kao, W. J., Heideman, W., and Peterson, R. E. (2007). Developmental toxicity of low generation PAMAM dendrimers in zebrafish. *Toxicol. Appl. Pharmacol.*, **225**(1), 70–79.

108. Schins, R. P., Duffin, R., Höhr, D., Knaapen, A. M., Shi, T., Weishaupt, C., et al. (2002). Surface modification of quartz inhibits toxicity, particle uptake, and oxidative DNA damage in human lung epithelial cells. *Chem. Res. Toxicol.*, **15**(9), 1166–1173.

109. El Badawy, A. M., Silva, R. G., Morris, B., Scheckel, K. G., Suidan, M. T., and Tolaymat, T. M. (2010). Surface charge-dependent toxicity of silver nanoparticles. *Environ. Sci. Technol.*, **45**(1), 283–287.

110. Arts, J. H., Muijser, H., Duistermaat, E., Junker, K., and Kuper, C. F. (2007). Five-day inhalation toxicity study of three types of synthetic amorphous silicas in wistar rats and post-exposure evaluations for up to 3 months. *Food Chem. Toxicol.*, **45**(10), 1856–1867.

111. Reuzel, P., Bruijntjes, J., Feron, V., and Woutersen, R. (1991). Subchronic inhalation toxicity of amorphous silicas and quartz dust in rats. *Food Chem. Toxicol.*, **29**(5), 341–354.

112. Chompoosor, A., Saha, K., Ghosh, P. S., Macarthy, D. J., Miranda, O. R., Zhu, Z., et al. (2010). The role of surface functionality on acute cytotoxicity,

ROS generation and DNA damage by cationic gold nanoparticles. *Small*, **6**(20), 2246–2249.

113. Bhushan, B., Jung, Y. C., and Koch, K. (2009). Micro-, nano- and hierarchical structures for superhydrophobicity, self-cleaning and low adhesion. *Philos. Trans. A Math. Phys. Eng. Sci.*, **367**(1894), 1631–1672. doi: 10.1098/rsta.2009.0014.
114. Lafuma, A., and Quéré, D. (2003). Superhydrophobic states. *Nat. Mater.*, **2**(7), 457–460.
115. Warheit, D. B., Webb, T. R., Colvin, V. L., Reed, K. L., and Sayes, C. M. (2007). Pulmonary bioassay studies with nanoscale and fine-quartz particles in rats: toxicity is not dependent upon particle size but on surface characteristics. *Toxicol. Sci.*, **95**(1), 270–280. doi: kfl128 [pii].
116. Organisation for Economic Co-operation and Development (OECD). (2014). Report of the OECD expert meeting on the physical chemical properties of manufactured nanomaterials and test guidelines, No. ENV/JM/MONO(2014)15.
117. Kong, L., and Zepp, R. G. (2012). Production and consumption of reactive oxygen species by fullerenes. *Environ. Toxicol. Chem.*, **31**(1), 136–143.
118. Gorham, J. M., MacCuspie, R. I., Klein, K. L., Fairbrother, D. H., and Holbrook, R. D. (2012). UV-induced photochemical transformations of citrate-capped silver nanoparticle suspensions. *J. Nanopart. Res.*, **14**(10), 1–16.
119. Pycke, B. F., Chao, T., Herckes, P., Westerhoff, P., and Halden, R. U. (2012). Beyond nC60: strategies for identification of transformation products of fullerene oxidation in aquatic and biological samples. *Anal. Bioanal. Chem.*, **404**(9), 2583–2595.
120. Lundqvist, M., Stigler, J., Elia, G., Lynch, I., Cedervall, T., and Dawson, K. A. (2008). Nanoparticle size and surface properties determine the protein corona with possible implications for biological impacts. *Proc. Natl. Acad. Sci. U. S. A.*, **105**(38), 14265–14270. doi: 10.1073/pnas.0805135105.
121. Monopoli, M. P., Walczyk, D., Campbell, A., Elia, G., Lynch, I., Baldelli Bombelli, F., et al. (2011). Physical-chemical aspects of protein corona: relevance to in vitro and in vivo biological impacts of nanoparticles. *J. Am. Chem. Soc.*, **133**(8), 2525–2534.
122. Lundqvist, M., Sethson, I., and Jonsson, B. (2004). Protein adsorption onto silica nanoparticles: conformational changes depend on the particles' curvature and the protein stability. *Langmuir*, **20**(24), 10639–10647.

123. Wangoo, N., Suri, C. R., and Shekhawat, G. (2008). Interaction of gold nanoparticles with protein: a spectroscopic study to monitor protein conformational changes. *Appl. Phys. Lett.*, **92**(13), 133104.

124. Wasdo, S. C., Barber, D. S., Denslow, N. D., Powers, K. W., Palazuelos, M., Jr., S. M. S., et al. (2008). Differential binding of serum proteins to nanoparticles. *Int. J. Nanotechnol.*, **5**(1), 92. doi: 10.1504/IJNT.2008.016550.

125. Deng, Z. J., Mortimer, G., Schiller, T., Musumeci, A., Martin, D., and Minchin, R. F. (2009). Differential plasma protein binding to metal oxide nanoparticles. *Nanotechnology*, **20**(45), 455101. doi: 10.1088/0957-4484/20/45/455101.

126. Ruh, H., Kühl, B., Brenner-Weiss, G., Hopf, C., Diabaté, S., and Weiss, C. (2012). Identification of serum proteins bound to industrial nanomaterials. *Toxicol. Lett.*, **208**(1), 41–50. doi: 10.1016/j.toxlet.2011.09.009.

127. Tenzer, S., Docter, D., Rosfa, S., Wlodarski, A., Kuharev, J., Rekik, A., et al. (2011). Nanoparticle size is a critical physicochemical determinant of the human blood plasma corona: a comprehensive quantitative proteomic analysis. *ACS Nano*, **5**(9), 7155–7167. doi: 10.1021/nn201950e.

128. Cedervall, T., Lynch, I., Lindman, S., Berggard, T., Thulin, E., Nilsson, H., et al. (2007). Understanding the nanoparticle-protein corona using methods to quantify exchange rates and affinities of proteins for nanoparticles. *Proc. Natl. Acad. Sci. U. S. A.*, **104**(7), 2050–2055.

129. Casals, E., Pfaller, T., Duschl, A., Oostingh, G. J., and Puntes, V. (2010). Time evolution of the nanoparticle protein corona. *ACS Nano*, **4**(7), 3623–3632. doi:10.1021/nn901372t.

130. Nowack, B., Ranville, J. F., Diamond, S., Gallego-Urrea, J. A., Metcalfe, C., Rose, J., et al. (2012). Potential scenarios for nanomaterial release and subsequent alteration in the environment. *Environ. Toxicol. Chem.*, **31**(1), 50–59.

131. Ichimura, S. (2010). Current activities of ISO TC229/WG2 on purity evaluation and quality assurance standards for carbon nanotubes. *Anal. Bioanal. Chem.*, **396**(3), 963–971.

132. Tombácz, E., and Szekeres, M. (2006). Surface charge heterogeneity of kaolinite in aqueous suspension in comparison with montmorillonite. *Appl. Clay Sci.*, **34**(1), 105–124.

Chapter 5

Physicochemical Properties of Engineered Nanomaterials and Their Importance in Assessing Relevant Metrics of Inhalation Exposures in Occupational Settings

Aleksandr B. Stefaniak*

National Institute for Occupational Safety and Health, 1095 Willowdale Road, Morgantown, WV 26505, USA

AStefaniak@cdc.gov

5.1 Introduction

Nanotechnology seeks to exploit the novel and unique properties that materials exhibit as their size is reduced from the micron scale to the nanoscale (approximately 1–100 nm). Nanoscale materials that are designed for a specific purpose or function are termed

***Disclaimer:** The findings and conclusions in this report are those of the author and do not necessarily represent the views of the National Institute for Occupational Safety and Health.

Physicochemical Properties of Nanomaterials
Edited by Richard C. Pleus and Vladimir Murashov

ISBN 978-981-4774-80-2 (Hardcover), 978-1-351-16860-1 (eBook)
www.panstanford.com

"engineered nanomaterials" (ENMs). ENMs can be categorized as nanoparticles (all three dimensions in the nanoscale), nanofibers (two dimensions in the nanoscale), and nanoplates (one external dimension in the nanoscale). Nanofibers are further subdivided into electrically conducting nanowires, hollow nanotubes, and rigid nanorods [1]. Naturally occurring (e.g., sea spray, volcanic dust) or anthropogenic (e.g., diesel combustion exhaust) nanoscale materials present in the atmosphere are referred to as incidental nanomaterials to distinguish them from ENMs.

By design, ENMs possess properties that are intentionally exploited to improve existing products or develop new products that are technically superior to existing ones. Exploitation of many size- and structure-dependent properties (high surface-to-volume ratio, which increases the available surface area for reactions; increased reactivity of surface atoms) of materials has led to the availability of over 1600 nanotechnology-enabled products in the commercial marketplace [2]. Among ENMs, commercialization at this time is high for silver, carbons (nanotubes and fullerenes), zinc, silica, titanium dioxide, and gold [3–7]. Silver is a potent antimicrobial agent that is used as a coating for disinfecting appliance surfaces, water treatment, textiles, children's products (bottles, teething rings), food packaging and processing, personal care products (shampoo, conditioner), household products (cleaners, paints), and medical devices (to prevent biofilm growth). Carbon-based ENMs such as single- and multiwalled carbon nanotubes (SWCNTs and MWCNTs) possess low density, high strength, and excellent electrical conductivity, which has led to their use in electronics and computers, polymer composites, energy storage, and sensors. Zinc oxide and titanium dioxide have high refractive indices, which make them excellent materials for scattering ultraviolet (UV) light. Additionally, their nanoscale size permits more homogeneous dispersion in liquid than micron-scale forms, which, in turn, allows for a more uniform application of the materials on the skin and for more visually appealing topical products such as sunscreens, personal care products, and cosmetics. The facile surface modifiability of gold nanoparticles makes them a useful material for development of highly selective sensors for detecting environmental contaminants and pathogenic bacteria in food and water, as well as useful platforms for drug delivery.

With any new technology, workers are the first people to be exposed to the products, and nanotechnology is no exception. As such, responsible development of ENMs requires knowledge of risk and understanding exposure is a key component of risk assessment [2]. In occupational environments, the inhalation pathway is often considered the primary exposure route, and regulatory and other organizations have developed many occupational exposure limits (OELs) for comparison to monitoring results. Only a few OELs exist for inhalation exposure to ENMs (e.g., titanium dioxide, carbon nanotubes [CNTs], and carbon nanofibers [CNFs]).

Aerosols containing ENMs may be generated unintentionally in a number of ways. A few examples are during production and handling of ENMs [8, 9]; normal use of nanotechnology products such as spray cleaners [10–12], or machining [13, 14], abrading [15–17], degrading [18], or burning [19] of polymer composites; from sanding paints [20]; and during disposal of ENMs by incineration [21, 22]. Dermal exposures may also be a relevant pathway for ENMs [23, 24], although there are no OELs for skin exposure and few standardized monitoring approaches. The ingestion pathway generally receives less attention in occupational exposure assessments, unless there is evidence of hand-to-mouth contact from activities such as smoking or high levels of contamination in break rooms where food is consumed.

Given the importance of the inhalation route of exposure for ENMs, the purpose of this chapter is to review current approaches to occupational inhalation exposure assessments for airborne ENMs in workplaces and critically discuss relevant metrics for exposure and toxicity. In Section 5.2, common metrics and exposure assessment techniques are discussed and compared to published literature. In Section 5.3, the interrelationship of occupational exposure assessment metrics and toxicological endpoint metrics is critically evaluated using titanium dioxide (TiO_2) and CNTs and CNFs as examples.

5.2 Commonly Measured Airborne Particle Properties in Occupational Settings

It is well established that accurate characterization of ENM physicochemical properties is required for accurate understanding of exposure, toxicity, and risk. However, agreement on which specific ENM properties should be measured is lacking [25]. Additionally, Chapter 4 discusses and contrasts examples of physicochemical parameter lists for ENM properties from various sources and provides descriptions of commonly cited parameters.

5.2.1 ENM Physicochemical Properties Important for Occupational Inhalation Exposures

As summarized in Table 5.1, for occupational inhalation exposures, metrics of interest include both physical and chemical properties. Specific physical properties are particle size, size distribution, and morphology because all are important for understanding regional deposition in the respiratory tract. Generally, particles with aerodynamic diameter less than about 4 μm have high probability of depositing in the nonciliated alveolar (gas exchange) region of the human lung, particles with aerodynamic diameter less than 10 μm are capable of depositing in the conducting airways and alveolar regions, and particles with aerodynamic diameter less than 100 μm are capable of depositing throughout the respiratory tract (head airways, conducting airways, and alveolar regions). Particles with diameter less than about 30 nm are preferentially deposited by diffusion in the upper airways of the human lung before they are able to reach the lower airways, but agglomerates of such particles will behave according to their agglomerate size rather than their primary particle size. For more detailed information on particle lung deposition, the reader is referred to Maynard and Kuempel [26].

Particle volume is also an important metric because if too many particles deposit in the lung alveoli, it can overwhelm the macrophage-mediated clearance response, leading to a decrease in the clearance rate, referred to as particle overload [27]. Once deposited in the respiratory tract, the residence time of particles will depend on their rates of mechanical clearance (mucociliary mediated in the conducting airways, cell mediated in the alveoli) and chemical clearance via dissolution (the act of a particle dissolving into ionic or molecular species) in airway lining fluid (conducting airways) and inside phagolysosomes of phagocytic cells (residing in the alveoli). The dissolution rate is influenced by the properties of the particles themselves as well as the properties of the biological fluid or tissue in which they are in contact. Specific particle properties that influence dissolution include particle bulk chemistry (the atomic element(s) of which an ENM is composed), surface chemistry (elemental and/ or molecular constituents on particle surfaces), crystallinity (3D order at the level of molecular dimensions) and surface area. The dissolution rate is important because it can influence the biological mode of toxicity; the capacity of some inhaled particles to cause adverse health effects in the lung is strongly related to residence time, whereas for other materials it is the release of ions that drive toxicity. Particles that deposit in the lung and resist clearance through mechanical and chemical processes will remain in the particulate state and can result in chronic adverse health effects such as inflammation, fibrosis, and cancer. As such, for chronic diseases the mass of poorly soluble material that deposits in the lung is also important because it influences bioaccumulation of a lung burden [28]. Particles that are cleared quickly by mechanical means may present less of a chronic disease hazard; however, material that is highly amenable to dissolution may release components into the lungs, which can contribute to acute adverse health effects in the lungs or in other organs to which the components may be distributed [29].

For occupational inhalation exposure assessment, numerous ENM properties, including size, size distribution, morphology, surface area, and mass, as well as bulk and surface chemistry and crystallinity, may be important for exposure and toxicity [26] (Table 5.1); however, for other exposed populations the properties of interest are not all the same. The divergence in metrics is related to differences in exposure pathways and target organs among various populations [30]. For consumers and the general public, the ingestion pathway is considered highly important because ENMs are intentionally added to some products [30] or can leach from containers into food [31]. In a review of physicochemical properties deemed important for characterization in various settings, six commonly agreed-upon metrics for risk assessment of ENMs in foods were identified: size, morphology, surface area, bulk and surface chemistry, and surface charge [28]. Oral exposures to ENMs in food occur via ingestion and passage through the gastrointestinal (GI) tract. As such, ENM properties that influence dissolution (surface area, chemistry) are important because available ions can be absorbed from the small intestine into the bloodstream. Properties such as particle size, size distribution, and surface charge are important metrics that influence uptake of particles across the small intestine and into the bloodstream [30]. The oral pathway is also important for therapeutic drug delivery where ENMs such as graphene, gold, or metal oxides are used as drug carriers. When using ENMs as drug carriers, examples of particle properties that are important include surface functionality for drug loading using gold nanoparticles [32] and magnetic properties for drug delivery using superparamagnetic iron oxide nanoparticles [33].

The dermal exposure pathway is important for consumers and the general public for intentionally applied topical products such as cosmetics or sunscreens that contain, for example, TiO_2 nanoparticles [30] or garments in close contact with the skin that contain, for example, silver nanoparticles [34]. For cosmetics and sunscreens, particle size is an important physicochemical property that could influence penetration across skin. While particle penetration across intact skin is controversial for intact skin [30], it is well established that compromised skin facilitates penetration of nanoparticles [35, 36]. Additionally, ENM properties that influence dissolution are important for the dermal exposure pathway. When some ENMs come in contact with skin surface liquids (sweat), will undergo dissolution to yield water-soluble ions that can readily penetrate skin [35, 36]. While the previous discussion focused on the ingestion and dermal exposure pathways, it is important to note that the inhalation exposure pathway is also relevant for consumers because ENMs (e.g., silver nanoparticles) are used in some household products such as spray cleaners [12].

5.2.2 Exposure Monitoring

Techniques for occupational inhalation exposure assessment can be categorized as real time, which provide near-instantaneous results, or time integrated, which collect material on a substrate over time and require subsequent off-line analysis. In the following sections, techniques commonly used for exposure assessment are briefly reviewed. For a more in-depth discussion of these specific techniques, the reader is referred to Bello et al. [13, 14], Brouwer et al. [37], Kuhlbusch et al. [38], Leskinen et al. [39], and Park et al. [40]. For details and guidance on sampling strategies, the reader is referred to Brouwer et al. [41], Eastlake et al. [42], Evans et al. [43], and Ramachandran et al. [44].

5.2.2.1 Real-time instruments

Real-time instruments offer the advantage that the user is provided with near-instantaneous results, which make these instruments useful for identifying process emission sources or work tasks and practices with elevated concentrations for further characterization and, if necessary, control. The main disadvantage of real-time instruments is that few of them are specific to particles of a distinct composition and therefore cannot discriminate an ENM of interest from incidental nanoparticles in a workplace atmosphere. Some promising methods to meet this limitation include the material-specific aerosol multi-element spectrometer [45], which combines elemental analysis by atomic emission spectroscopy with particle sizing using size-selective inlets, and a similar device called the aerosol mass spectrometer (AMS), which permits online characterization of both airborne particle size and chemical content [46].

The simplest real-time instruments measure a single particle metric (number, mass, surface area). The most common type of instrument to measure particle number concentration is the condensation nuclei counter (CNC) or condensation particle counter (CPC). These instruments aspirate aerosol particles into a chamber containing a saturated water or isopropyl alcohol atmosphere, and the vapor condenses on particle surfaces to grow the size to the optical range, where it can be counted using light scattering. Depending on the device and manufacturer, these instruments are capable of counting particles in the size range from about 10 nm to 3 μm [47]. Instruments that measure particle mass concentration include aerosol photometers (APs) (sold commercially, for example, as DustTrak® and SidePak® by TSI Inc., Shoreview, MN), which operate on the principle of light scattering, and the tapered element oscillating microbalance (TEOM™), which contains a cantilever that oscillates at a natural frequency (proportional to mass and therefore losses in oscillation frequency from sensed particles can be expressed in terms of mass concentration). These instruments often have a size-selective inlet to limit measurement of particulate matter to that with aerodynamic diameter less than 1, 2.5, or 10 μm. Instruments that measure outer (or envelope) surface area concentration are based on the attachment rate of unipolar ions to nanoparticles and include the epiphaniometer and diffusion charger (DC) [48].

Several types of instruments are available that measure both airborne particle size and number to provide information on size distribution. Instruments that use light scattering are referred to as optical particle counters (OPCs); however, because of the relative scale of the wavelength of visible light to the size of a nanoparticle, these instruments are limited to detecting particles in the submicron to micron scale. An example of a commercially available OPC device is the GRIMM (Grimm Aerosoltechnik, Ainring, Germany), which sizes and counts particles in 15 channels between 0.3 and >20 μm. Another instrument that resolves the number and size of submicron- to micron-scale particles is the aerodynamic particle sizer (APS), which aerodynamically classifies particles from >0.5 μm to 20 μm (TSI Inc.). Instruments that contain both a mobility analyzer and a CNC (such as the scanning mobility particle sizer [SMPS] or the fast mobility particle sizer [FMPS]; TSI Inc.) are capable of determining mobility size distributions for particles from a few nanometers to hundreds of nanometers. Nano-ID™ (model NPS500, Naneum, UK) is a portable SMPS that measures size distribution over the range 5 nm to 5 μm. The nanoTracer (Philips Aerasense, Eindhoven, the Netherlands) is an instrument that uses the principle of diffusion charging to determine particle number concentration from 10 to 300 nm and mean particle (mobility) diameter [49] and has been used in workplace exposure assessments [23, 50]. A similar instrument is the diffusion size classifier (DiSC) and its handheld version, DiSCmini (Matter Aerosol, Wohlen, Switzerland), which can determine particle number concentration from 20 to 240 nm and mean particle (mobility) diameter [51].

Some instruments combine several measurement principles for particle measurement to simultaneously provide information on multiple metrics. Examples include the wide-range aerosol spectrometer (WRAS, Grimm Aerosoltechnik) and wide-range particle spectrometer (WRPS, MSP Corp.), both of which combine an SMPS (mobility analyzer and CPC) with an OPC and are capable of evaluating particle size distributions from the nanoscale to the micron scale, and the electrical low-pressure impactor (ELPI, Dekati Ltd., Kangasala, Finland), which has a range from 6.8 nm to 10 μm. A further advantage of the ELPI is that particles are collected on substrates that can be weighed to determine mass as a function of size and subjected to additional analyses such as elemental mass using mass spectroscopy or morphological and chemical examination by electron microscopy.

With regard to surface area, a variation of the DC is size-resolved surface area measurements combined with a particle lung deposition algorithm (usually the International Commission on Radiological Protection [ICRP]) to estimate surface area concentration that would deposit in the tracheobronchial and/or alveolar regions of the lung of a reference worker. Examples of instruments to estimate the deposited surface area in the lung include the nanoparticle surface area monitor (NSAM) (TSI Inc.), the modified electrical aerosol detector (MEAD) [52], and AeroTrak9000™ (TSI Inc.). Additionally, surface area concentrations can be calculated from CPC (TSI Inc.), SMPS (TSI Inc.), APS (TSI Inc.), OPC (Grimm Aerosoltechnik), or any other size distribution data [53] or automatically determined by the DiSC (Matter Aerosol) and nanoTracer (Philips Aerasense) instruments from size data. These indirect calculations assume spherical particle geometry and are weighted using the ICRP lung deposition curves in order to estimate the deposited surface area in the lung.

5.2.2.2 Time-integrated sampling

Time-integrated sampling techniques in combination with off-line analysis offer the advantage of specificity, meaning that an ENM of interest can be differentiated from incidental nanoparticles in a workplace atmosphere. The main disadvantages of time-integrated techniques is that they are insensitive to rapid fluctuations in particle concentrations (peaks), results are not known until after a task or activity is completed, and there is potential for bias from sample preparation or analysis. All time-integrated approaches entail using a pump to aspirate particles from the workplace atmosphere onto a substrate (filters, membranes, grids). With regard to particle collection onto filter substrates, various sampling heads are available and include plastic cassettes for "total" dust independent of size (e.g., 25 or 37 mm cassettes) as well as size-selective heads such as "respirable" cyclones (50% collection efficiency for particles with aerodynamic diameter of 4 μm) to collect particles that may deposit in the lung alveoli and "inhalable" samplers (50% collection efficiency for particles with aerodynamic diameter of 100 μm) to collect particles that may deposit anywhere in the respiratory tract. Additionally, impactors can be used to separate particles into multiple size fractions. Examples of impactors include personal multistage impactors, Berner impactors, and micro-orifice uniform deposit impactors (MOUDI™, MSP Corp., Shoreview, MN). Depending on the instrument model, MOUDI impactors are capable of size-separating particles over the size range of 10 nm to >18 μm. The wide-range aerosol sampling system (WRASS, Naneum, Ltd., UK) is a device that consists of a cascade impactor in-line with a diffusion battery to collects particles from 20 μm down to 25 nm (impactor) onto glass substrates for spectroscopy or microscopy analysis and from 250 nm down to 2 nm (diffusion battery) onto screens, with real-time counting of particles between each stage of collection [14].

The choice of substrate is critical and a substrate must be selected specifically for the intended analysis. For filter-based sampling, many standard analytical methods (e.g., *NIOSH Manual of Analytical Methods*) prescribe the appropriate filter type for sample collection and should be consulted before sampling. Mixed cellulose ester (MCE) is usually prescribed to quantify elemental mass using inductively coupled plasma (ICP) mass spectroscopy. Polyvinyl chloride (PVC) filters are weight-stable and therefore used for determination of dust mass (independent of chemical composition) by gravimetric techniques. Quartz fiber (QF) filters are used to quantify elemental carbon (EC), used as a surrogate for CNFs and CNTs, by thermal-optical analysis. If the intent is to determine particle morphology by electron microscopy, the above-mentioned sampling heads can be used with polycarbonate (PC) filters, which have a smooth appearance that makes it easy to visualize collected particles using scanning electron microscopy (SEM). Particle collection onto filters for SEM analysis requires sectioning the filter, mounting it on a stub, and coating with gold/palladium or other conductive material prior to analysis. Sectioning introduces an opportunity for sample selection bias that may be present if particles are not uniformly deposited across a filter and the conductive coating can increase particle size, which may be relevant for very small nanoparticles such as quantum dots. Note that in addition to information on particle morphology and size, SEM analysis can be supplemented with various chemical detectors such as energy-dispersive X-ray analysis (EDX) to determine elemental composition. A precipitator is a device that collects particles directly onto a 3 mm transmission electron microscopy (TEM) grid. There are two main types, electrostatic precipitators (ESPs), which collect particles onto which an electrostatic charge has been placed [54], and thermophoretic precipitators (TPs), which collect particles on a substrate using a thermal gradient [55]. The main advantage of precipitator-based collection is that the electron microscope grid or other substrate can be removed from the sampler and placed directly into TEM or SEM without manipulation or preparation, thereby eliminating the potential for sample preparation artefacts. TEM can also be supplemented with EDX or electron diffraction analysis to obtain information on elemental and crystalline composition, respectively.

5.2.3 Summary of Occupational Exposure Literature

Table 5.1 is a summary of published occupational exposure assessment studies for ENMs. This table lists only workplace studies or simulations of actual work tasks; studies performed in a specialized laboratory setting to evaluate release are excluded. Consistent with the high commercialization of silver, CNTs, and metal oxides, the majority of workplace assessments focus on evaluation of these ENMs. Most evaluations have investigated task-based influences on aerosol concentrations such as ENM production, harvesting, handling, packaging, and manipulation (e.g., machining composites). In nearly all exposure assessments listed in the table, investigators have utilized a combination of real-time and time-integrated techniques. Common approaches include real-time instruments to evaluate size distribution and usually another metric such as number (or mass or surface area) concentration and membrane-based time-integrated sampling for quantification of elements or electron microscopy characterization to identify the ENM of interest. In the following section, a critical comparison is made between metrics of exposure determined in occupational environments using the techniques identified in Table 5.1 and metrics of exposure utilized in toxicology studies.

5.3 Comparison of ENM Metrics of Workplace Exposure to Toxicological Metrics of Response

When the initial exposure assessment studies for ENMs were conducted in the early 2000s [56, 57], there was little understanding of toxicological mechanisms for adverse health effects. At that time, limited data were available from studies of ultrafine TiO_2 particles, which indicated that surface area was an important metric for pulmonary inflammatory responses in rats [58, 59]. Additionally, it was recognized that because of their small size, individual ENM particles had little mass, so historical approaches of measuring mass alone would be insufficient and it would be necessary to consider alternative metrics for ENMs, such as particle number and surface area. As such, multimetric approaches for particle size/distribution, concentration (number, mass, surface area), morphology, and bulk chemical composition were deemed most appropriate for assessing ENM exposures in workplace settings (Table 5.1).

5.3.1 Biological Relevance of Workplace Exposure Measurements

Toxicological studies provide information on the disease mechanisms and exposure–response relationships necessary for risk assessment and development of OELs. In toxicology studies, often a large mass of powder is available (relative to amounts airborne in workplace atmospheres) and the physicochemical properties are characterized using pristine material rather than actual workplace exposure particles. Hence, it is important to recognize that many measurement techniques used for characterization of ENM physicochemical properties for laboratory toxicology studies often differ from those used in occupational exposure assessments. Potential for disconnect between occupational exposure metrics (size, size distribution, morphology, surface area, and mass, as well as bulk and surface chemistry and crystallinity) and toxicological response metrics are described in the following sections. For additional details on physicochemical characterization of ENMs, see Chapters 3 and 4.

5.3.1.1 Size/size distribution/morphology

In workplace atmospheres, particle size distribution is determined using real-time instruments such as the APS, FMPS, OPC, SMPS, etc. The FMPS and SMPS provide a measure of electrical mobility diameter (diameter of a unit density spherical particle moving through air at the same velocity in an electric field as an irregular-shaped particle of interest), whereas the APS measures aerodynamic diameter (diameter of a unit density spherical particle that has the equivalent settling velocity in air as an irregular-shaped particle of interest) and the OPC physical diameter. Time-integrated sampling with an appropriate substrate followed by off-line analysis using electron microscopy can be used to determine size (and size distribution) of ENMs in workplace atmospheres. Similarly, electron microscopy is often used to determine the size/distribution of as-received ENM powder for toxicology studies. Dynamic light scattering is a laboratory technique for determination of hydrodynamic diameter (diameter of a hard sphere that diffuses at the same speed in a specified medium as the particle of interest), an intensity-weighted (light scattering is proportional to radius to the sixth power) equivalent diameter calculated from the diffusion coefficient of particles in a liquid. In some toxicology studies, an ENM is placed in a liquid vehicle, it is dispersed by ultrasonic agitation, and size distribution is measured using dynamic light scattering prior to dosing animals via intratracheal instillation or pharyngeal aspiration. Inhalable and respirable particle sizes in experimental models (rats, mice) are much smaller than in humans [60], making dispersion of agglomerated or aggregated nanomaterials by sonication necessary studies so that they can enter the rodent respiratory tract; however, the energy input from ultrasonic agitation may influence morphology by dispersing particles that would normally be present as agglomerates in workplace atmospheres. In summary, all techniques mentioned before provide a measure of size, though the measurement is method dependent and therefore not directly comparable among techniques.

5.3.1.2 Surface area

Surface area is also an example where measurement techniques differ between workplace exposure assessments and laboratory toxicology studies. As discussed previously, surface area of airborne nanoparticles in workplaces is measured using (i) real-time DCs, which measure the active surface area (area of the particle that interacts with the surrounding gas or ions and is accessible only from the outside) [48]; (ii) electrical mobility analyzers (or other real-time instruments), which calculate the spherical-equivalent diameter, which, in turn, can be converted to mobility-based surface area using geometric relationships [53]; or (iii) collection of airborne particles on a substrate (filter, grid, etc.) and selective measurement of the external dimensions of the ENM of interest using electron microscopy and conversion to area using geometric relations. Measures of surface area by real-time DCs and calculations from particle external dimensions do not account for porosity, cracks, and other surface irregularities on particles and therefore may provide inaccurate estimates of surface area [28, 61]. Further, these real-time techniques are nonspecific and cannot discriminate the surface area of an ENM of interest from other nanoscale particles in the workplace atmosphere. In laboratory toxicology studies, the total surface area (external area plus internal pores and crevices) of as-received powder is measured using inert gas adsorption (e.g., N_2, Kr) and the Brunauer–Emmett–Teller (BET) method. In the previously mentioned studies in which the TiO_2 surface area was a better predictor of pulmonary retention and inflammatory responses than mass, the powder's total surface area was measured using the BET method [58, 59]. For situations in which dissolution or free-radical generation drives the underlying toxicological mechanism, calculating the powder's total surface area by the BET method, representing all possible area in contact with solvent or available for reacting, may be the more appropriate metric. In contrast, for situations in which toxicity is driven by particle–membrane interactions, active (external, excluding pores) surface area may be more appropriate. Thus, particle surface area as measured in workplace atmospheres by DCs (external) or calculated from SMPS measurements (mobility) is not the same property as surface area measured by the BET method (total), and there can be important differences between metrics that may be relevant to toxicological exposure responses and metrics that may be reliably measured during real-world exposure assessments [62].

5.3.1.3 Bulk/surface chemistry

In general, determination of bulk particle chemistry using ICP analysis should provide similar results for a given ENM collected on a substrate in a workplace atmosphere and the same material in the form of as-received powder for a toxicology study. However, differences could exist if the element of interest is not homogeneously dispersed across all particle sizes. For example, if the workplace assessment technique employed a size-selective sampling head such as a respirable cyclone and the element of interest was disproportionately segregated in larger particles (diameters greater than the aerodynamic cut-off of the sampler), the mass concentration of collected particles would be biased low, whereas a representative sample of as-received ENM powder will include all particle sizes in the material and therefore a higher mass concentration.

Surface chemistry is an important ENM physicochemical property because the proportion of atoms on a particle surface relative to its core increases as particle size decreases in the nanoscale and surface-driven reactions such as dissolution or free-radical generation are controlled by the chemistry of surface atoms. Workplace atmospheres are complex environments that contain not only the ENM of interest but also other particles and gases and vapors. Depending on particle number concentration, airborne ENMs can agglomerate with non-ENMs (or incidental nanoparticles) in workplace air and/or bind gases and vapors on their surfaces. As such, upon deposition in the respiratory tract, the surface chemistry of an ENM initially "seen" by the lung will constitute atoms of the ENM plus surface-adsorbed molecules from the general workplace atmosphere. In contrast, for animal inhalation toxicology experiments, ENM surface chemistry is determined using the as-delivered powder and represents a pristine surface relative to the same ENM in a workplace atmosphere (it is assumed that the surface chemistry of the as-received powder is representative of the ENM particles as-delivered to the animals in the exposure chamber). For intratracheal instillation or pharyngeal aspiration toxicology studies, a representative sample of as-received ENM is placed in a liquid vehicle prior to dosing animals. Common liquid vehicles include animal bronchoalveolar lavage fluid (BAL), phosphate-buffered saline (PBS), and dispersion media (DM). PBS often contains salts such as phosphate. DM is a synthetic mixture based in PBS or saline that is designed to mimic the fluid that lines the lungs. It contains a protein that is compatible with the test species (e.g., mouse or rat albumin to mimic the surfactant proteins in the lung fluid) and synthetic dipalmitoyl phosphotidyl choline (DPPC), the major lipid in the lung lining fluid that is believed to decrease surface tension in the lung. Importantly, salts and proteins in these vehicles will quickly bind to ENM surfaces to form a corona surface coating, thereby changing the surface chemistry, reactivity, hydrophobicity/hydrophilicity, and charge [63]. As such, the surface chemistry of an ENM in a workplace atmosphere can differ considerably from the surface chemistry of an ENM that is used in a toxicology study to understand exposure–response relationships for a given toxicological mechanism.

5.3.1.4 Crystallinity

For workplace exposure assessments, time-integrated sampling with an appropriate substrate, followed by off-line analysis using TEM, can be used to determine crystalline properties of ENMs in workplace atmospheres. Specifically, TEM with selected area electron diffraction (TEM-SAED) analysis is a useful technique to determine whether a material is crystalline or not. TEM-SAED is rapid (requiring only a few minutes to collect a diffraction pattern) and can be performed on individual particles or small groups of particles, which makes this technique particularly useful for analysis of airborne particles collected on substrates from workplace atmospheres. However, there is high potential for bias because only a small group of particles is analyzed and the results assumed to be representative of the particle distribution as a whole in the workplace. Interestingly, none of the exposure assessment studies summarized in Table 5.1 included determination of ENM crystallinity. Generally, if large masses (mg to g quantities) of powder are available, X-ray diffraction (XRD) is the preferred method to determine crystallinity of a powder. For toxicology studies, XRD is performed on the as-received ENM powder and offers the advantage of integrating counting statistics from millions of particles thereby improving accuracy. Disadvantages of XRD is that measurement time is on the order of several hours (even days) and it is insensitive to crystalline constituents present in low amounts (approximately less than 0.1%), which may be relevant for toxicological responses. Understanding crystallinity of ENM particles in workplace atmospheres and as-received powders for toxicology studies is an important consideration for risk assessment. For example, if an as-received ENM powder used in a toxicology study is a final product crystalline powder, its atomic order could differ from that of airborne ENMs of the same type in a workplace atmosphere if the emission source is an intermediary process step. In this scenario, the ENM in the workplace atmosphere may have no (amorphous) or less atomic order, which, in turn, will influence dissolution behavior and therefore residence time in the lung alveoli [64].

In summary, there are likely differences between exposure metrics measured in occupational environments and characterized exposure metrics associated with toxicological responses in laboratory studies. Unfortunately, no quantitative comparisons of ENM properties (e.g., surface chemistry) in workplace atmospheres and animal toxicology exposure chambers have been reported, so it is difficult to determine how significant any differences may be. Additionally, as noted before, some differences in properties (e.g., size/size distribution) may be required for equivalent internal doses in humans and experimental rodent models [60]. Nonetheless, the state of ENMs encountered in workplace atmospheres (agglomerated, containing surface-adsorbed gases and vapors, etc.) differs from the state of ENMs used in toxicology studies (pristine for inhalation experiments, surface protein corona for aspiration studies, etc.). Investigators recognize that these disconnects limit our risk assessments and are beginning to address these important gaps by developing new models for obtaining representative real-world ENM samples for toxicology studies [65]. In the remaining sections, examples of two ENMs with recommended OELs (CNFs/CNTs, TiO_2) are reviewed and a critical comparison made between metrics of workplace exposure (from Table 5.1) and metrics associated with toxicological endpoints used in the risk assessment to set the limits.

5.3.2 Carbon Fibers and Nanotubes

CNFs are ENMs that consist of a rolled graphene sheet. An important subset of nanofibers is hollow nanotubes. If the graphene plane and fiber axis do not align, the structure is defined as a CNF; however, when the plane and fiber axis are parallel, the structure is referred to as a CNT [1]. CNTs can be further categorized as SWCNTs, consisting of a single rolled graphene sheet; double-walled carbon nanotubes (DWCNTs), consisting of two single-walled tubes concentrically one inside the other; and MWCNTs, consisting of many single-walled tubes arranged concentrically one inside the other. Both CNFs and CNTs possess many desirable properties, including mechanical strength, flexibility, lightweight, heat resistance, and high electrical conductivity [57]. These properties are exploited in numerous commercial applications, including, but not limited to, electronics, batteries, composites, and polymer coatings in telecommunication, aerospace, construction and defense industries [13, 14, 66, 67].

5.3.2.1 Toxicological endpoints for occupational exposure limits

As part of their risk assessment for CNFs/CNTs, the US National Institute for Occupational Safety and Health (NIOSH) systematically reviewed available animal toxicology data (i.e., intratracheal, aspiration, and inhalation) [68]. In these studies, lung exposures to CNTs (i.e., various types of MWCNTs and SWCNTs, purified and unpurified, dispersed or agglomerated, and with different metal content) were observed to cause early-stage noncancerous adverse health effects such as pulmonary inflammation, granulomas, alveolar septal thickening, and pulmonary fibrosis. NIOSH concluded that the best data to use for a quantitative risk assessment were the nonmalignant pulmonary data from two subchronic (90-day) rat inhalation studies [69, 70] and five other studies conducted by other routes or for other durations. On the basis of the risk assessment, NIOSH proposed a recommended exposure limit (REL) of 1 μg/m^3 EC as an 8-hour time-weighted average (TWA) respirable mass concentration. The intent of the NIOSH REL was to reduce the potential risk for pulmonary inflammation and fibrosis. Note that NIOSH is not a regulatory agency and the REL is not a legally enforceable OEL.

In addition to NIOSH, several other groups have proposed OELs for CNTs [68]. The first OEL proposed for CNTs was from the British Standards Institute; it suggested a limit of 0.01 fibers/cm^3 (i.e., one-tenth of the asbestos exposure limit). Using data from a subchronic rat inhalation study [69], the producers of Nanocyl® MWCNTs derived an OEL of 2.5 μg/m^3 for an 8-hour TWA. In another study, investigators reviewed the Ma-Hock et al. [69] and Pauluhn [70] studies and proposed two OELs: 1 μg/m^3 for Nanocyl® MWCNTs and 2 μg/m^3 for Baytube® MWCNTs. Subsequently, Bayer Material Science, the maker of Baytube® MWCNTs, derived an OEL of 50 μg/m^3 as an 8-hour TWA exposure for this material [71]. Finally, the Japanese National Institute of Advance Industrial Science and Technology derived an OEL of 30 μg/m^3 for CNTs based on rat data. Variability among these OELs may include differences in the toxicity of materials as well as differences in the risk assessment methods and assumptions in interpreting animal toxicology data [68].

5.3.2.2 Relevant exposure metrics for carbon nanofibers/nanotubes

In its risk assessment, NIOSH [68] acknowledged that in addition to mass, other metrics of CNF/CNT exposure associated with adverse lung responses in animal studies included particle volume, size (length) number, and surface area; structural defects; surface modification, functionalization, and coatings; and degree of agglomeration [68]. However, a mass-based REL was chosen because mass of CNFs/CNTs was associated with lung responses in all animal studies in the risk assessment and because mass is typically used to measure airborne exposure in the workplace (see Table 5.1).

Pauluhn [72] used a modeling approach to understand the mechanisms underlying observed adverse lung effects from MWCNT exposures in rats as a means to elucidate relevant dose metrics. Using a modeling approach (with similarities but also differences to that used by NIOSH), Pauluhn [72] reanalyzed data from a previous rat inhalation study of Baytube® MWCNTs [70], as well as available published data from rat inhalation studies of Nanocyl® MWCNTs [69]. On the basis of this modeling approach, Pauluhn advocated that two modes of action were relevant for MWCNT-induced noncancerous pulmonary effects [72]. The first mode of action was acute effects on the lung surfactant related to MWCNT surface activity and surface area that occurred upon particle deposition in the lung. MWCNTs that deposit in the lung surfactant will adsorb proteins and other biomolecules, thereby temporarily destabilizing the surfactant and cause transient dysfunction of the air–blood barrier. The second mode of action was chronic accumulation of a MWCNT lung burden, which produced pulmonary inflammation that was dependent on the cumulative particle volumetric lung burden. In this mode of action, if the accumulated particle displacement volume of deposited MWCNTs within the pool of alveolar macrophages exceeded the kinetic overload threshold of the lungs (6%), clearance was impaired, resulting in inflammation. MWCNTs have very low density; as such the particle displacement volume increases rapidly relative to mass and therefore development of pulmonary inflammation [72]. Hence, the key metric for cumulative particle displacement volume of the highly agglomerated MWCNTs appeared to be the apparent density of deposited particles. Note that this metric may not be applicable for rigid, fiber-like MWCNTs.

5.3.2.3 Occupational exposure assessment and laboratory toxicology

In the *Current Intelligence Bulletin on Carbon Nanotubes and Nanofibers* [68], NIOSH stated that its REL uses respirable EC mass concentration as the exposure metric. This REL was set at the optimal limit of quantification of the analytical method for EC (NIOSH Method 5040). The respirable particle size fraction was chosen because adverse health effects in the animal studies used in their risk assessment were observed in the alveolar region. However, NIOSH does acknowledge that in the future, new data may become available that indicate other metrics of exposure would be more effective in protecting workers' health and the REL could be updated to reflect that information [68].

As noted in Section 5.2 of this chapter, various time-integrated sampling devices are available to size-selectively sample for the respirable aerosol fraction, including cyclones; these devices have collection characteristics intended to meet the respirable sampling convention, a target specification for sampling instruments when the respirable fraction is the fraction of interest (i.e., aerodynamic diameter from 0 to 10 μm with 50% collection efficiency at 4 μm). Air samples for CNFs/CNTs are collected by aspirating air through quartz fiber filters, followed by off-line analysis using NIOSH Method 5040 to determine EC content. If it is known that a workplace atmosphere contains negligible amounts of incidental sources of EC, such as diesel soot, then an elevated airborne EC concentration relative to background (environmental and in nonprocess areas in the workplace) can be used as a reasonable indicator of exposure to CNTs or CNFs [68]. However, if appreciable sources of incidental EC are present in a workplace atmosphere, additional analytical techniques such as TEM equipped with an energy dispersive X-ray spectroscopy detector will be required to discriminate exposures to CNFs/CNTs from incidental contributors to EC mass levels on filters. Hence, if a workplace atmosphere is free of incidental sources of EC or if the contribution of CNFs/CNTs can be discriminated from incidental EC, then existing occupational exposure assessment techniques can provide an estimate of this metric as it was used in animal toxicology experiments to derive the REL.

Pauluhn [72] advocated that two modes of action were relevant for MWCNT-induced noncancerous pulmonary effects. As noted in Section 5.3.1.3, upon deposition in the respiratory tract, the surface chemistry of an ENM will quickly change because of adsorption of biomolecules in surfactant. As such, the surface chemistry of an ENM in a workplace atmosphere could differ from that of pristine material used in a toxicology study. Currently, there are no techniques to measure ENM surface activity/area in workplace atmospheres in a manner that would mimic in vivo (first mode of action). In the Baytube® MWCNT inhalation toxicology study [70], the key exposure metric for particle displacement volume was apparent density of lung-deposited particles in rats (second mode of action). Apparent density is defined as the mass of a powder divided by the total volume of the sample (including closed and inaccessible pores) and differs from "true" density, defined as the ratio of material mass to volume occupied by that mass (excluding pores or internal voids) [73]. Pauluhn determined the apparent density of Baytubes® using mercury pycnometry of as-received material and TEM analysis of airborne MWCNTs collected on substrates in the inhalation exposure chamber [70]. It is important to note that apparent density is dependent upon the structure of the airborne MWCNT assemblies (agglomerates) and is not an intrinsic particle property; rather it will change depending upon the technique used to aerosolize a material [74]. Determination of apparent density of airborne particles is highly complex and requires specialized measurement instruments and knowledge. For example, Ku and Kulkarni determined apparent densities of SWCNTs and MWCNTs under laboratory conditions using a tandem differential mobility analyzer-aerosol mass analyzer system [74]. While their system was useful for laboratory studies, the lack of specificity of real-time instruments for an ENM of interest in an atmosphere that also contains incidental nanoparticles precludes its use to determine the apparent density of dispersed CNT agglomerates in complex workplace atmospheres. As such, under the mode of action hypothesis by Pauluhn [72], there is disconnect between biologically relevant metrics of exposure derived from animal toxicology studies and current abilities to measure the same metric in workplace atmospheres.

5.3.3 Titanium Dioxide

TiO_2 is a metal oxide with numerous industrial applications (e.g., pigments, cosmetics, catalysts). The most common forms of TiO_2 are crystalline anatase and rutile, with the rutile form being used in pigment applications (e.g., paints and plastics) and a mixture of the two forms (usually 80% anatase, 20% rutile) used in photoactive applications (e.g., catalysts, sunscreens). TiO_2 particles are often categorized by size as pigment grade (250 to 400 nm) or ultrafine/nanoparticles (<100 nm) and may have surface coatings to impart specific properties [75].

5.3.3.1 Toxicological endpoints for occupational exposure limits

NIOSH conducted a risk assessment of TiO_2 [76]. In its risk assessment, NIOSH concluded that the most relevant data for assessing the health risk to workers were the results from a chronic animal inhalation study with ultrafine TiO_2 in which a statistically significant increase in adenocarcinomas was observed, literature that supported a pattern of TiO_2-induced persistent pulmonary inflammation in rats and mice and cancer responses for several poorly soluble low-toxicity (PSLT) particles such as TiO_2 and carbon black. On the basis of the data supporting formation of adenocarcinomas and the pattern of pulmonary inflammatory responses for PSLT particles, NIOSH determined that "exposure to ultrafine TiO_2 should be considered a potential occupational carcinogen" [76]. NIOSH cited evidence that a plausible mechanism for TiO_2-induced cancer in rats can be described as the accumulation of TiO_2 in the lungs to the point that it overloads lung clearance mechanisms, which, in turn, results in increased pulmonary inflammation and oxidative stress (reactive oxygen species [ROS] generation), cellular proliferation, and, at higher doses, tumorigenesis. According to evidence cited by NIOSH, the weight of evidence suggested that the tumor response observed in rats exposed to ultrafine TiO_2 was the result of a secondary genotoxic mechanism involving chronic inflammation and cell proliferation, not the genotoxicity of TiO_2 itself. Using lung cancer as the toxicological endpoint, NIOSH developed a REL of 0.3 mg/m^3 for ultrafine (including ENMs) TiO_2 as a time-weighted average concentration for up to 10 hours per day during a 40-hour work week for all forms of ultrafine TiO_2. DuPont, a manufacturer of ultrafine TiO_2, using different methods and assumptions than NIOSH in its risk assessment, developed two OELs for ultrafine TiO_2 on the basis of transient pulmonary inflammation as the relevant toxicological endpoint, not lung cancer [75]. The DuPont OELs are 1 mg/m^3 for high-surface-reactivity anatase/rutile forms and 2 mg/m^3 for low-surface-reactivity rutile forms. Other OELs for ultrafine TiO_2 include the Japanese Institute of Advanced Industrial Science and Technology value of 0.61 mg/m^3 [77, 78]; the Japanese Society for Occupational Health value of 0.3 mg/m^3 [79]; the German MAK general dust respirable fraction of 0.3 mg/m^3 [80]; and a value of 0.017 mg/m^3 derived by Aschberger et al. [81].

Table 5.1 Summary of metrics of ENM aerosol physicochemical properties characterized in occupational exposure assessment

ENM[a]	Tasks	Metrics (techniques)		Reference
		Real time[c]	Time integrated[d]	
Metallic				
Ag	Production, harvesting	Size distribution (OPC, SMPS)	Metals by ICP (MCE) Morphology by STEM (MCE)	[83]
Ag	Production	None	Metals by ICP (MCE)	[84]
Ag	Production, drying, grinding product	Size distribution (SMPS)	Morphology by TEM (grid in ESP)	[85]
Ag	Handling powders	Size distribution (FMPS)	Morphology by STEM (grid on PC)	[86]
Ag	Production	Size distribution (OPC, SMPS)	Metals by ICP (MCE) Morphology by STEM (MCE)	[87]
Ag	Cleaning reactor	Size distribution (OPC) $\#/cm^3$ (CPC)	Metals by ICP (MCE) Morphology by TEM (MCE)	[88]
Ag	Cleaning reactor	Size distribution (ELPI, OPC, SMPS) $\#/cm^3$ (CPC)	Metals by ICP (MCE) Morphology by TEM (MCE)	[89]
Ag	Cleaning reactor	Size distribution (OPC) $\#/cm^3$ (CPC)	Metals by ICP (MCE) Morphology by TEM (MCE)	[90]

		Metrics (techniques)		
ENM[a]	Tasks	Real time[c]	Time integrated[d]	Reference
Pb	Operating epitaxy furnace	Size distribution (FMPS, OPC, SMPS)	Metals by ICP, XRF (filters)	[91]
Pt	Workplace simulation	Size distribution (OPC, SMPS) #/cm^3 (CPC)	None	[92]
Unspecified	Production, cleaning, packaging product	Size distribution (OPC, SMPS) #/cm^3 (CPC) M/cm^3 (AP)	None	[93]
Various	Production	Size distribution (SMPS) #/cm^3 (CPC) SA/cm^3 (NSAM)	Mass by weighing (PC) Morphology by SEM (PC)	[94]
Various	Maintenance	Size distribution (APS) #/cm^3 (CPC) M/cm^3 (AP) Size and chemistry (LV-AMS)	Morphology by SEM (PC)	[46]
Metal oxides				
Al_2O_3	Compounding composites	Size distribution (FMPS)	Morphology by STEM (grid on PC)	[95]

(*Continued*)

Table 5.1 (*Continued*)

		Metrics (techniques)		
ENM[a]	**Tasks**	**Real time**[c]	**Time integrated**[d]	**Reference**
Al_2O_3	Compounding composites	Size distribution (FMPS)	Morphology by STEM (grid on PC)	[96]
Al_2O_3	Handling powders	Size distribution (FMPS)	Morphology by STEM (grid on PC)	[86]
Al_2O_3	Compounding composites	Size distribution (FMPS)	None	[97]
Al_2O_3	Handling powders	Size distribution (APS, FMPS)	None	[98]
Al_2O_3	Compounding composites	Size distribution (APS, FMPS)	Morphology by TEM (grid on PC)	[99]
Al_2O_3	Handling powders	#/cm^3 (CPC)	None	[100]
Al_2O_3	Production, separating, packaging	Size distribution (SMPS) #/cm^3 (CPC) M/cm^3 (AP) SA/cm^3 (DC)	Morphology by SEM (Al) Size distribution by weighing (Al in impactor)	[101]
Al_2O_3, TiO_2	Production, drying, filtering, milling, bagging powders	Size distribution (FMPS, SMPS) M/cm^3 (TEOM™)	Mass by weighing (QF) Morphology by SEM (carbon in ESP)	[102]

ENM[a]	Tasks	Metrics (techniques)		Reference
		Real time[c]	Time integrated[d]	
Al_2O_3, Fe_2O_3	Production	Size distribution (SMPS) #/cm^3 (CPC) M/cm^3 (AP) SA/cm^3 (DC)	Mass by weighing (Al) Morphology by SEM (Al)	[103]
$CaCO_3$	Production, drying, packaging	#/cm^3 (CPC) SA/cm^3 (DC)	Mass by weighing (TF)	[104]
$CaCO_3$	Production, drying, packaging	Size distribution (OPC) #/cm^3 (CPC)	Mass by weighing (TF) Morphology by SEM (TF)	[105]
$CaCO_3$	Simulated production failures	#/cm^3 and mobility size (DiSC)	None	[106]
$CaCO_3$, SiO_2	Mixing composites, bagging	Size distribution (SMPS)	Mass by weighing (Al, TF) Metals by ICP (MCE, TF)	[107]
CeO_2	Production	Size distribution (ELPI, SMPS) #/cm^3 (CPC) M/cm^3 (TEOM™)	Morphology by SEM, TEM (grid in ESP)	[108]
Fe_2O_3	Calcining, drying, operating process	Size distribution (APS, SMPS) #/cm^3 (CPC) M/cm^3 (AP)	None	[109]

(*Continued*)

Table 5.1 (*Continued*)

ENM[a]	Tasks	Metrics (techniques)		Reference
		Real time[c]	Time integrated[d]	
ITO, ZnO	Mixing, recovering product, spraying	Size distribution (APS, SMPS) #/cm^3 (CPC)	Metals by ICP (filters) Morphology by SEM (filters)	[110]
SiO_2	Mixing, stirring, drying, packaging	Size distribution (SMPS) SA/cm^3 (NSAM)	Mass by weighing (PC) Morphology by TEM (grid in ESP) Silica by FTIR (PC)	[111]
SiO_2	Milling, packaging	Size distribution (SMPS) #/cm^3 (DiSC)	Mass by weighing (PC) Morphology by TEM (grid in ESP)	[112]
ITO	Production, maintenance	Size distribution (OPC)	Metals by ICP (TF) Morphology by SEM (PC)	[113]
LTO	Wet milling, spray drying, calcining, sifting powders	Size distribution (OPC) #/cm^3 (CPC)	Mass by weighing (PVC) Metals by ICP (PVC) Morphology by TEM, SEM (MCE)	[114]
TiO_2	Production, harvesting	Size distribution (OPC, SMPS)	Metals by ICP (MCE) Morphology by STEM (MCE)	[83]

ENM[a]	Tasks	Metrics (techniques)		Reference
		Real time[c]	Time integrated[d]	
TiO_2	Production, harvesting, packaging, maintenance	Size distribution (SMPS) #/cm^3 (CPC)	Morphology by SEM (grids)	[115]
TiO_2	Production, opening and cleaning reactor, harvesting	Size distribution (OPC, WRAS) #/cm^3 (CPC)	Morphology by SEM (Au, grid in TP)	[116]
TiO_2	Simulating construction tasks	Size distribution (SMPS)	Morphology by TEM (grid in ESP)	[117]
TiO_2	Packaging	Size distribution (ELPI, SMPS, WRAS) #/cm^3 (CPC) M/cm^3 (TEOM™)	Morphology by TEM (grid on PC)	[118]
TiO_2	Production, fabricating, applying, drilling and demolishing mortars	Size distribution (ELPI, OPC) #/cm^3 (CPC)	Metals by ICP (filters) Morphology by SEM (filters)	[119]
TiO_2	Powder milling	Size distribution (WRPS)	Mass by weighing (filters) Ti mass by UV-Vis (wet sampler)	[120]
TiO_2	Powder milling	Size distribution (WRPS)	Morphology by SEM (filters)	[121]

(*Continued*)

Table 5.1 (*Continued*)

		Metrics (techniques)		
ENM[a]	**Tasks**	**Real time**[c]	**Time integrated**[d]	**Reference**
TiO_2	Weighing, pressing, drilling, packaging	Size distribution (ELPI) #/cm^3 (CPC)	None	[122]
TiO_2	Production, calcining, micronizing, coating	Size distribution (APS, SMPS) #/cm^3 (CPC) M/cm^3 (AP)	None	[123]
TiO_2	Production, packaging	Size distribution (FMPS)	Size distribution from dust by weighing (TF in cyclone or impactor) Size distribution from metals by ICP (MCE in cyclone or impactor)	[124]
TiO_2	Packaging	Size distribution (OPC) #/cm^3 (CPC)	Size distribution from dust by weighing (filters) Metals by ICP (PC)	[125]
Various	Adding salts to reactor, changing spray dryer drum	Size distribution (ELPI, OPC, SMPS) #/cm^3 (CPC)	Metals by ICP (MCE) Morphology by TEM (MCE)	[89]

		Metrics (techniques)		
ENM[a]	Tasks	Real time[c]	Time integrated[d]	Reference
Various	Cleaning reactor	Size distribution (OPC) #/cm^3 (CPC)	Metals by ICP (MCE) Morphology by TEM (MCE)	[88]
Various	Production	Size distribution (SMPS) #/cm^3 (CPC) M/cm^3 (AP)	None	[126]
Various	Cleaning reactor	Size distribution (OPC) #/cm^3 (CPC)	Metals by ICP (MCE) Morphology by TEM (MCE)	[90]
Various	Production, harvesting, bagging	Size distribution (ELPI, OPC) #/cm^3 (CPC)	Morphology by SEM (PC)	[127]
Various	Production, handling	Size distribution (OPC) #/cm^3 (CPC) SA/cm^3 (DC)	Mass by weighing (PVC) Metals by ICP (PVC) Morphology by TEM (MCE) Size distribution from metals by ICP (MCE in impactor)	[128]
Various	Production	Size distribution (SMPS) #/cm^3 (CPC) SA/cm^3 (NSAM)	Mass by weighing (PC) Morphology by SEM (PC)	[94]

(*Continued*)

Table 5.1 (*Continued*)

ENM[a]	Tasks	Metrics (techniques) Real time[c]	Time integrated[d]	Reference
Various	Handling, abrading, spraying, heating, machining	#/cm^3 (nanoTracer) SA/cm^3 (calculated from nanoTracer)	None	[50]
Various	Maintenance and cleanout	Size distribution (ELPI, FMPS, SMPS) #/cm^3 (CPC)	Morphology by SEM (Al)	[129]
Various	Production, handling, packaging	Size distribution (APS, ELPI, SMPS) #/cm^3 (CPC) M/cm^3 (AP) SA/cm^3 (DC, NSAM)	Morphology by TEM (grid in TP, grid on PC)	[47]
Various	Chemical mechanical planarization	Size distribution (SMPS, OPC) #/cm^3 (CPC)	Mass by weighing (filters) Morphology by TEM (PC)	[130]
Various	Laser ablation, pouring, weighing, blending, bagging, brushing, rolling, spraying, sonication, drying, sawing, cleaning	Size distribution (Nano-ID™) #/cm^3 (nanoTracer)	Morphology by SEM (PC)	[131]

		Metrics (techniques)		
ENM[a]	Tasks	Real time[c]	Time integrated[d]	Reference
Various	Chemical mechanical planarization	Size distribution (SMPS, OPC) #/cm^3 (CPC)	Mass by weighing (filters) Metals by ICP (filters) Morphology by TEM or SEM (PC)	[132]
Quantum dots				
CdS, Au	Spraying	Size distribution (SMPS) #/cm^3 (CPC)	Morphology by AFM (mica disc in TP) Morphology by STEM (grids)	[133]
CdZnSe	Production	Size distribution (ELPI, OPC, SMPS) #/cm^3 (CPC)	Metals by ICP (MCE) Morphology by TEM (MCE)	[89]
Clays				
Montmorillonite, talc	Shredding	Size distribution (FMPS, OPC) #/cm^3 (UCPC) M/cm^3 (AP) SA/cm^3 (NSAM)	Morphology by SEM (PC in impactor)	[134]
Montmorillonite	Compounding composites	Size distribution (APS, FMPS)	Morphology by TEM (grid on PC)	[100]

(*Continued*)

Table 5.1 (*Continued*)

		Metrics (techniques)		
ENM[a]	Tasks	Real time[c]	Time integrated[d]	Reference
Carbon-based				
C60	Packaging	Size distribution (OPC, SMPS)	Morphology by SEM (QF)	[135]
C60, CNTs	Production, cleaning	Size distribution (SMPS) M/cm^3 (AP)	None	[136]
C60, CB, MWCNT	Handling powders	Size distribution (OPC) #/cm^3 (CPC)	Morphology by TEM (MCE)	[137]
CB	Packaging	Size distribution (APS, SMPS) M/cm^3 (TEOM™)	EC by thermal-optical technique (QF)	[56]
CB	Production, pelletizing	Size distribution (APS, SMPS) M/cm^3 (TEOM™)	EC by thermal-optical technique (QF)	[138]
CB	Pelletizing, packaging, and warehousing	Size distribution (SMPS) SA/cm^3 (MEAD, NSAM)	None	[52]
CB	Bagging	Size distribution (SMPS)	Mass by weighing (Al) EC by thermal-optical technique (QF)	[107]
CB, CNTs, Graphene	Harvesting, pouring, weighing, blending, bagging, sonication, molding, cleaning	Size distribution (Nano-ID™) #/cm^3 (nanoTracer)	Morphology by SEM (PC)	[129]

		Metrics (techniques)		
ENM[a]	Tasks	Real time[c]	Time integrated[d]	Reference
Cellulose	Grinding, spray drying	Size distribution (SMPS) #/cm^3 (CPC)	None	[139]
Cellulose	Production, handling	None	Metals by ICP (MCE)	[140]
CNFs	Composite production, handling	Size distribution (ELPI) #/cm^3 (CPC) M/cm^3 (AP) SA/cm^3 (DC)	EC by thermal-optical technique (QF) Morphology by TEM (grid in ESP)	[68]
CNFs	Handling powders, machining composites	Size distribution (OPC) #/cm^3 (CPC) M/cm^3 (AP)	EC by thermal-optical technique (QF) Morphology by TEM (MCE)	[141]
CNFs	Drying, harvesting, packaging	Size distribution (ELPI, FPSS) #/cm^3 (CPC) M/cm^3 (AP) SA/cm^3 (DC)	None	[43]
CNFs	Production	None	EC by thermal-optical technique (QF in cassette, impactor) Metals by ICP (QF) Morphology by TEM (grid in ESP, impactor)	[67]

(*Continued*)

Table 5.1 (*Continued*)

ENM[a]	Tasks	Metrics (techniques)		Reference
		Real time[c]	Time integrated[d]	
CNFs, CNTs	Drilling composites	Size distribution (APS, FMPS) #/cm^3 (CPC) M/cm^3 (AP) SA/cm^3 (DC)	Metals by ICP (glass slides in WRASS) Morphology by SEM (MCE) Morphology by TEM (grid in TP, ESP)	[14]
CNFs, CNPs, MWCNTs	Production, harvesting	Size distribution (ELPI, OPC, SMPS) #/cm^3 (CPC)	EC by thermal-optical technique (QF) Metals by ICP (MCE) Morphology by TEM (MCE)	[89]
CNFs, DWCNTs, MWCNTs, SWCNTs	Production, harvesting, blending, sonicating, weighing	None	EC by thermal-optical technique (QF) Morphology by TEM (MCE)	[142]
CNFs, DWCNTs, MWCNTs, SWCNTs	Production, harvesting, blending, sonicating, weighing	#/cm^3 (CPC) M/cm^3 (AP) SA/cm^3 (DC)	EC by thermal-optical technique (QF) Morphology by TEM (MCE)	[143]
CNFs, DWCNTs, MWCNTs, SWCNTs	Production, harvesting, blending, sonicating, weighing	None	EC by thermal-optical technique (QF) Morphology by TEM (MCE)	[144]

		Metrics (techniques)		
ENM[a]	Tasks	Real time[c]	Time integrated[d]	Reference
CNFs, CNTs, BNTs	Production, harvesting, handling, blending, weighing, transferring, spraying, grinding, cleaning	Size distribution (OPC) #/cm^3 (CPC)	EC by thermal-optical technique (QF) Morphology by TEM, SEM (MCE)	[145]
CNFs, MWCNTs, SWCNTs	Production, handling, packaging	Size distribution (APS, ELPI, SMPS) #/cm^3 (CPC) M/cm^3 (AP) SA/cm^3 (DC, NSAM)	Morphology by TEM (grid in TP, grid on PC)	[128]
CNTs	Production, harvesting	Size distribution (FMPS) #/cm^3 (CPC)	Morphology by TEM (grid in TP, ESP; MCE)	[8]
CNTs	Dry and wet machining composites	Size distribution (APS, FMPS) #/cm^3 (CPC) M/cm^3 (AP)	Morphology by TEM (grid in TP) Morphology by SEM (MCE)	[13]
CNTs	Weighing, mixing, grinding	Size distribution (ELPI, SMPS) #/cm^3 (CPC)	Morphology by TEM (grids)	[9]

(*Continued*)

Table 5.1 (*Continued*)

		Metrics (techniques)		
ENM[a]	Tasks	Real time[c]	Time integrated[d]	Reference
CNTs	Production, handling, cutting (ENM and composites)	Size distribution (APS, FMPS) M/cm^3 (AP)	Morphology by TEM (grid on PC)	[146]
CNTs, graphene	Production, harvesting, weighing, mixing, cleaning	Size distribution (FMPS) M/cm^3 (AP)	None	[147]
MWCNTs	Production, blending, weighing	Size distribution (APS, SMPS)	Morphology by STEM (MCE)	[148]
MWCNTs	Production, handling, packaging	Size distribution (OPC, SMPS) #/cm^3 (UCPC)	Morphology by STEM (MCE)	[149]
MWCNTs	Weighing tubes, sanding composites	Size distribution (OPC) #/cm^3 (CPC)	Morphology by TEM (grid on PC)	[15]
MWCNTs	Handling	Spectral identification (LIBS)	Morphology by SEM, TEM (grid in ESP)	[150]
MWCNTs	Packaging powder, weaving composite fibers	Size distribution (OPC, SMPS) #/cm^3 (CPC) M/cm^3 (AP)	EC by thermal-optical technique (QF) Morphology by SEM (PC)	[151]
MWCNTs	Packaging powder, weaving composite fibers	None	EC by thermal-optical technique (QF) Morphology by SEM (PC)	[152]

		Metrics (techniques)		
ENM[a]	Tasks	Real time[c]	Time integrated[d]	Reference
MWCNTs	Production, handling, purifying, functionalizing	Mobility size (nanoTracer) #/cm^3 (CPC, nanoTracer) M/cm^3 (AP)	EC by thermal-optical technique (QF) Mass by weighing (MCE) Morphology by SEM (PC)	[23]
MWCNTs	Production	Size distribution (APS, FMPS)	Morphology by TEM (grids) Morphology by STEM (CA, GF, QF)	[153]
MWCNTs	Production, harvesting, cleaning	Size distribution (OPC, SMPS)	EC by thermal-optical technique (QF) Mass by weighing (MCE) Metals by ICP (MCE) Morphology by SEM (MCE)	[65]
MWCNTs, SWCNTs	Operating reactor	Size distribution (APS, FMPS)	Morphology by TEM (grid on PC)	[154]
SWCNTs	Production, harvesting	Size distribution (OPC) #/cm^3 (CPC)	Metals by ICP (MCE) Morphology by SEM (PC)	[58]
SWCNTs	Production, harvesting	Size distribution (APS, OPC, SMPS) #/cm^3 (CPC)	Morphology by SEM (PC)	[155]

(Continued)

Table 5.1 (*Continued*)

		Metrics (techniques)		
ENM[a]	**Tasks**	**Real time**[c]	**Time integrated**[d]	**Reference**
SWCNTs	Production, harvesting, packaging	Size distribution (OPC) #/cm^3 (CPC) M/cm^3 (AP)	Morphology by SEM (PC) EC by thermal-optical technique (QF)	[156, 157]
Unspecified	Production, compounding polymers	Size distribution (WRAS) #/cm^3 (CPC)	None	[158]

[a]ENM, engineered nanomaterial; Ag, silver; Al_2O_3, aluminum oxide; Au, gold; BNTs, boron nitride tubes; C60, fullerenes; $CaCO_3$, calcium carbonate; CB, carbon black; CdS; cadmium selenide; CdZnSe; cadmium zinc selenide; CeO_2; cerium dioxide; CNFs; carbon nanofibers; CNPs; carbon nanopearls; CNTs; carbon nanotubes; DWCNTs; double-walled carbon nanotubes; Fe_2O_3; iron oxide; ITO; indium tin oxide; LTO; lithium titanate; MWCNTs; multiwalled carbon nanotubes; Pb; lead; Pt; platinum; SiO_2; silicon dioxide; SWCNTs; single-walled carbon nanotubes; TiO_2; titanium dioxide; Unspecified; composition of ENM not given in study; Various; numerous different chemical compositions of ENMs; ZnO; zinc oxide.

[b]#/cm^3 = particle number concentration; M/cm^3 = particle mass concentration; SA/cm^3 = particle surface area concentration.

[c]Real time: AP, aerosol photometer; APS, aerodynamic particle sizer; CPC, condensation particle counter; DC, diffusion charger; DiSC, diffusion size classifier; ELPI, electrical low-pressure impactor; FMPS, fast mobility particle sizer; FPSS, fast particle size spectrometer; LIBS, laser-induced breakdown spectroscopy; LV-AMS, laser vaporization-aerosol mass spectrometer; MEAD, modified electrical aerosol detector ; nanoTracer, diffusion charger; Nano-ID®, portable SMPS; OPC, optical particle counter; SMPS, scanning mobility particle sizer; TEOM™, tapered element oscillating microbalance; NSAM, nanoparticle surface area monitor; UCPC, ultrafine CPC; WRAS, wide-range aerosol spectrometer; WRPS, wide-range particle spectrometer.

[d]Time integrated: Al, aluminum substrate; AFM, atomic force microscopy; Au, gold filter; CA, cellulose acetate filter; EC, elemental carbon; ESP, electrostatic precipitator; FTIR, Fourier transform infrared; ICP, inductively coupled plasma; MCE, mixed cellulose ester filter; PC, polycarbonate; PVC, polyvinyl chloride; QF, quartz fiber; SEM, scanning electron microscopy; STEM, scanning transmission electron microscopy; TEM, transmission electron microscopy; TF, Teflon® filter; TP, thermophoretic precipitator; UV-Vis, ultraviolet-visible; WRASS, wide-range aerosol sampling system; XRF, X-ray fluorescence spectroscopy.

5.3.3.2 Relevant exposure metrics for ultrafine TiO_2

In its risk assessment, NIOSH noted that the REL of 0.3 mg/m^3 for ultrafine TiO_2 was based on chronic inhalation studies in rats that were used to predict lung tumor risks in humans and that the higher potency of ultrafine TiO_2 compared to fine (pigment-scale) TiO_2 was associated with the greater surface area of ultrafine particles for a given mass. NIOSH also considered the crystal structure of ultrafine TiO_2 as a modifying factor in its carcinogenicity and inflammation because of reported differences in ROS generated on the surface of different crystal structures of TiO_2 (e.g., anatase, rutile, or mixtures) in cell-free systems, differences in cytotoxicity among in vitro studies, and differences in inflammation and cell proliferation in vivo in rats [76]. However, in subchronic inhalation studies using rats, there was no difference in pulmonary inflammation response between fine and ultrafine TiO_2 particles with different crystal structure (i.e., 99% rutile vs. 80% anatase/20% rutile) when the inhaled dose was expressed as particle surface area, nor was there any difference in lung tumor response at a given surface area dose. NIOSH also evaluated whether surface coatings on TiO_2 particles were relevant metrics that modify the toxicity. While toxicity of TiO_2 has been shown to increase after coating with various substances [75], it has not been shown to be attenuated by application of coatings. Therefore, NIOSH concluded that its TiO_2 risk assessment could be used as a reasonable floor for potential toxicity, recognizing that toxicity may be substantially increased by particle treatment and process modification. NIOSH concluded that the available scientific evidence supported surface area as the critical metric for occupational inhalation exposure to ultrafine TiO_2. In addition to surface area, other recognized metrics that may influence toxicity include crystal structure, particle size distribution in relevant media, presence of surface coatings, surface reactivity, method of ultrafine TiO_2 synthesis, and presence of impurities [75, 76].

5.3.3.3 Occupational exposure assessment and laboratory toxicology

In its *Current Intelligence Bulletin on Titanium Dioxide*, NIOSH states, "It would be a better reflection of the entire body of available data to set RELs as the inhaled surface area of the particles rather than the mass of the particles. This would be consistent with the scientific evidence showing an increase in potency with increase in particle surface area (or decrease in particle size) of TiO_2 and other PSLT particles. For this reason, the basis of the RELs for fine and ultrafine TiO_2 is the rat dose-response data for particle surface area dose and pulmonary response." However, as noted earlier in this chapter and in the NIOSH risk assessment, in the toxicology studies in which TiO_2 surface area was a better predictor of adverse lung responses than mass, the powder's total surface area was measured using the BET method. Further, results from a cell-free study [82] suggest that ROS generation, which is a step in the proposed tumorgenesis pathway, was associated with the number of surface defects per unit area. Hence, surface area itself may be a surrogate metric for a surface defects metric.

As discussed in Section 5.3, measures of airborne particle surface area in occupational environments by real-time instruments such as diffusion chargers or calculations from particle external dimensions do not account for porosity, cracks, and other surface irregularities on particles and therefore may provide inaccurate estimates of surface area [28, 61, 62]. Further, real-time techniques are nonspecific and cannot discriminate the surface area of ultrafine TiO_2 particles (or any ENM) from incidental nanoscale particles in the workplace atmosphere. In laboratory toxicology studies, the total surface area (external area plus internal pores and crevices) of as-received powder is measured using inert gas adsorption (e.g., N_2, Kr) and the BET method. Hence, the same type of particle surface area, upon which the NIOSH REL for ultrafine TiO_2 is based, cannot be measured by existing field sampling equipment in workplace settings. NIOSH acknowledged that this technology does not exist and instead recommended sampling using airborne mass concentration of TiO_2 as the appropriate exposure metric for two broad primary particle size categories, fine (<10 μm) and ultrafine (<0.1 μm), until more appropriate measurement techniques can be developed. NIOSH recommends that personal exposures to fine (pigment) and ultrafine (including ENMs) TiO_2 be determined gravimetrically using a respirable cyclone (described previously in Section 5.2.2) or equivalent particle size–selective sampler to collect most ultrafine TiO_2 particles and agglomerates. In work environments with chemically heterogeneous atmospheres or where the relative size distributions of fine and ultrafine TiO_2 is unknown, additional exposure metrics may need to be characterized, including total metals analysis for titanium using ICP and/or filter-based sampling followed by off-line analysis using electron microscopy with energy dispersive X-ray analysis (see Section 5.2.2 and Table 5.1) to specifically measure and identify ultrafine TiO_2 particles. Once the percentage of TiO_2 (by particle size) has been determined from electron microscopy, adjustments can be made to the mass concentration to assess whether it complies with the NIOSH REL ultrafine TiO_2.

5.4 Summary

Nanotechnology is a rapidly growing area of scientific exploration that will continue to yield ENM with novel properties for commercial applications that impact virtually all facets of our daily life, including food, medicine, transportation, clothing, and shelter. As these novel materials are developed and put into commerce, workers will be the first to experience exposure to them and are at greatest initial risk for development of adverse health effects. There are many real-time and time-integrated techniques available to characterize various metrics of ENM exposure in occupational settings; a combination of both types of techniques is almost always necessary to discriminate an ENM of interest from incidental nanoparticles in workplace atmospheres. Laboratory toxicology studies often utilize commercially available ENMs that may not represent workplace exposure materials. Further, techniques used to characterize the physicochemical properties of study materials (surface area, surface chemistry, size, size distribution, etc.) often yield metrics that cannot be determined in workplaces with existing technology. Future efforts should be made to unify metrics across these disciplines.

References

1. International Organization for Standardization. (2008). Nanotechnologies: Terminology and Definitions for Nano-objects; Nanoparticle, Nanofibre and Nanoplate. Geneva, Switzerland, ISO/TS 27687:2008.

2. Schulte, P. A., Iavicoli, I., Rantanen, J. H., Dahmann, D., Iavicoli, S., Pipke, R., Guseva Canu, I., Boccuni, F., Ricci, M., Polci, M. L., Sabbioni, E., Pietroiusti, A., and Mantovani, E. (2016). Assessing the protection of the nanomaterial workforce. *Nanotoxicology*, **10**(7), 1013–1019.
3. Faunce, T., and Watal, A. (2010). Nanosilver and global public health: international regulatory issues. *Nanomedicine*, **5**, 617–632.
4. Hansen, S. F., Michelson, E. S., Kamper, A., Borling, P., Stuer-Lauridsen, F., and Baun, A. (2008). Categorization framework to aid exposure assessment of nanomaterials in consumer products. *Ecotoxicology*, **17**, 438–447.
5. Hendren, C. O., Mesnard, X., Dröge, J., and Wiesner, M. R. (2011). Estimating production data for five engineered nanomaterials as a basis for exposure assessment. *Environ. Sci. Technol.*, **45**, 2562–2569.
6. Lorenz, C., Tiede, K., Tear, S., Boxall, A., Von Goetz, N., and Hungerbühler, K. (2010). Imaging and characterization of engineered nanoparticles in sunscreens by electron microscopy, under wet and dry conditions. *Int. J. Occup. Environ. Health*, **16**, 406–428.
7. Meyer, D. E., Curran, M. A., and Gonzalez, M. A. (2009). An examination of existing data for the industrial manufacture and use of nanocomponents and their role in the life cycle impact of nanoproducts. *Environ. Sci. Technol.*, **43**, 1256–1263.
8. Bello, D., Hart, A. J., Ahn, K., Hallock, M., Yamamoto, N., Garcia, E. J., Ellenbecker, M. J., and Wardle, B. L. (2008). Particle exposure levels during CVD growth and subsequent handling of vertically-aligned carbon nanotube films. *Carbon*, **46**, 974–977.
9. Fleury, D., Bomfim, J. A. S., Vignes, A., Girard, C., Metz, S., Muñoz, F., R'mili, B., Ustache, A., Guiot, A., and Bouillard, J. X. (2013). Identification of the main exposure scenarios in the production of CNT-polymer nanocomposites by melt-moulding process. *J. Cleaner Prod.*, **53**, 22–36.
10. Bekker, C., Brouwer, D. H., Van Duuren-Stuurman, B., Tuinman, I. L., Tromp, P., and Fransman, W. (2014). Airborne manufactured nano-objects released from commercially available spray products: temporal and spatial influences. *J. Exposure Sci. Environ. Epidemiol.*, **24**, 74–81.
11. Nazarenko, Y., Han, T. W., Lioy, P. J., and Mainelis, G. (2011). Potential for exposure to engineered nanoparticles from nanotechnology-based consumer spray products. *J. Exposure Sci. Environ. Epidemiol.*, **21**, 515–528.
12. Quadros, M. E., and Marr, L. C. (2010). Environmental and human health risks of aerosolized silver nanoparticles. *J. Air Waste Manage. Assoc.*, **60**, 770–781.

13. Bello, D., Wardle, B. L., Yamamoto, N., Guzman Devilloria, R., Garcia, E. J., Hart, A. J., Ahn, K., Ellenbecker, M. J., and Hallock, M. (2009). Exposure to nanoscale particles and fibers during machining of hybrid advanced composites containing carbon nanotubes. *J. Nanopart. Res.*, **11**, 231–249.

14. Bello, D., Wardle, B. L., Zhang, J., Yamamoto, N., Santeufemio, C., Hallock, M., and Virji, M. A. (2010). Characterization of exposures to nanoscale particles and fibers during solid core drilling of hybrid carbon nanotube advanced composites. *Int. J. Occup. Environ. Health*, **16**, 434–450.

15. Cena, L. G., and Peters, T. M. (2011). Characterization and control of airborne particles emitted during production of epoxy/carbon nanotube nanocomposites. *J. Occup. Environ. Hyg.*, **8**, 86–92.

16. Giraldo, L. F., Brostow, W., Devaux, E., López, B. L., and Pérez, L. D. (2008). Scratch and wear resistance of polyamide 6 reinforced with multiwall carbon nanotubes. *J. Nanosci. Nanotech.*, **8**, 3176–3183.

17. Gläsel, H. J., Bauer, F., Ernst, H., Findeisen, M., Hartmann, E., Langguth, H., Mehnert, R., and Schubert, R. (2000). Preparation of scratch and abrasion resistant polymeric nanocomposites by monomer grafting onto nanoparticles, 2a: characterization of radiation-cured polymeric nanocomposites. *Macromol. Chem. Phys.*, **201**, 2765–2770.

18. Busquets-Fité, M., Fernandez, E., Janer, G., Vilar, G., Vázquez-Campos, S., Zanasca, R., Citterio, C., Mercante, L., and Puntes, V. (2013). Exploring release and recovery of nanomaterials from commercial polymeric nanocomposites. *J. Phys. Conf. Ser.*, **429**, 012048.

19. Beyer, G. (2002). Short communication: carbon nanotubes as flame retardants for polymers. *Fire Mater.*, **26**, 291–293.

20. Golanski, L., Gaborieau, A., Guiot, A., Uzu, G., Chatenet, J., and Tardif, F. (2011). Characterization of abrasion-induced nanoparticle release from paints into liquids and air. *J. Phys. Conf. Ser.*, **304**, 012062.

21. Derrough, S., Raffin, G., Locatelli, D., Nobile, P., and Durand, C. (2013). Behaviour of nanoparticles during high temperature treatment (incineration type). *J. Phys. Conf. Ser.*, **429**, 012047.

22. Sotiriou, G. A., Singh, D., Zhang, F., Wohlleben, W., Chalbot, M. C. G., Kavouras, I. G., and Demokritou, P. (2015). An integrated methodology for the assessment of environmental health implications during thermal decomposition of nano-enabled products. *Environ. Sci. Nano*, **2**, 262–272.

23. Hedmer, M., Ludvigsson, L., Isaxon, C., Nilsson, P. T., Skaug, V., Bohgard, M., Pagels, J. H., Messing, M. E., and Tinnerberg, H. (2014). Detection of

multi-walled carbon nanotubes and carbon nanodiscs on workplace surfaces at a small-scale producer. *Ann. Occup. Hyg.*, **59**, 836–852.

24. Platten, W. E., Sylvest, N., Warren, C., Arambewela, M., Harmon, S., Bradham, K., Rogers, K., Thomas, T., and Luxton, T. P. (2016). Estimating dermal transfer of copper particles from the surfaces of pressure-treated lumber and implications for exposure. *Sci. Total Environ.*, **548–549**, 441–449.
25. Stefaniak, A. B., Hackley, V. A., Roebben, G., Ehara, K., Hankin, S., Postek, M. T., Lynch, I., Fu, W. E., Linsinger, T. P., and Thunemann, A. F. (2013). Nanoscale reference materials for environmental, health and safety measurements: needs, gaps and opportunities. *Nanotoxicology*, **7**, 1325–1337.
26. Maynard, A. D., and Kuempel, E. D. (2005). Airborne nanostructured particles and occupational health. *J. Nanopart. Res.*, **7**, 587–614.
27. Morrow, P. E. (1988). Possible mechanisms to explain dust overloading of the lungs. *Fundam. Appl. Toxicol.*, **10**, 369–384.
28. Stefaniak, A. B., Hoover, M. D., Dickerson, R. M., Peterson, E. J., Day, G. A., Breysse, P. N., Kent, M. S., and Scripsick, R. C. (2003). Surface area of respirable beryllium metal, oxide, and copper alloy aerosols and implications for assessment of exposure risk of chronic beryllium disease. *Am. Ind. Hyg. Assoc. J.*, **64**, 297–305.
29. Brunner, T. J., Wick, P., Manser, P., Spohn, P., Grass, R. N., Limbach, L. K., Bruinink, A., and Stark, W. J. (2006). In vitro cytotoxicity of oxide nanoparticles: comparison to asbestos, silica, and the effect of particle solubility. *Environ. Sci. Technol.*, **40**, 4374–4381.
30. Warheit, D. B., and Donner, E. M. (2015). Risk assessment strategies for nanoscale and fine-sized titanium dioxide particles: recognizing hazard and exposure issues. *Food Chem. Toxicol.*, **85**, 138–147.
31. Addo Ntim, S., Thomas, T. A., Begley, T. H., and Noonan, G. O. (2015). Characterisation and potential migration of silver nanoparticles from commercially available polymeric food contact materials. *Food Addit. Contam. A*, **32**, 1003–1011.
32. Rizk, N., Christoforou, N., and Lee, S. (2016). Optimization of anti-cancer drugs and a targeting molecule on multifunctional gold nanoparticles. *Nanotechnology*, **27**, 185704.
33. Agiotis, L., Theodorakos, I., Samothrakitis, S., Papazoglou, S., Zergioti, I., and Raptis, Y. S. (2016). Magnetic manipulation of superparamagnetic nanoparticles in a microfluidic system for drug delivery applications. *J. Magn. Magn. Mater.*, **401**, 956–964.

34. Tulve, N. S., Stefaniak, A. B., Vance, M. E., Rogers, K., Mwilu, S., Lebouf, R. F., Schwegler-Berry, D., Willis, R., Thomas, T. A., and Marr, L. C. (2015). Characterization of silver nanoparticles in selected consumer products and its relevance for predicting children's potential exposures. *Int. J. Hyg. Environ. Health*, **218**, 345–357.

35. Larese-Filon, F., D'agostin, F., Crosera, M., Adami, G., Renzi, N., Bovenzi, M., and Maina, G. (2009). Human skin penetration of silver nanoparticles through intact and damaged skin. *Toxicology*, **255**, 33–37.

36. Larese Filon, F., Crosera, M., Timeus, E., Adami, G., Bovenzi, M., Ponti, J., and Maina, G. (2013). Human skin penetration of cobalt nanoparticles through intact and damaged skin. *Toxicol. in Vitro*, **27**, 121–127.

37. Brouwer, D. H., Gijsbers, J. H. J., and Lurvink, M. W. M. (2004). Personal exposure to ultrafine particles in the workplace: exploring sampling techniques and strategies. *Ann. Occup. Hyg.*, **48**, 439–453.

38. Kuhlbusch, T. A. J., Asbach, C., Fissan, H., Göhler, D., and Stintz, M. (2011). Nanoparticle exposure at nanotechnology workplaces: a review, *Part. Fibre Toxicol.*, **8**, 22.

39. Leskinen, J., Joutsensaari, J., Lyyränen, J., Koivisto, J., Ruusunen, J., Järvelä, M., Tuomi, T., Hämeri, K., Auvinen, A., and Jokiniemi, J. (2012). Comparison of nanoparticle measurement instruments for occupational health applications. *J. Nanopart. Res.*, **14**, 718.

40. Park, J., Kwak, B. K., Bae, E., Lee, J., Choi, K., Yi, J., and Kim, Y. (2009a). Exposure assessment of engineered nanomaterials in the workplace. *Kor. J. Chem. Eng.*, **26**, 1630–1636.

41. Brouwer, D., Berges, M., Virji, M. A., Fransman, W., Bello, D., Hodson, L., Gabriel, S., and Tielemans, E. (2012). Harmonization of measurement strategies for exposure to manufactured nano-objects: report of a workshop. *Ann. Occup. Hyg.*, **56**, 1–9.

42. Eastlake, A. C., Beaucham, C., Martinez, K. F., Dahm, M. M., Sparks, C., Hodson, L. L., and Geraci, C. L. (2016). Refinement of the nanoparticle emission assessment technique into the nanomaterial exposure assessment technique (NEAT 2.0). *J. Occup. Environ. Hyg.*, **13**(9), 708–717.

43. Evans, D. E., Ku, B. K., Birch, M. E., and Dunn, K. H. (2010). Aerosol monitoring during carbon nanofiber production: mobile direct-reading sampling. *Ann. Occup. Hyg.*, **54**, 514–531.

44. Ramachandran, G., Ostraat, M., Evans, D. E., Methner, M. M., O'shaughnessy, P., D'arcy, J., Geraci, C. L., Stevenson, E., Maynard, A., and

Rickabaugh, K. (2011). A strategy for assessing workplace exposures to nanomaterials. *J. Occup. Environ. Hyg.*, **8**, 673–685.

45. Diwakar, P. K., and Kulkarni, P. (2012). Measurement of elemental concentration of aerosols using spark emission spectroscopy. *J. Anal. At. Spectrom.*, **27**, 1101–1109.
46. Nilsson, P. T., Isaxon, C., Eriksson, A. C., Messing, M. E., Ludvigsson, L., Rissler, J., Hedmer, M., Tinnerberg, H., Gudmundsson, A., Deppert, K., Bohgard, M., and Pagels, J. H. (2013). Nano-objects emitted during maintenance of common particle generators: direct chemical characterization with aerosol mass spectrometry and implications for risk assessments. *J. Nanopart. Res.*, **15**, 2052.
47. Brouwer, D. H., Van Duuren-Stuurman, B., Berges, M., Bard, D., Jankowska, E., Moehlmann, C., Pelzer, J., and Mark, D. (2013). Workplace air measurements and likelihood of exposure to manufactured nano-objects, agglomerates, and aggregates. *J. Nanopart. Res.*, **15**, 2090.
48. Keller, A., Fierz, M., Siegmann, K., and Siegmann, H. C. (2001). Surface science with nanosized particles in a carrier gas. *J. Vac. Sci. Technol. A*, **19**, 1–8.
49. Marra, J., Voetz, M., and Kiesling, H. J. (2010). Monitor for detecting and assessing exposure to airborne nanoparticles. *J. Nanopart. Res.*, **12**, 21–37.
50. Van Broekhuizen, P., Van Broekhuizen, F., Cornelissen, R., and Reijnders, L. (2012). Workplace exposure to nanoparticles and the application of provisional nanoreference values in times of uncertain risks. *J. Nanopart. Res.*, **14**, 770.
51. Fierz, M., Houle, C., Steigmeier, P., and Burtscher, H. (2011). Design, calibration, and field performance of a miniature diffusion size classifier. *Aerosol Sci. Technol.*, **45**, 1–10.
52. Wang, Y. F., Tsai, P. J., Chen, C. W., Chen, D. R., and Hsu, D. J. (2010). Using a modified electrical aerosol detector to predict nanoparticle exposures to different regions of the respiratory tract for workers in a carbon black manufacturing industry. *Environ. Sci. Technol.*, **44**, 6767–6774.
53. Park, J. Y., Ramachandran, G., Raynor, P. C., and Olson Jr, G. M. (2010). Determination of particle concentration rankings by spatial mapping of particle surface area, number, and mass concentrations in a restaurant and a die casting plant. *J. Occup. Environ. Hyg.*, **7**, 466–476.
54. Cardello, N., Volckens, J., Tolocka, M. P., Wiener, R., and Buckley, T. J. (2002). Technical note: performance of a personal electrostatic precipitator particle sampler. *Aerosol Sci. Technol.*, **36**, 162–165.

55. Miller, A., Marinos, A., Wendel, C., King, G., and Bugarski, A. (2012). Design optimization of a portable thermophoretic precipitator nanoparticle sampler. *Aerosol Sci. Technol.*, **46**, 897–904.

56. Kuhlbusch, T. A. J., Neumann, S., and Fissan, H. (2004). Number size distribution, mass concentration, and particle composition of PM_1, $PM_{2.5}$, and PM_{10} in bag filling areas of carbon black production. *J. Occup. Environ. Hyg.*, **1**, 660–671.

57. Maynard, A. D., Baron, P. A., Foley, M., Shvedova, A. A., Kisin, E. R., and Castranova, V. (2004). Exposure to carbon nanotube material: aerosol release during the handling of unrefined single-walled carbon nanotube material. *J. Toxicol. Environ. Health A*, **67**, 87–107.

58. Oberdörster, G., Ferin, J., Gelein, R., Soderholm, S. C., and Finkelstein, J. (1992). Role of the alveolar macrophage in lung injury: studies with ultrafine particles. *Environ. Health Perspect.*, **97**, 193–199.

59. Oberdörster, G., Ferin, J., Soderholm, S., Gelein, R., Cox, C., Baggs, R., and Morrow, P. E. (1994). Increased pulmonary toxicity of inhaled ultrafine particles: due to lung overload alone?. *Ann. Occup. Hyg.*, **38**, 295–302.

60. Shang, Y., Dong, J., Inthavong, K., and Tu, J. (2015). Comparative numerical modeling of inhaled micron-sized particle deposition in human and rat nasal cavities. *Inhalation Toxicol.*, **27**, 694–705.

61. Weibel, A., Bouchet, R., Boulc'h, F., and Knauth, P. (2005). The big problem of small particles: a comparison of methods for determination of particle size in nanocrystalline anatase powders. *Chem. Mater.*, **17**, 2378–2385.

62. Lebouf, R. F., Ku, B. K., Chen, B. T., Frazer, D. G., Cumpston, J. L., and Stefaniak, A. B. (2011). Measuring surface area of airborne titanium dioxide powder agglomerates: relationships between gas adsorption, diffusion and mobility-based methods. *J. Nanopart. Res.*, **13**, 7029–7039.

63. Lynch, I., Cedervall, T., Lundqvist, M., Cabaleiro-Lago, C., Linse, S., and Dawson, K. A. (2007). The nanoparticle-protein complex as a biological entity; a complex fluids and surface science challenge for the 21st century. *Adv. Colloid Interface Sci.*, **134–135**, 167–174.

64. Shin, H. U., Stefaniak, A. B., Stojilovic, N., and Chase, G. G. (2015). Comparative dissolution of electrospun Al_2O_3 nanofibres in artificial human lung fluids. *Environ. Sci. Nano*, **2**, 251–261.

65. Pal, A. K., Watson, C. Y., Pirela, S. V., Singh, D., Chalbot, M. C. G., Kavouras, I., and Demokritou, P. (2015). Linking exposures of particles released from nano-enabled products to toxicology: an integrated methodology

for particle sampling, extraction, dispersion, and dosing. *Toxicol. Sci.*, **146**, 321–333.

66. Birch, M. E., Ku, B. K., Evans, D. E., and Ruda-Eberenz, T. A. (2011). Exposure and emissions monitoring during carbon nanofiber production. Part I: Elemental carbon and iron-soot aerosols. *Ann. Occup. Hyg.*, **55**, 1016–1036.
67. Methner, M. M., Birch, M. E., Evans, D. E., Ku, B. K., Crouch, K., and Hoover, M. D. (2007). Identification and characterization of potential sources of worker exposure to carbon nanofibers during polymer composite laboratory operations. *J. Occup. Environ. Hyg.*, **4**, D125–130.
68. NIOSH. (2013). Current intelligence bulleting 65: occupational exposure to carbon nanotubes and nanofibers. DHHS, Cincinnati, OH.
69. Ma-Hock, L., Treumann, S., Strauss, V., Brill, S., Luizi, F., Mertler, M., Wiench, K., Gamer, A. O., Van Ravenzwaay, B., and Landsiedel, R. (2009). Inhalation toxicity of multiwall carbon nanotubes in rats exposed for 3 months. *Toxicol. Sci.*, **112**, 468–481.
70. Pauluhn, J. (2009). Subchronic 13-week inhalation exposure of rats to multiwalled carbon nanotubes: toxic effects are determined by density of agglomerate structures, not fibrillar structures. *Toxicol. Sci.*, **113**, 226–242.
71. Pauluhn, J. (2010). Multi-walled carbon nanotubes (Baytubes®): approach for derivation of occupational exposure limit. *Regul. Toxicol. Pharm.*, **57**, 78–89.
72. Pauluhn, J. (2014). The metrics of MWCNT-induced pulmonary inflammation are dependent on the selected testing regimen. *Regul. Toxicol. Pharm.*, **68**, 343–352.
73. Lowell, S., Shields, J., Thomas, M., and Thommes, M. (2004). *Characterization of Porous Solids and Powders: Surface Area, Pore Size and Density* (Kluwer Academic, Dordrecht, the Netherlands).
74. Ku, B. K., and Kulkarni, P. (2015). Measurement of transport properties of aerosolized nanomaterials. *J. Aerosol Sci.*, **90**, 169–181.
75. Warheit, D. B. (2013). How to measure hazards/risks following exposures to nanoscale or pigment-grade titanium dioxide particles. *Toxicol. Lett.*, **220**, 193–204.
76. NIOSH. (2011). Current intelligence bulletin 63: occupational exposure to titanium dioxide. DHHS, Cincinnati, OH.
77. Gamo, M. (2011). Risk assessment of manufactured nanomaterials: titanium dioxide (TiO_2). Institute of Advanced Industrial Science and Technology, Tsukuba, Japan.

78. Nakanishi, J. (2011). Risk assessment of manufactured nanomaterials: "approaches" - overview of approaches and results. National Institute of Advanced Industrial Science, Tsukuba, Japan.

79. JSFOH. (2013). Recommendation of occupational exposure limits (2013–2014). *J. Occup. Health*, **55**, 422–441.

80. MAK. (2015). *List of MAK and BAT Values 2015* (Wiley-VCH Bonn, Germany).

81. Aschberger, K., Micheletti, C., Sokull-Klüttgen, B., and Christensen, F. M. (2011). Analysis of currently available data for characterising the risk of engineered nanomaterials to the environment and human health: lessons learned from four case studies. *Environ. Int.*, **37**, 1143–1156.

82. Jiang, J., Oberdörster, G., Elder, A., Gelein, R., Mercer, P., and Biswas, P. (2008). Does nanoparticle activity depend upon size and crystal phase?. *Nanotoxicology*, **2**, 33–42.

83. Lee, J. H., Kwon, M., Ji, J. H., Kang, C. S., Ahn, K. H., Han, J. H., and Yu, I. J. (2011). Exposure assessment of workplaces manufacturing nanosized TiO_2 and silver. *Inhalation Toxicol.*, **23**, 226–236.

84. Lee, J. H., Mun, J., Park, J. D., and Yu, I. J. (2012b). A health surveillance case study on workers who manufacture silver nanomaterials. *Nanotoxicology*, **6**, 667–669.

85. Park, J., Kwak, B. K., Bae, E., Lee, J., Kim, Y., Choi, K., and Yi, J. (2009b). Characterization of exposure to silver nanoparticles in a manufacturing facility. *J. Nanopart. Res.*, **11**, 1705–1712.

86. Tsai, S.-J., Ada, E., Isaacs, J. A., and Ellenbecker, M. J. (2009a). Airborne nanoparticle exposures associated with the manual handling of nanoalumina and nanosilver in fume hoods. *J. Nanopart. Res.*, **11**, 147–161.

87. Lee, J. H., Ahn, K., Kim, S. M., Jeon, K. S., Lee, J. S., and Yu, I. J. (2012a). Continuous 3-day exposure assessment of workplace manufacturing silver nanoparticles. *J. Nanopart. Res.*, **14**, 1134.

88. Methner, M. M. (2008). Engineering case reports. Effectiveness of local exhaust ventilation (LEV) in controlling engineered nanomaterial emissions during reactor cleanout operations. *J. Occup. Environ. Hyg.*, **5**, D63–69.

89. Methner, M., Hodson, L., Dames, A., and Geraci, C. (2010). Nanoparticle emission assessment technique (NEAT) for the identification and measurement of potential inhalation exposure to engineered nanomaterials--Part B: Results from 12 field studies. *J. Occup. Environ. Hyg.*, **7**, 163–176.

90. Methner, M. M. (2010). Effectiveness of a custom-fitted flange and local exhaust ventilation (LEV) system in controlling the release of nanoscale metal oxide particulates during reactor cleanout operations. *Int. J. Occup. Environ. Health*, **16**, 475–487.

91. Artous, S., Zimmermann, E., Douissard, P. A., Locatelli, D., Motellier, S., and Derrough, S. (2015). Strategy for the lowering and the assessment of exposure to nanoparticles at workspace: case of study concerning the potential emission of nanoparticles of lead in an epitaxy laboratory. *J. Phys. Conf. Ser.*, **617**, 012007.

92. Seipenbusch, M., Binder, A., and Kasper, G. (2008). Temporal evolution of nanoparticle aerosols in workplace exposure. *Ann. Occup. Hyg.*, **52**, 707–716.

93. Demou, E., Peter, P., and Hellweg, S. (2008). Exposure to manufactured nanostructured particles in an industrial pilot plant. *Ann. Occup. Hyg.*, **52**, 695–706.

94. Ham, S., Yoon, C., Lee, E., Lee, K., Park, D., Chung, E., Kim, P., and Lee, B. (2012). Task-based exposure assessment of nanoparticles in the workplace. *J. Nanopart. Res.*, **14**, 1126.

95. Tsai, S.-J., Ashter, A., Ada, E., Mead, J. L., Barry, C. F., and Ellenbecker, M. J. (2008a). Airborne nanoparticle release associated with the compounding of nanocomposites using nanoalumina as fillers. *Aerosol Air Qual. Res.*, **8**, 160–177.

96. Tsai, S.-J., Ashter, A., Ada, E., Mead, J. L., Barry, C. F., and Ellenbecker, M. J. (2008b). Control of airborne nanoparticles release during compounding of polymer nanocomposites. *Nano*, **3**, 301–309.

97. Ashter, A., Tsai, S. J., Lee, J. S., Ellenbecker, M. J., Mead, J. L., and Barry, C. F. (2010). Effects of nanoparticle feed location during nanocomposite compounding. *Polym. Eng. Sci.*, **50**, 154–164.

98. Tsai, S.-J., Huang, R. F., and Ellenbecker, M. J. (2010). Airborne nanoparticle exposures while using constant-flow, constant-velocity, and air-curtain-isolated fume hoods. *Ann. Occup. Hyg.*, **54**, 78–87.

99. Tsai, C. S. J., White, D., Rodriguez, H., Munoz, C. E., Huang, C. Y., Tsai, C. J., Barry, C., and Ellenbecker, M. J. (2012). Exposure assessment and engineering control strategies for airborne nanoparticles: an application to emissions from nanocomposite compounding processes. *J. Nanopart. Res.*, **14**, 989.

100. Dunn, K. H., Tsai, C. S. J., Woskie, S. R., Bennett, J. S., Garcia, A., and Ellenbecker, M. J. (2014). Evaluation of leakage from fume hoods using tracer gas, tracer nanoparticles and nanopowder handling test methodologies. *J. Occup. Environ. Hyg.*, **11**, D164–D173.

101. Xing, M., Zou, H., Gao, X., Chang, B., Tang, S., and Zhang, M. (2015). Workplace exposure to airborne alumina nanoparticles associated with separation and packaging processes in a pilot factory. *Environ. Sci. Process. Impacts*, **17**, 656–666.

102. Kaminski, H., Beyer, M., Fissan, H., Asbach, C., and Kuhlbusch, T. (2015). Measurements of nanoscale TiO_2 and Al_2O_3 in industrial workplace environments – methodology and results. *Aerosol Air Qual. Res.*, **15**, 129–141.

103. Zou, H., Zhang, Q., Xing, M., Gao, X., Zhou, L., Tollerud, D. J., Tang, S., and Zhang, M. (2015). Relationships between number, surface area, and mass concentrations of different nanoparticles in workplaces. *Environ. Sci. Process. Impacts*, **17**, 1470–1481.

104. Zhao, P., Tang, S. C., Liu, J. M., Wang, Y. Q., and Yu, Z. (2014a). Occupational exposure assessment of $CaCO_3$ nanoparticles using a multi-metrics approach. *Adv. Mater. Res.*, **886**, 271–274.

105. Zhao, P., Tang, S. C., Wang, Y. Q., Yu, Z., and Liu, J. M. (2014b). Exposure assessment of nano-$CaCO_3$ manufacturing workplaces. *Adv. Mater. Res.*, **850–851**, 38–44.

106. Walser, T., Hellweg, S., Juraske, R., Luechinger, N. A., Wang, J., and Fierz, M. (2012). Exposure to engineered nanoparticles: model and measurements for accident situations in laboratories. *Sci. Total Environ.*, **420**, 119–126.

107. Tsai, C.-J., Huang, C.-Y., Chen, S.-C., Ho, C.-E., Huang, C.-H., Chen, C.-W., Chang, C.-P., Tsai, S.-J., and Ellenbecker, M. J. (2011). Exposure assessment of nano-sized and respirable particles at different workplaces. *J. Nanopart. Res.*, **13**, 4161–4172.

108. Leppanen, M., Lyyranen, J., Jarvela, M., Auvinen, A., Jokiniemi, J., Pimenoff, J., and Tuomi, T. (2012). Exposure to CeO_2 nanoparticles during flame spray process. *Nanotoxicology*, **6**, 643–651.

109. Pelclova, D., Zdimal, V., Kacer, P., Fenclova, Z., Vlckova, S., Syslova, K., Navratil, T., Schwarz, J., Zikova, N., Barosova, H., Turci, F., Komarc, M., Pelcl, T., Belacek, J., Kukutschova, J., and Zakharov, S. (2016). Oxidative stress markers are elevated in exhaled breath condensate of workers exposed to nanoparticles during iron oxide pigment production. *J. Breath Res.*, **10**, 016004.

110. Möhlmann, C., Welter, J., Klenke, M., and Sander, J. (2009). Workplace exposure at nanomaterial production processes. *J. Phys. Conf. Ser.*, **170**, 012004.

111. Kim, B., Kim, H., and Yu, I. J. (2014). Assessment of nanoparticle exposure in nanosilica handling process: including characteristics of nanoparticles leaking from a vacuum cleaner. *Ind. Health*, **52**, 152–162.

112. Oh, S., Kim, B., and Kim, H. (2014). Comparison of nanoparticle exposures between fumed and sol-gel nano-silica manufacturing facilities. *Ind. Health*, **52**, 190–198.

113. Choi, K. M., and An, H. C. (2016). Characterization and exposure measurement for indium oxide nanofibers generated as byproducts in the LED manufacturing environment. *J. Occup. Environ. Hyg.*, **13**, D23–D30.

114. Peters, T. M., Elzey, S., Johnson, R., Park, H., Grassian, V. H., Maher, T., and O'shaughnessy, P. (2009). Airborne monitoring to distinguish engineered nanomaterials from incidental particles for environmental health and safety. *J. Occup. Environ. Hyg.*, **6**, 73–81.

115. Sahu, M., and Biswas, P. (2011). Single-step processing of copper-doped titania nanomaterials in a flame aerosol reactor. *Nanoscale Res. Lett.*, **6**, 1–14.

116. Plitzko, S. (2009). Workplace exposure to engineered nanoparticles. *Inhalation Toxicol.*, **21**(Suppl 1), 25–29.

117. Dylla, H., and Hassan, M. M. (2012). Characterization of nanoparticles released during construction of photocatalytic pavements using engineered nanoparticles. *J. Nanopart. Res.*, **14**, 825.

118. Koivisto, A. J., Lyyränen, J., Auvinen, A., Vanhala, E., Hämeri, K., Tuomi, T., and Jokiniemi, J. (2012). Industrial worker exposure to airborne particles during the packing of pigment and nanoscale titanium dioxide. *Inhalation Toxicol.*, **24**, 839–849.

119. Vaquero, C., Gelarza, N., De Ipiña, J. L. L., Gutierrez-Cañas, C., Múgica, I., Aragón, G., Jaen, M., Pina, R., Larraza, I., Esteban-Cubillo, A., Thompson, D., and Pui, D. Y. H. (2015). Occupational exposure to nano-TiO_2 in the life cycle steps of new depollutant mortars used in construction. *J. Phys. Conf. Ser.*, **617**, 012006.

120. Yang, Y., Mao, P., Xu, C. L., Chen, S. W., Zhang, J. H., and Wang, Z. P. (2011). Distribution characteristics of nano-TiO_2 aerosol in the workplace. *Aerosol Air Qual. Res.*, **11**, 466–472.

121. Yang, Y., Mao, P., Wang, Z. P., and Zhang, J. H. (2012). Distribution of nanoparticle number concentrations at a nano-TiO_2 plant. *Aerosol Air Qual. Res.*, **12**, 934–940.

122. López De Ipiña J. M., Vaquero, C., Gutierrez-Cañas, C., and Pui, D. Y. H. (2015). Analysis of multivariate stochastic signals sampled by on-

line particle analyzers: application to the quantitative assessment of occupational exposure to NOAA in multisource industrial scenarios (MSIS). *J. Phys. Conf. Ser.*, **617**, 012003.

123. Pelclova, D., Barosova, H., Kukutschova, J., Zdimal, V., Navratil, T., Fenclova, Z., Vlckova, S., Schwarz, J., Zikova, N., Kacer, P., Komarc, M., Belacek, J., and Zakharov, S. (2015). Raman microspectroscopy of exhaled breath condensate and urine in workers exposed to fine and nano TiO_2 particles: a cross-sectional study. *J. Breath Res.*, **9**, 036008.

124. Huang, C. H., Tai, C. Y., Huang, C. Y., Tsai, C. J., Chen, C. W., Chang, C. P., and Shih, T. S. (2010). Measurements of respirable dust and nanoparticle concentrations in a titanium dioxide pigment production factory. *J. Environ. Sci. Health. A*, **45**, 1227–1233.

125. Ichihara, S., Li, W., Omura, S., Fujitani, Y., Liu, Y., Wang, Q., Hiraku, Y., Hisanaga, N., Wakai, K., Ding, X., Kobayashi, T., and Ichihara, G. (2016). Exposure assessment and heart rate variability monitoring in workers handling titanium dioxide particles: a pilot study. *J. Nanopart. Res.*, **18**, 1–14.

126. Demou, E., Stark, W. J., and Hellweg, S. (2009). Particle emission and exposure during nanoparticle synthesis in research laboratories. *Ann. Occup. Hyg.*, **53**, 829–838.

127. Ogura, I., Sakurai, H., and Gamo, M. (2011a). Onsite aerosol measurements for various engineered nanomaterials at industrial manufacturing plants. *J. Phys. Conf. Ser.*, **304**, 012004.

128. Curwin, B., and Bertke, S. (2011). Exposure characterization of metal oxide nanoparticles in the workplace. *J. Occup. Environ. Hyg.*, **8**, 580–587.

129. Zimmermann, E., Derrough, S., Locatelli, D., Durand, C., Fromaget, J. L., Lefranc, E., Ravanel, X., and Garrione, J. (2012). Results of potential exposure assessments during the maintenance and cleanout of deposition equipment. *J. Nanopart. Res.*, **14**, 1209.

130. Shepard, M. N., and Brenner, S. (2014). An occupational exposure assessment for engineered nanoparticles used in semiconductor fabrication. *Ann. Occup. Hyg.*, **58**, 251–265.

131. Bekker, C., Kuijpers, E., Brouwer, D. H., Vermeulen, R., and Fransman, W. (2015). Occupational exposure to nano-objects and their agglomerates and aggregates across various life cycle stages: a broad-scale exposure study. *Ann. Occup. Hyg.*, **59**, 681–704.

132. Brenner, S. A., Neu-Baker, N. M., Caglayan, C., and Zurbenko, I. G. (2015). Occupational exposure to airborne nanomaterials: an assessment of worker exposure to aerosolized metal oxide nanoparticles in

semiconductor wastewater treatment. *J. Occup. Environ. Hyg.*, **12**, 469–481.

133. Jankovic, J. T., Hollenbeck, S. M., and Zontek, T. L. (2010). Ambient air sampling during quantum-dot spray deposition. *Int. J. Occup. Environ. Health*, **16**, 388–398.

134. Raynor, P. C., Cebula, J. I., Spangenberger, J. S., Olson, B. A., Dasch, J. M., and D'arcy, J. B. (2012). Assessing potential nanoparticle release during nanocomposite shredding using direct-reading instruments. *J. Occup. Environ. Hyg.*, **9**, 1–13.

135. Fujitani, Y., Kobayashi, T., Arashidani, K., Kunugita, N., and Suemura, K. (2008). Measurement of the physical properties of aerosols in a fullerene factory for inhalation exposure assessment. *J. Occup. Environ. Hyg.*, **5**, 380–389.

136. Yeganeh, B., Kull, C. M., Hull, M. S., and Marr, L. C. (2008). Characterization of airborne particles during production of carbonaceous nanomaterials. *Environ. Sci. Technol.*, **42**, 4600–4606.

137. Johnson, D. R., Methner, M. M., Kennedy, A. J., and Steevens, J. A. (2010). Potential for occupational exposure to engineered carbon-based nanomaterials in environmental laboratory studies. *Environ. Health Perspect.*, **118**, 49–54.

138. Kuhlbusch, T. A. J., and Fissan, H. (2006). Particle characteristics in the reactor and pelletizing areas of carbon black production. *J. Occup. Environ. Hyg.*, **3**, 558–567.

139. Vartiainen, J., Pohler, T., Sirola, K., Pylkkanen, L., Alenius, H., Hokkinen, J., Tapper, U., Lahtinen, P., Kapanen, A., Putkisto, K., Hiekkataipale, P., Eronen, P., Ruokolainen, J., and Laukkanen, A. (2011). Health and environmental safety aspects of friction grinding and spray drying of microfibrillated cellulose. *Cellulose*, **18**, 775–786.

140. Martinez, K. F., Eastlak, A., Rudie, A., and Geraci, C. (2013). Occupational exposure characterization during the manufacture of cellulose nanomaterials, In: Postek, M., Moon, R. J., Rudie, A. W., and Bilodeau, M. A. (eds.), *Production and Applications of Cellulose Nanomaterials* (TAPPI Press, Peachtree Corners, GA), pp. 61–64.

141. Methner, M., Crawford, C., and Geraci, C. (2012b). Evaluation of the potential airborne release of carbon nanofibers during the preparation, grinding, and cutting of epoxy-based nanocomposite material. *J. Occup. Environ. Hyg.*, **9**, 308–318.

142. Dahm, M. M., Evans, D. E., Schubauer-Berigan, M. K., Birch, M. E., and Fernback, J. E. (2012). Occupational exposure assessment in carbon

nanotube and nanofiber primary and secondary manufacturers. *Ann. Occup. Hyg.*, **56**, 542–556.

143. Dahm, M. M., Evans, D. E., Schubauer-Berigan, M. K., Birch, M. E., and Deddens, J. A. (2013). Occupational exposure assessment in carbon nanotube and nanofiber primary and secondary manufacturers: mobile direct-reading sampling. *Ann. Occup. Hyg.*, **57**, 328–344.

144. Dahm, M. M., Schubauer-Berigan, M. K., Evans, D. E., Birch, M. E., Fernback, J. E., and Deddens, J. A. (2015). Carbon nanotube and nanofiber exposure assessments: an analysis of 14 site visits. *Ann. Occup. Hyg.*, **59**, 705–723.

145. Methner, M., Beaucham, C., Crawford, C., Hodson, L., and Geraci, C. (2012a). Field application of the nanoparticle emission assessment technique (NEAT): task-based air monitoring during the processing of engineered nanomaterials (ENM) at four facilities. *J. Occup. Environ. Hyg.*, **9**, 543–555.

146. Lo, L.-M., Tsai, C.-J., Dunn, K., Hammond, D., Marlow, D., Topmiller, J., and Ellenbecker, M. J. (2015). Performance of particulate containment at nanotechnology workplaces. *J. Nanopart. Res.*, **17**, 435.

147. Heitbrink, W. A., Lo, L. M., and Dunn, K. H. (2015). Exposure controls for nanomaterials at three manufacturing sites. *J. Occup. Environ. Hyg.*, **12**, 16–28.

148. Han, J. H., Lee, E. J., Lee, J. H., So, K. P., Lee, Y. H., Bae, G. N., Lee, S.-B., Ji, J. H., Cho, M. H., and Yu, I. J. (2008). Monitoring multiwalled carbon nanotube exposure in carbon nanotube research facility. *Inhalation Toxicol.*, **20**, 741–749.

149. Lee, J. H., Lee, S.-B., Bae, G. N., Jeon, K. S., Yoon, J. U., Ji, J. H., Sung, J. H., Lee, B. G., Lee, J. H., Yang, J. S., Kim, H. Y., Kang, C. S., and Yu, I. J. (2010). Exposure assessment of carbon nanotube manufacturing workplaces. *Inhalation Toxicol.*, **22**, 369–381.

150. R'mili, B., Dutouquet, C., Sirven, J., Aguerre-Chariol, O., and Frejafon, E. (2011). Analysis of particle release using LIBS (laser-induced breakdown spectroscopy) and TEM (transmission electron microscopy) samplers when handling CNT (carbon nanotube) powders. *J. Nanopart. Res.*, **13**, 563–577.

151. Takaya, M., Ono-Ogasawara, M., Shinohara, Y., Kubota, H., Tsuruoka, S., and Koda, S. (2012). Evaluation of exposure risk in the weaving process of MWCNT-coated yarn with real-time particle concentration measurements and characterization of dust measurements. *Ind. Health*, **50**, 147–155.

152. Ono-Ogasawara, M., Takaya, M., Kubota, H., Shinohara, Y., Koda, S., Akiba, E., Tsuruoka, S., and Myojo, T. (2013). Approach to the exposure assessment of MWCNT by considering size distribution and oxidation temperature of elemental carbon. *J. Phys. Conf. Ser.*, **429**, 012004.

153. Lee, J., Choi, Y., Shin, J., Lee, J., Lee, Y., Park, S., Baek, J., Park, J., Ahn, K., and Yu, I. J. (2015). Health surveillance study of workers who manufacture multi-walled carbon nanotubes. *Nanotoxicology*, **9**, 802–811.

154. Tsai, C.-J., Hofmann, M., Hallock, M., Ellenbecker, M. J., and Kong, J. (2015). Assessment of exhaust emissions from carbon nanotube production and particle collection by sampling filters. *J. Air Waste Manage. Assoc.*, **65**, 1376–1385.

155. Tsai, S.-J., Hofmann, M., Hallock, M., Ada, E., Kong, J., and Ellenbecker, M. (2009b). Characterization and evaluation of nanoparticle release during the synthesis of single-walled and multiwalled carbon nanotubes by chemical vapor deposition. *Environ. Sci. Technol.*, **43**, 6017–6023.

156. Ogura, I., Sakurai, H., Mizuno, K., and Gamo, M. (2011b). Release potential of single-wall carbon nanotubes produced by super-growth method during manufacturing and handling. *J. Nanopart. Res.*, **13**, 1265–1280.

157. Ogura, I., Kotake, M., Hashimoto, N., Gotoh, K., and Kishimoto, A. (2013). Release characteristics of single-wall carbon nanotubes during manufacturing and handling. *J. Phys. Conf. Ser.*, **429**, 012057.

158. Manodori, L., and Benedetti, A. (2009). Nanoparticles monitoring in workplaces devoted to nanotechnologies. *J. Phys. Conf. Ser.*, **170**, 012001.

Chapter 6

Physicochemical Properties and Their Importance in the Environment: Current Trends in Nanomaterial Exposure

Justin M. Kidd and Paul Westerhoff

School of Sustainable Engineering and the Built Environment, Arizona State University, Tempe, Arizona 85287-3005, USA

Justin.Kidd@asu.edu, P.Westerhoff@asu.edu

The rapid advances in engineered nanomaterial synthesis and manufacturing, combined with their use and eventual disposal, have resulted in the release of nanomaterials into the environment. The objectives of this chapter are to provide a review of the state of science surrounding nanomaterial exposure, explore the methods and data available for nanomaterial releases from products across their life cycle, consider what tools are used to detect and quantify nanomaterial exposure, discuss future steps to understand nanomaterial exposure, and summarize critical data gaps and methods that could advance nanomaterial exposure analysis in the environment.

Physicochemical Properties of Nanomaterials
Edited by Richard C. Pleus and Vladimir Murashov

ISBN 978-981-4774-80-2 (Hardcover), 978-1-351-16860-1 (eBook)
www.panstanford.com

6.1 Introduction

Engineered nanomaterials (ENMs) are used in a wide range of applications, including healthcare, energy, agriculture, and personal care products. Projections for both the range and the volume of ENM applications show continuous exponential growth. This rapid growth in the manufacturing of nanomaterial-based technologies, combined with their commercial and individual use, has resulted in the release of nanomaterials into the environment from multiple pathways. Point source emissions, such as those from industrial systems or from urban wastewater treatment plants, emit ENMs to air, water, and soil. Diffuse source emissions (throughout the product life cycle) also release ENMs into the environment during synthesis, manufacturing, use, recycling, and end of life. These releases and their dilution in the environment can lead to human and ecosystem exposures.

There are various ENM physicochemical properties that have implications on these exposure pathways. One particular challenging issue is that multiple forms of the same ENM manufactured, even of the same chemistry, can have different unique properties. For example, quantum dots are semiconducting ENMs commonly used in transistors and light-emitting diodes (LEDs). The alteration in particle diameter by even 1 nm, even with the same metal core, surface chemistry, and shape, can alter its optoelectronic properties such that it emits a unique photoluminescence [1]. This variation creates challenges in regulating nanomaterials. A second challenge is that ENMs undergo biogeochemical transformations and association with surfaces, including sediment and suspended particulate matter [2]. Tracking transformations of ENMs is analytically very difficult in environmental systems. ENM surface properties determine their transformation and aggregation behavior, thus influencing their mobility, interaction with, and bioavailability to organisms.

Models developed for chemical fate and transport (F&T) may not be appropriate for ENMs; however, such models are crucial to develop in order to describe the state of ENMs in the environment. A major obstacle has been uncertainty as to which exposure metric is most suited to ENMs: mass concentration, size distribution, shape, surface versus core composition, etc. The ENM material properties differ to those generated for bulk chemical substances, which have relatively few surface ions relative to its bulk density [3–5]. Significant advances in how to use exposure data in risk assessment ENM models remain ill-defined.

This chapter first provides a general review of the state of science in nanomaterial exposure, specifically on the current trends in ENM exposure, dosimetry challenges, and concentration levels of concern. Second, we explore the methods and data available for ENM releases from products across their life cycle, explicitly the diversity of ENMs and their transformations in the environment. Third, we consider what tools are used to detect and quantify ENM exposures, while also highlighting ENM sample preparation challenges. Fourth, we discuss data streams and their role in taking future steps to understand ENM exposure. Finally, we summarize critical data gaps and methods that could advance ENM exposure analysis in the environment.

6.2 The State of Science in Nanomaterial Exposure

6.2.1 Nanoparticle Nomenclature

The common definition of "nanomaterial" loosely revolves around structures that are less than 100 nm in at least one of their dimensions, while also exhibiting unique properties. Over the past decade, there have been numerous attempts at developing a universal definition for nanomaterials, but regulatory groups have been giving unique definitions to different entities that manufacture and use nanomaterials in their products [6, 7]. For instance, the European Union (EU) regulations surrounding nano-enhanced products have at least three times given a unique definition for nanomaterials used in three different products. In 2009, the EU's regulation on cosmetics required nanomaterials to be insoluble or biopersistent and intentionally manufactured. In 2011, its regulation on food labeling required nanomaterials to be intentionally manufactured but also to be less than 100 nm in one dimension. In 2012, its regulation on biocidal products required nanomaterials to be natural or manufactured and required that at least half of these nanomaterials must have one or more dimensions less than 100 nm. This lack of a sound definition is problematic moving forward, as the majority of the public is unaware of what nanomaterials really are. This uncertainty means that the state of science surrounding nanomaterials is still at an infant phase and will need refinement in order to address the concerns surrounding its further development.

6.2.2 Nanomaterial Manufacturing

There are two approaches for the manufacturing of nanomaterials: the top-down approach and the bottom-up approach [8, 9]. The top-down approach involves the breakdown of bulk materials to generate nanostructures from them. This is a common method when manufacturing interconnected and integrated structures (i.e., electronic circuitry). Synthesis techniques include solid-phase techniques like mechanical attrition through either milling or mechanochemical processing. The bottom-up approach utilizes atoms and molecules to assemble larger nanostructures. This method allows for precise reproducibility of simple, identical nanostructures. Synthesis techniques include vapor-phase techniques like flame pyrolysis, molecular condensation, arc discharge generation, laser ablation, plasma, and chemical vapor deposition. Liquid-phase techniques include sol–gel, solvothermal methods, and sonochemical methods.

6.2.3 Nanomaterial Release from Industry

The physicochemical properties of nanomaterials allow for them to have transformative benefits to individuals and society through applications including but not limited to enhanced food products, improved energy storage, antimicrobial fabrics, and water purification. Estimations for the value of the engineered nanotechnology sector range in the hundreds of billions of dollars [10–12]. As nanomaterial manufacturing continues to rise, it is imperative to understand how nanomaterial properties can enhance release potential. The presence of ENMs in the environment is thought to occur from the increase in production of nanomaterials of all natures, thus increasing the potential for their release and subsequent effects on ecosystem health [13]. Potential releases of ENMs, shown in Table 6.1, can come from a variety of release scenarios, including release during production, manufacturing, and use of products.

Table 6.1 Products and applications shown to cause direct or indirect release of ENMs into the environment

Type of release	Example products/applications	Likely mode of release	Ref.
Direct	Nano-aerosols	Inhalation	[14]
	Food additives	Digestion	[15]
	Nanopaint	Weathering	[16]
Indirect	Nanosunscreens	Application to skin	[17]
	Automotive fuel	Combustion	[18]
	Nanotextiles	Abrasion/washing	[19]

6.2.4 Natural Sources of Nanomaterials

There are many physical, chemical, and biological processes that occur naturally and form nanomaterial byproducts. These can include volcanic ash, ocean spray, fine dust and sand, erosion, and biological matter. These are diverse nanomaterials that can rival their synthetically engineered counterparts and are found in soil, aquatic, and atmospheric systems. The most abundant nanomaterials in soil systems are layer silicate nanoclays, metals, and metal hydroxides [20]. Nanoclays are formed by three unique abiotic weathering processes. Microorganisms can form metal nanostructures due to their negatively charged peptidoglycan cell wall and their high surface-area-to-volume ratio. Cationic metals accumulate along their surface and combine with anions in the surrounding media, resulting in nanoscale mineral formations [21].

Nanomaterial distribution in various aquatic environments is influenced by the hydrodynamic and morphological characteristics of rivers and coastal zones [22]. A common occurrence of nanomaterials in aquatic systems results from the increase in temperature and evaporation over water bodies. Increases in water temperature reduce the solubility of mineral basins, causing the formation and precipitation of nanomaterials and their eventual release as sea salt aerosols [23]. Natural organic matter (NOM) in surface waters can interact with metal salts or ions via photochemical-generated reactive oxygen species (ROS), causing the formation of metal-based nanomaterials [24–26]. Metal ions and sulfur in the ocean can be emitted by hydrothermal vents on the ocean floor, where they react with each other and form metal-bearing sulfide nanomaterials [25].

Nanomaterials in the atmosphere may be present by either primary emission (direct release from source) or secondary emission (atmospheric reactions). Over half of atmosphere-produced nanomaterials come from terrestrial dust storms [27–29]. These nanomaterials are lifted into the atmosphere via air currents and distributed globally through dust migration across the continents, demonstrating the reach and influence of environmental nanomaterials. Forest fires can also spread ash and smoke over thousands of miles, increasing nanoparticulate matter in the atmosphere. Volcanoes are another source for naturally occurring atmospheric nanoparticles. Volcanic eruptions throw basaltic lava into the atmosphere, which is rich in magnesium and iron nanoparticles. As the ash spreads into the atmosphere, the gas temperature lowers, leading to the accumulation and deposition of nanoparticles into clusters due to electrostatic forces of attraction [30]. Nanoparticles in the atmosphere may linger there for years or accumulate, decompose, or react to enter food chains. A major challenge is detecting the amount and characteristics of what may be relatively small amounts of engineered ENMs within this group of natural ENMs.

6.2.4.1 The methods and data available for releases from products across the life cycle

6.2.4.1.1 *Nanomaterial concentration levels of concern in the environment*

Identification of nanomaterial waste streams often relies on use patterns, estimates of manufacturing volumes, and laboratory models. Measurement methods and instrumentation are nonspecific, making it difficult to differentiate between naturally occurring and engineered particles. Detecting nanoparticles is complex, both in gases and in liquids. Nanomaterials are so small that they cannot be detected by optical microscopes. Chemical analysis of individual nanomaterials in gases and liquids has been limited because of their low mass. Only recently have analytical instruments and methods become available for this purpose, and as a result, nanomaterials as small as 1 nm can be detected [31, 32]. While the instruments used are not themselves size selective, they can be coupled with other instruments covering specific size ranges. Table 6.2 highlights the current methods and their subsequent generalized detection limits for an array of different nanomaterial natures.

Table 6.2 Common detection methods and analytical tools used for engineered nanomaterials. Detection limits for each analytical tool are given

Method	Nanomaterial type	Generalized detection limit comments
Light scattering (UV-Vis)	Any	>1 mg/L in water 0.05 mg/L with HPLC of nanomaterial extract
ICP-MS TOF-MS (emerging)	Metals	>10 ppt in water (total metal concentration)
LC-MS	C_{60}	~1 ppt
Thermal combustion or microwave thermal analysis	MWCNT and SWCNT	~1 ppb
Isotopes	^{13}C metal isotopes	<1 ppb by scintillation counting isotopic ratios

UV-Vis, ultraviolet-visible; ICP-MS, inductively coupled plasma mass spectrometry; TOF-MS, time-of-flight mass spectrometry; LC-MS, liquid chromatography–mass spectrometry; MWCNT, multiwalled carbon nanotube; SWCNT, single-walled carbon nanotube.

6.2.4.1.2 *The big 10 nanomaterials*

In 2013, Keller et al. published on the global life cycle releases of ENMs (metric tons/year) from manufacturing, applications, disposal, and release into the environment, with some consideration of the high range of production estimates and releases [33]. From this analysis we term the "big 10 nanomaterials" as the top 10 ENMs that are currently being released into the environment: (i) titanium dioxide, (ii) silver, (iii) iron oxides, (iv) zinc oxide, (v) copper oxides, (vi) aluminum oxide, (vii) cerium oxide, (viii) nanoclays, (ix) carbon nanotubes (CNTs), and (x) silicon dioxide. They are used in a variety of manufactured applications (i.e., cosmetics, paints, electronics, food, etc.). The majority of these ENMs end up disposed in landfills (up to 90%), soil (up to 28%), water (up to 7%), or the atmosphere (up to 1.5%). In specific cases, the ENMs are released and flow through wastewater treatment plants (WWTPs) or waste incineration plants (WIPs) before they reach their eventual environmental endpoint. Figure 6.1 shows the global material emission distributions for the big 10 nanomaterials in 2010 to the environment.

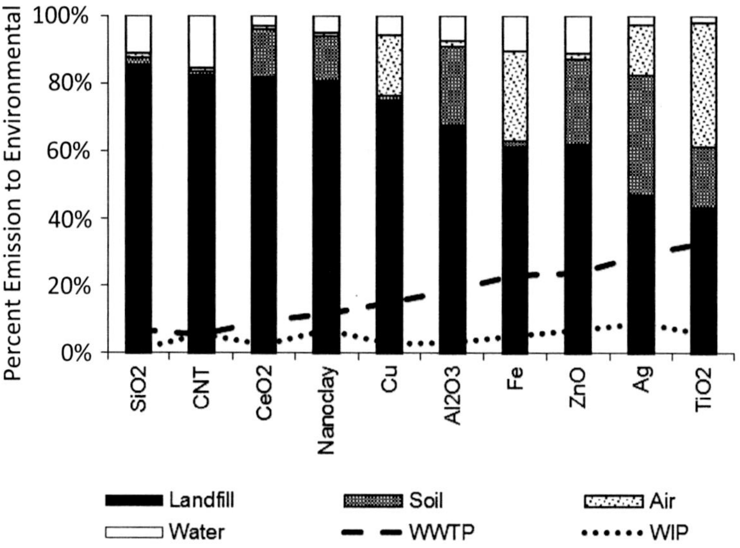

Figure 6.1 Big 10 engineered nanomaterials in 2010 to the environment. The majority of these ENMs are released to landfills before or after flow through wastewater treatment plants (WWTPs) or waste incineration plants (WIPs), which are not considered endpoints. The dashed lines depict the percentage of total nanoparticle emissions through each plant before translocation to one of the four environmental compartments. Data reconstructed from Keller et al. 2013.

6.2.4.1.3 *The impact of ENM properties on their environmental release*

ENMs that release into the environment are guided by their material properties, but isolating and determining the specific material property responsible for the release is a complex task because nanomaterials fall into a "gray area," where they can behave either like small particles or like large solutes. To complicate it further, currently there are no techniques able to distinguish ENMs from naturally formed nanomaterials in the environment. In this section we will examine different nanomaterial properties to determine whether they influence the release of ENMs into the environment.

Even though studies have shown a release of ENMs from an anthropogenic product (i.e., Ag ENMs on textiles released during washing), very few of these studies have explored further to determine the relationship between nanomaterial properties and release potential.

The most common material properties found to influence ENM release are dissolution and aggregation. However, these are chemical and physical transformation processes, which we will discuss later in the chapter. While dissolution will release metal oxide ENMs into the external environment, they end up as cationic ions and can no longer be called nanomaterials. Abrasion of textiles can lead to aggregation of ENMs, but this physical transformation converts the once nanomaterials into the microscale. Nanomaterial properties studied that show release potential, while keeping the ENM intact are few and far between. One study found that size can potentially play a role as smaller quantum dots (<10 nm) were released in greater amounts than those with 30 nm diameter from hydrogels [34]; however, hydrogel mesh size variability could influence these results. Another study found that the aspect ratio of ENMs plays a role in colloid transport, where nanomaterials with higher aspect ratios show a decrease in electric double-layer (EDL) thickness and display greater biological cell retention [35]. This has been commonly observed in studies that focus on ENM translocation through biological matrices, where smaller, spherical ENMs have greater translocation through cell membranes and more release into interstitial regions than larger, rod-shaped ENMs [35]. This is a relatively untouched area of nanoscience, and the uncertainty surrounding the influence of ENM properties on environmental release potential is a major challenge moving forward. It should be a priority to reduce the knowledge gaps in this area.

6.2.5 The Diversity of Nanotechnology Products

ENM applications are very diverse. Figure 6.2 highlights the technological applications of the big 10 nanomaterials and the unique material properties that make them an effective technology. Current application product lines involving ENMs can be broken down into four product lines: (i) the dispersion of ENMs into liquids that are used in industrial manufacturing (i.e., polishing agents), (ii) the dispersion of ENMs into products (i.e., foods), (iii) the embedding of ENMs into composite polymers (i.e., thermoplastics, membranes for water filtration), and (iv) the coating of ENMs on the surfaces of flexible polymeric materials (i.e., textiles). These product lines utilize nanomaterial functionality to optimize their application, as seen in Fig. 6.2. The *y* axis in the figure corresponds to the reactivity of ENMs in the four product lines. Product lines A and D utilize the reactive properties of ENMs during product design and synthesis (i.e., redox activity, hydrophilicity), while product lines B and C utilize ENMs for structural support and product stability (i.e., mechanical strength). The *x* axis in the figure corresponds to the physical relationship of the ENMs and the products. Product lines A and B contain ENMs that either do not reside in the final consumer product or are loosely bound to the surface of the product (i.e., food coating). Product lines C and D contain ENMs that are embedded within the product and are unlikely to be released during their use or disposal. These can include ENMs in polymers or floor coating.

Product line A includes polishing agents like chemical-mechanical polishing (CMP) fluids. Over 5500 tons per year of CMPs are used [36]. We can realistically estimate that in urban locations, there is between 0.1 and 1.0 mg ENMs/L that flow through a WWTP at any given time that originate from CMP fluids [36]. In the semiconductor industry there are concerns surrounding workplace exposure and monitoring and the lack of on-site CMP industrial treatment. Product line B includes nanomaterials in foods. ENMs are added to food for a variety of reasons, including texture, anticaking, color, oxygen barrier, abrasives, and antimicrobial properties [11]. Unfortunately, there is little confirmed occurrence and exposure data available. Product line C includes embedded nanomaterials throughout polymers. This includes formed plastics, where ENMs are added for strength [37]. Product line D includes nano-enabled textiles, which are used because of their "self-cleaning," flame retardancy, and antimicrobial properties [38]. Table 6.3 highlights the variety of technological applications that utilize ENMs for their unique material properties.

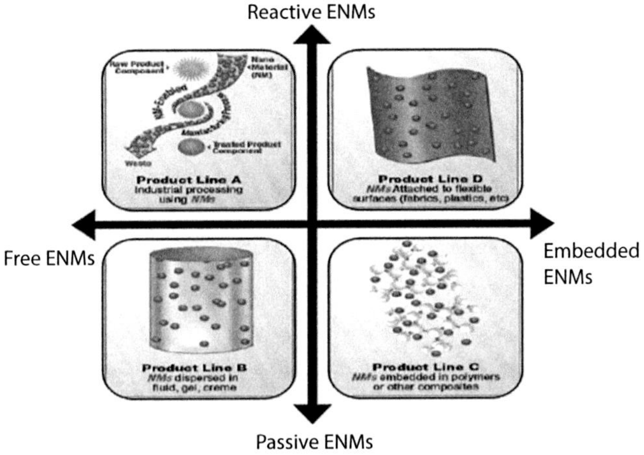

Figure 6.2 Conceptualization of the generalizable relationships for the state of ENMs and their release potential across product lines and commercial products.

6.2.6 Transformations of ENMs Have an Impact on Exposures

Current research efforts toward understanding nanomaterial fate, transport, and reactivity in the environment have focused on testing pristine ENMs that have had no prior contact with the environment. The truth is that the physicochemical properties of ENMs make them highly reactive in environmental systems, resulting in transformations that will greatly influence their behavior. These properties, coupled with the complex and random nature of environmental systems, greatly complicate our understanding of risks associated with the release of ENMs in the environment.

Oxidation and reduction reactions, dissolution, aggregation, and adsorption of macromolecules all readily occur in the environment [53], but there is still uncertainty surrounding the role these transformations play on both exposure and impacts across the whole life cycle of ENMs. In this section, we will discuss chemical, physical, and macromolecule-influenced transformations of ENMs in the environment and the hazards associated with ENM release.

Table 6.3 Material properties and their subsequent technological applications of the big 10 nanomaterials

ENM	Material property	Technological applications	Ref.
TiO_2	Photocatalysis	Sunscreen, pigments	[39]
	Texture	Food, toothpaste	[40]
Ag	Antimicrobial	Healthcare, textiles	[41]
Fe	Magnetism	Groundwater treatment	[42]
ZnO	Photocatalysis	Sunscreen, pigments	[43]
	Luminescence	Electronics, displays	[44]
CuO	Catalysis	Gas sensors, lithium cells	[45]
Al_2O_3	Strength	Filler for rubber	[46]
CeO_2	UV absorption	Sunscreen	[47]
Nanoclay	Strength	Reinforced plastics	[48]
CNT	Antimicrobial	Antifouling membranes	[49]
	Strength	Sporting equipment	[50]
SiO_2	Resistance	Glass, optics	[51]
	Texture	Food	[52]

6.2.6.1 Chemical transformations

Reduction and oxidation (redox) reactions are coupled processes that involve the transfer of electrons between two entities. Redox processes are also the basis of various precipitation and dissolution reactions that influence the sequestration and mobility of inorganic metals. Thus, redox reactions might be important for the transformation and fate of ENMs. ENMs can contain material properties that will undergo reduction, oxidation, or both in the environment [54]. Aquatic conditions with high dissolved oxygen exist in many well-mixed surface waters. Low-oxygen-containing environments exist in carbon-rich sediments and groundwater, hypolimnionic reservoirs, WWTPs that implement denitrification, etc. Tidal zones can have cycling between redox states. Sunlight can induce catalyzed redox reactions (photo-oxidation and photoreduction), which can effect ENM coatings, oxidation states, generation of ROS, and ENM persistence in the environment [25].

Dissolution occurs when molecules of the dissolving ENM migrate from the ENM surface to the bulk solution through a diffusion layer, where the concentration gradient between the ENM surface and the bulk solution acts as the driving force. The rate of dissolution depends on ENM properties (i.e., size, surface coating, aggregation potential), combined with the mass/molar concentration, which determines the concentration of ENM surface area available for dissolution reactions and water quality [55, 56]. For example, nanosilver (Ag^0) equilibrium with dissolved silver ions behaves more like a redox equilibrium than a solubility equilibrium because oxidation proceeds Ag^+ release. As Ag^+ is released in a closed system, the equilibrium changes [57, 58].

Metal oxide nanomaterials can undergo proton-promoted dissolution in aqueous matrices. In this mechanism, protons are bound to oxide ions closest to the surface of the nanoparticle [59]. The protons polarize the bonds between the oxide and metal ions. Because sorption of protons to the ENM surface is fast, the rate of dissolution is proportional to the concentration of the nanomaterial. However, if there is a ligand attachment on the ENM surface, the reaction can be inhibited [60]. This occurs because ligands form surface complexes with metal oxide ENMs. More importantly, the dissolution kinetics of ENMs are strongly influenced by the water chemistry of the aqueous media, such as pH, redox potential, and the type of concentration of inorganic and organic ligands [61]. The presence of some inorganic ligands (i.e., phosphate, sulfide, carbonate) can induce the transformation of soluble ENMs to less soluble minerals (ZnO ENMs to zinc sulfides), thus decreasing dissolved metal concentrations [62]. Like redox reactions, dissolution of ENMs varies significantly with environmental matrices. While it is still relatively uncertain, we can begin to conclude that the environment to which ENMs are released may be just as important in their release as the intrinsic physicochemical properties of the ENMs.

6.2.6.2 Physical transformations

The aggregation of ENMs occurs when their surfaces come in contact with each other and close-range thermodynamic interactions drive particle–particle attachment. For ENMs <100 nm in size, Brownian diffusion controls the forces between individual particles, causing random collisions, resulting in their attachment or repulsion. The thermodynamic interactions that control this can be understood through Derjaguin–Landau–Verwey–Overbeek (DLVO) theory. This theory predicts the probability of two particles sticking together by the summation of van der Waals (vdW) and EDL potentials to determine whether forces are net attractive or net repulsive. For example, in Fig. 6.3, vdW and EDL potentials are plotted as a function of separation distance between the particles. Summation of these curves demonstrates that particles can have a net attraction in a primary or a secondary well. Primary well particles are irreversibly aggregated, whereas secondary well particles are reversibly aggregated.

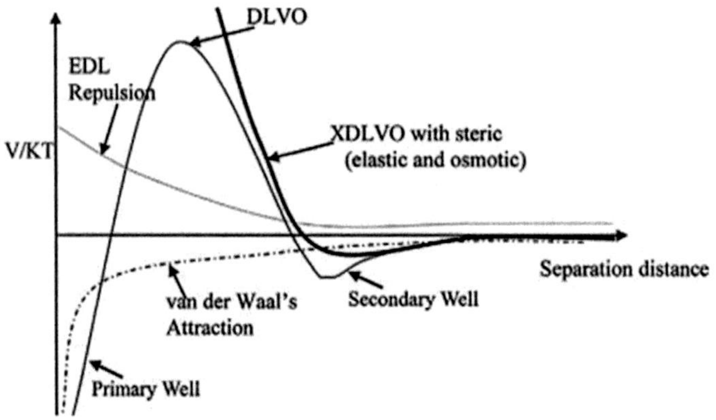

Figure 6.3 Van der Waals force, EDL force, total DLVO forces, and elastic force plotted together to find the total potential as a function of separation distance. XDLVO is extended DLVO. *V*/*KT* is the potential energy divided by Boltzmann's constant and absolute temperature. Reprinted from Ref. [63] with permission from American Society of Agronomy.

DLVO forces alone are not sufficient to accurately predict ENM aggregation behavior. Steric repulsion forces occurring from ENM coatings or NOM makes it so these particles might only have a net attraction in the secondary well [64]. This means that coated ENMs can aggregate reversibly, which plays a major role in the release, fate, transport, and bioavailability of ENMs in the environment. These additional forces are summed with DLVO, resulting in extended DLVO (XDLVO).

If we apply these concepts to aggregation in the environment, it becomes clear that there are two types of aggregation that are important: homoaggregation and heteroaggregation. Homoaggregation refers to the aggregation of two similar particles. This is observed in homogenous suspensions of particles that are typically studied in the lab to correlate research with DLVO theory. Homoaggregation is primarily influenced by diffusion potential at the colloidal scale, the radius of particle collisions, mixing conditions, and properties of ENMs (i.e., zeta potential, Hamaker constants). Experimental studies have a vast knowledge of the fundamentals of homoaggregation theory and its mechanisms [65]; however, environmental systems contain natural particles in numbers far greater than the number of manufactured ENMs, so we assume that homoaggregation has a minimal impact on ENMs in the environment. Heteroaggregation refers to aggregation of dissimilar particles in terms of their chemical composition, electrical charge, size, or shape. Nanomaterial interaction in complex environmental systems is likely to be influenced by physicochemical properties and background chemical conditions [63]. Heteroaggregation of ENMs with low-density natural colloids may facilitate the stabilization or disaggregation of ENMs, which would increase their residence times in water bodies, making the aggregation state of ENMs more difficult to predict. Heteroaggregation with bacteria, NOM, or mobile colloids could enhance ENM stability, but heteroaggregation to large enough particles could also destabilize ENM dispersions [66].

Recently there have been a handful of new studies that have tried to create a framework to determine the heteroaggregation rates for collisions between ENMs and NOM, as well as ENMs and natural nanomaterials (NNMs). While not validated, a working theory suggests that we can develop aggregation rate constants for heteroaggregation using Eq. 6.1 [67]:

$$k_{\text{het}} = K \times \alpha, \tag{6.1}$$

where k_{het} is the aggregation rate constant for heteroaggregation, K is the product of collision frequency, and α is the attachment efficiency (stickiness factor). However, it is important to note that this rate constant provides estimates for the average behavior of ENMs and is not indicative of all potential release and transformation scenarios. This is further complicated when investigating ENMs with structural deformations or complex matrices, as this theory has only been utilized in ideal systems with spherical ENMs. The complexities of natural systems and uncertainties surrounding ENM release and subsequent transformation by aggregation need further refinement, and it may be necessary to develop unique aggregation constants for specific ENMs and specific natural systems, as a universal constant applicable to all aggregation scenarios is highly unlikely.

6.2.6.3 Macromolecule-induced transformations

The adsorption of macromolecules (i.e., NOM) on ENMs can occur in all environments. Once released into the environment, both uncoated and coated ENMs can become transformed through interactions with NOM, whose concentrations are typically orders of magnitude higher in concentration than manufactured ENMs, resulting in the significant modification of ENM properties and behaviors. Most ENM–NOM interactions will involve the displacement of weakly bound coatings on the particle surface to form thin monolayer, thick monolayer, or multilayer surface coatings of NOM with varying coherence. The consistency and thickness of the ENM–NOM interactions depends on the ENM properties, and the matrix conditions (e.g., pH and ionic strength) during interaction negatively affect homoaggregation and heteroaggregation. In addition to changes in aggregation, ENM–NOM complexes have been shown to reduce short-term bacterial toxicity for metal-based nanomaterials [68]. It is thought that NOM prohibited the effect of the ENMs, either by directly coating the surface or by minimizing dissolution.

6.2.7 Hazards of Nanomaterial Release

There is potential for nanomaterials to be toxic in the environment. However, despite over a decade of findings surrounding ENM physicochemical properties and their associated biological health effects, uncertainties remain on universal frameworks, such as those that exist for traditional chemicals to a priori predict ENM toxicity. As the number of ENM-enhanced technologies increases, release and exposure of ENMs into soil, water, and atmospheric systems can lead to hazardous conditions. Nanotoxicity is complicated further by the number of ENM transformations that occur in the environment. Alterations in ionic strength, the ENM surface chemistry, or contact with NOM can change the aggregation potential and size of the nanoparticles, leading to bioaccumulation within organisms, thus increasing body burdens and stress [69–71]. For some ENMs with smaller diameters, their chemical reactivity is high, which, in turn, can result in the increased production of ROS, causing toxicity in biological organisms [72]. Some nanoparticles, like silver (Ag), are susceptible to surface reactions with oxygen and sulfur atoms, while other nanomaterials can experience dissolution to ions or chemical reactions [58], which can be more toxic than the nanomaterial itself (i.e., cadmium quantum dots to cadmium ions). All of these scenarios impact ENM physicochemical properties that can ultimately drive the toxicity, bioavailability, and even bioaccumulation of nanoparticles within the environment.

In the environment, bacteria play an integral role in nutrient cycling, in photosynthesis, and as a food source. While it has been shown that some ENMs are toxic to bacteria, the exact toxic pathway is somewhat controversial. Current research indicates that both ROS production and metal ion dissolution are potential causes of bacterial nanotoxicity [73], but more research needs to be conducted to verify working theories. In some cases, photocatalytic ROS production under ultraviolet (UV) light has been shown to produce electron–hole pairs that cause reduction/oxidation of nearby biological species [57]. In other cases, increases in metal ion concentrations intensify nanotoxicity toward bacterial species by causing the formation of oxidative radicals [74]. At this time, there have not been enough studies to correlate nanoparticle physicochemical properties to specific bacterial nanotoxicity, leaving much to be desired in this field of research. Advances in real-time biological assays and linkage of nanotoxicity/gene expression will contribute to reducing these knowledge gaps.

There is some evidence for plant toxicity due to nanoparticles. Studies have shown that plants facilitate translocation of nanoparticles from their roots to their leaves via the upward transport water system [75], but there is a lack of analytical tools to allow visualization of nanoparticle–plant interactions (i.e., super-resolution microscopy), creating an expansive knowledge gap. Right now we rely on phenotypic assessments and standard assay kits, which are incapable of such detection. Some studies have shown that introduction of nanomaterials during plant germination have resulted in the impediment of plant growth [76]. However, these results are often contradictory, as nanoparticle type and plant type appear to play a significant impact in toxicity, with even some studies showing increases in plant and crop yields when introduced to nanoparticles [78].

Multicellular organisms have been used most to examine nanotoxicity. Common model aquatic organisms are the medaka (*Oryzias latipes*) and zebrafish (*Danio rerio*). The nanotoxic effects on the medaka are influenced by the nanomaterial nature and surface coating, where nanotoxicity is a function of concentration, not mass [79]. Specific mechanisms of toxicity involve increased oxidative stress and the down-regulation of genes coding for growth, cell proliferation, and differentiation. The nanotoxic effects on zebrafish can be related to the shape of the nanomaterial, as sharp-edged nanomaterials can lyse cell membranes [79]. A common model terrestrial organism is the earthworm (*Lumbricus terrestris*). The nanotoxicity impact for these organisms varies by the nature of the nanomaterial [80]. Inorganic nanoparticles each cause growth and reproductive damage at different concentrations, while carbon nanoparticles are likely to become sequestered in soil systems, reducing their bioavailability and toxicity to earthworms.

Species sensitivity distributions (SSDs) can be used to predict the potential impacts of ENMs on biological organisms when exposed to ENMs in natural environmental conditions by modeling the affected fraction of species that would be harmed when exposed to ENMs. Unfortunately, there are few exposure limits put into place for specific ENMs, and what currently exists may not be sufficient to effectively reduce the risks associated with ENM exposure. One research area currently working to better understand ENM exposures is the field of modeling, where the collection of data may lead to breakthroughs in identifying the driving parameters for ENM exposure and subsequent toxicity.

6.2.8 The Current State of Modeling Efforts on Nanomaterial Exposure in the Environment

Models are powerful tools for describing the behavior of contaminants in complex environmental systems. The aim of investigating the fate and behavior of nanomaterials is to determine whether they pose a risk to environmental and human health and to guide management strategies; however, the current detection of ENMs in environmental systems is very challenging and suitable analytical methods are still under development. Most ENM models have also been used for the identification of important fate processes or parameters via parametric analysis or sensitivity analysis, the estimation of potential for long-range transport, and the estimation of overall residence times. Two general modeling approaches for ENMs in the environment are material flow analysis (MFA) and process-based F&T.

6.2.8.1 Material flow analysis

The earliest approaches to ENM fate modeling relied on MFA, which is a specific assessment methodology used to track the amount and flow of substances into and between technological "compartments" and environmental "compartments" (i.e., air, water, soil, landfills, etc.). These models are not spatially explicit, but they do help conceptualize a material's life cycle. ENM size, shape, aggregation state, surface coatings, particle chemistry, and phase changes are not explicitly considered in this model framework [81]. Instead, they are implied factors. MFAs are not the most appropriate tool for predicting environmental concentrations or specific locations (i.e., downstream of WWTPs) but are helpful in understanding general use and fate patterns. Experimental research and heteroaggregation models show that ENMs typically associate strongly with solid phases, leading to sedimentation and the accumulation of ENMs in sediments at "hot spots" near points of release and exposure [82].

6.2.8.2 Process-based fate and transport analysis

Even though ENMs behave differently than larger particles and solutes in the environment, they are largely subject to the same F&T processes that have been modeled successfully for organic and ionic contaminants. Existing chemical F&T modeling frameworks are capable, with some adaptation, of describing all major ENM fate processes, but major assumptions are made with respect to model scale and spatial resolution, steady state or time variable, and whether transformations and heteroaggregation are expressed as dependent on ENM properties, environmental conditions, or both [81]. Some models conserve mass, while others conserve particle number. For example, some models compare the sizes of ENMs and use time-independent partitioning ratios for heteroaggregation and attachment of ENMs in different environmental compartments, using only one transformation parameter (i.e., dissolution), while neglecting the rest [83]. Other modeling efforts include colloidal science instead of partitioning to determine the fate of ENMs [84]. Such radically different assumptions can completely change predicted results. If we compare the two modeling analyses, process-based models can provide better estimates of ENM environmental concentrations than MFAs because they model relevant environmental processes at a higher spatial resolution than MFAs. However, there is a need to validate these models using field exposure measurements of predicted hotspots.

6.3 The Tools for Detection and Quantification of Nanomaterial Exposures

6.3.1 Measurement Exposures

Measurement methods and instrumentation are nonspecific, making it difficult to differentiate between naturally occurring and engineered nanoparticles. Furthermore, the background levels of naturally occurring nanomaterials are unknown. Due to the complexity surrounding the potential transformations of ENMs in the environment, it is important to determine the most appropriate metrics for detection and quantification of ENMs in environmental matrices. For instance, particle size is ambiguous but has multiple parameters that play a large role in ENM release and F&T. These parameters that need to be evaluated are particle diameter (electron microscopy), hydrodynamic diameter (dynamic light scattering), and radius (static light scattering). Each parameter is as equally important as the others, but we can only obtain each parameter with a unique analytical tool. Only determining one parameter may not be sufficient. Table 6.4 highlights different nanomaterial properties and the corresponding analytical methods or analysis required to fully characterize them.

Table 6.4 Analytical methods or analyses for ENMs in soil, sediment, and groundwater for size fraction and distribution, surface area, and phase and structure. Reconstructed from U.S. EPA (600/R-14/244, 2014) [85]

Metric	Analytical method or analysis
Size fractionation	Centrifugation Ultrafiltration: direct flow or tangential flow (TFF) Field flow fractionation (FFF) Capillary electrophoresis (CE) Size-exclusion chromatography (SEC)
Size distribution	Transmission electron microscopy (TEM) Scanning electron microscopy (SEM) Scanning probe microscopy (SPM) Dynamic light scattering (DLS) Laser-induced breakdown detection (LIBD) Small-/wide-angle X-ray scattering (SAXS/WAXS)
Surface area	Brunauer–Emmett–Teller (BET) method Calculation from TEM, atomic force microscopy (AFM) measurements, and particle nanocrystalline geometrics
Phase and crystalline structure	Electron diffraction X-ray diffraction (XRD) X-ray absorption spectroscopy (XAS) Raman spectroscopy

Source: US government.

6.3.1.1 Mass concentration–based approach

The method for expressing concentration of ENMs is influenced by the research question at hand and by the anticipated analytical methods. Mass concentrations (mass/vol) are generally used for nonparticulate contaminants and may also be appropriate metrics for some ENMs. For readily soluble ENMs, mass concentration may be the most important metric, because exposure is based on the soluble metal and uptake is based on the particle mass. Some analytical methods, such as transmission electron microscopy (TEM) and nanotracking analysis (NTA), rely on detecting and quantifying individual particles. Other methods such as field flow fractionation–inductively coupled plasma mass spectrometry (FFF-ICP-MS) determine the mass-to-size ratio using the integrated signal of the many thousands of particles present in any given elution volume. Information on ENP size, shape, and density allows conversion between mass- and number-based concentrations, at least for simple ENMs.

6.3.1.2 Surface area–based approach

Traditional measurements of surface area (i.e., N_2 deposition using Brunauer–Emmett–Teller [BET] analysis) cannot be performed for ENM solutions because these measurements must be conducted in nonaqueous environments. Nuclear magnetic resonance (NMR) spectroscopy techniques can provide surface area information in aqueous media, but the required concentration range (on the order of a few weight percent) makes it impractical for application to natural samples. Rather, surface area must generally be inferred indirectly from both geometric characterization (size, shape, porosity) and mass or number concentration. It can also be calculated from FFF or single-particle inductively coupled plasma mass spectrometry (spICP-MS) with assumptions of ENM density.

6.3.1.3 ICP-MS analytical approach

The fastest expanding technique is most likely ICP-MS, which, within a few years, had its status changed from an advanced technique to a routine analytical method, although ICP-MS and laser ablation ICP-MS are capable only of determining total elemental concentrations on a bulk or spatially resolved basis. ICP-MS techniques have microgram-per-kilogram sensitivity and can discriminate between different isotopes of the same element. This includes metallic ENMs and CNTs (using metal catalysts).

6.3.1.4 Thermal method analytical approach

Thermal methods can be used to quantify CNTs. One method is through microwave-induced heating, where rapid heating of CNTs from microwave absorption can be used to create a CNT mass-to-temperature relationship used in quantifying the amount of CNTs in biological samples [86]. Another method is through programmed thermal analysis (PTA), which relies on the thermal stability of CNTs. Organic carbon and CNTs have different thermal stability and as such will have a different analytical footprint [87]. This technique can also be used to determine whether changes in the thermal stability of CNTs occur if extracted from environmental or complex matrices.

6.3.1.5 X-ray analytical approach

A number of X-ray-based techniques, such as X-ray absorption and fluorescence, as well as their microfocused declinations, are applicable, in theory, to the entire periodic table [88]. Synchrotron-based X-ray absorption techniques also are able to probe chemical speciation and the local electronic structure of elements. Determining the local electronic structure of metal atoms can be used to identify ENMs in a sample [80]. Conversely, although X-ray–based techniques have milligram-per-kilogram sensitivity, sensitivity of X-ray–based techniques can be enhanced by using spatially resolved analysis, which exploits the occurrence of foci of elevated concentrations relative to the bulk sample that can correspond to isolated or aggregated nanoparticles [80]. X-ray photoelectron spectroscopy and related techniques are attractive in the sense that they provide element-specific information while probing the surface of nanoparticles or their aggregates.

6.3.2 Environmental Sample Preparation Challenges

Presently, there is a lack of techniques for collecting, preserving, and storing samples containing ENMs. Which techniques are appropriate will depend on the sample type, ENM property of interest, and analytical method to be used. ENM systems are extremely sensitive to agitation from factors such as pH, ionic strength, sunlight, bacterial growth, and temperature. Processes such as aggregation, dispersion, and dissolution may affect the environmental state of ENMs. It is therefore important to determine the most appropriate metrics for detection, quantification, and characterization of ENMs in environmental and biological media. In some cases, sample preservation may not be possible for a given property of interest that must be analyzed, such as aggregation state. In other cases, sample preparation steps may be taken to preserve sample fractions for subsequently measuring properties of interest, such as particle concentrations. For example, some ENMs are extremely redox active (i.e., Ag ENMs). Quantification of dissolved ions in liquid media does not allow for proper storage, because dissolution may not be at equilibrium [53]. Dissolved ions first must be separated from the system using techniques such as ultracentrifugation or ultrafiltration and then preserved for analysis. Ultrafiltration is a type of filtration where pressure or concentration gradients can lead to the size separation of ENMs. Large ENMs are retained by the filter, while smaller ENMs and potentially dissolved metal ions pass through the filter [90]. This technique can be used to separate nanomaterials from their complex environmental matrices. Another technique is through cloud point extraction (CPE) [91]. CPE utilizes nonionic surfactants to capture ENMs out of liquid phases by heating. As the temperature of the solution rises, the surfactants form micelles that surround ENMs. As the temperature increases above the cloud point, the micelles become dehydrated and aggregate. This leads to phase separation of the matrix and the surfactant, resulting in the extraction of ENMs from their complex matrix.

6.3.3 The Need for Multiple Lines of Evidence for Nanomaterial Detection

ENM systems are complex; thus, multiple orthogonal lines of evidence are needed to detect and physicochemically characterize nanoparticles in complex media. In traditional chemical analytical techniques, one must identify chemical species in at least two independent ways. ENM systems may have even more rigorous requirements for identification and quantification, relying on numerous techniques because they are not discrete molecular species. For example, identification of CeO_2 nanoparticles in a soil solution may require separation based on particle size, verification of separation using light-scattering techniques, chemical identification using ICP-MS, examination of particle size distribution, crystal structure, and chemical composition using TEM. Each ENM's nature must be taken into account, and independent measures of each physicochemical property of interest are needed for validation. Each analytical technique must be validated using standards, quality control procedures, and standard reference materials. However, for ENMs, very little standard reference materials are available for nanomaterials. To make things more challenging, current standards for ENMs in complex matrices are not available for ENMs because of the inherent instability of ENMs.

6.3.4 Functional Assays and Radar Plots

The physicochemical properties associated with a unique ENM functionality can also influence inherent hazard and potential exposure routes of an ENM. For example, a material whose beneficial function is to generate ROS may be inherently more toxic than a material that does not. Further, the ability to generate ROS may promote the ENM's release from the matrix in which it is encapsulated. Elucidating these parametric relationships through functional assays allows for the prediction of the efficacy and unintended consequences in a desired application. Functional assays are high-throughput screening tools designed to elucidate ENM property–exposure relationships from a life cycle perspective by parameterizing exposure models and by comparing ENMs or transformations of ENMs [92]. Although functional assays (i.e., octanol–water partitioning) for longevity and mobility have been developed for organic compounds, this is a relatively new concept for ENMs. These functional assays are developed to quantify the basic material properties of ENMs that are consistent with proxies for the risks of ENMs in the environment (i.e., exposure, hazard, reactivity, and distribution). These risk parameters can be summarized as mean values on a radar plot where data for a given ENM, or release of ENMs along a product value chain, are grouped together. Large scores in these parameters signal a higher potential risk. This can be observed in Fig. 6.4.

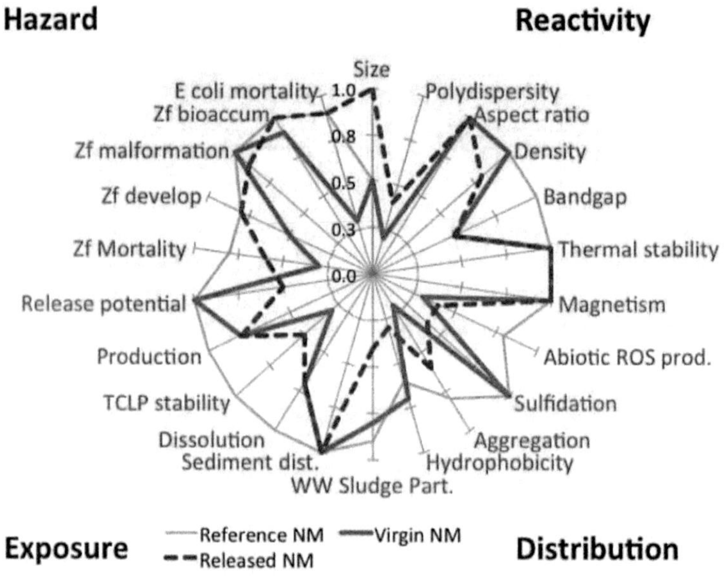

Figure 6.4 Risk-profiling radar plot. (Zf is the response to a high-throughput zebrafish embryo assay.)

Functional assays can also be used to quantify parameters that describe a specific process within a complex matrix. They can be used as predictors of ENM behaviors in the environment that will help determine the release, fate, and effects of ENMs [92]. There are three components to functional assays: The first component is that they can be used as standard protocols to determine ENM property parameter by differentiating between intrinsic physicochemical properties of ENMs and extrinsic, system-dependent properties. The second component is that they are reference systems for reporting ENM exposure data. Using functional assays and radar plots to compare different combinations of ENMs and environmental systems provides a backbone for the future standardization of ENMs. The third component is that they are key for predicting exposures. All of the potential transformations that can occur in an environment can be evaluated with functional assays. For instance, measuring the dissolution rate of an ENM in an environmental matrix can be compared with ENM bioavailability, toxicity, and persistence in the environment. Overall, functional assays provide a systematic path that will allow for more sustainable and rationale research, as well as aligning modeling efforts with lab-generated data.

6.4 What Does the Data Tell Us about Nanomaterial Exposure?

6.4.1 What Do We Know?

Current exposure measurements and models, while not perfect, have given insight into ENM exposure in the environment. The state of science pertaining to ENM exposure is still in the infant stage but is quickly developing. Intrinsic ENM properties and extrinsic, matrix-sensitive properties can create unique exposure scenarios that are currently too complex for available methodologies.

Currently, we are unable to determine whether specific ENM properties, or a combination of ENM properties, are responsible for ENM release and exposure in the environment. Quantification of ENMs and ENM material properties requires a number of different analytical tools because of a lack of analytical tools capable of conducting analysis on more than one specific parameter. ENM transformations in the environment (i.e., dissolution, aggregation) are key components in altering the release potential of ENMs in products. We can characterize feedstocks and pristine ENMs. Analysis of ENMs in complex matrices remains largely a purview of research labs. ENM manufacturers use both dry and wet ENM feedstocks, so it is difficult to distinguish between ENMs and NNMs. Few human studies track ENM distribution, availability, accumulation, or adverse outcomes released from consumer products.

6.4.2 What Should We Be Doing?

First, we should assess uncertainties surrounding common ENMs, like titanium dioxide and silicon dioxide. Some areas to address would involve answering the following questions:

- Should we remove these ENMs from concern?

- Do we really understand their consumer exposures?
- Are there sensitive consumer population or nanospecific adverse outcomes?

Second, we should apply functional assays to reduce uncertainties surrounding ENM use in products, as well as a guiding tool for life cycle exposures. We can utilize high-throughput screening assays to measure unique properties (optical, thermal, magnetic, etc.) and group products and exposure scenarios around ENM functional uses. Third, we should design studies across the life cycle of ENMs to validate models. In this way we can validate assumptions that pristine ENMs can be seen as precursors. Fourth, we can assess human exposures (workers, consumers) to measured ENM exposure levels (inhalation, oral, dermal), within biological fluids (nasal, urine, blood) and health outcomes. Finally, we should continue life cycle studies but compare efficacy versus exposure and toxicity risk and compare the risks of ENMs relative to use of other anthropogenic chemicals.

Acknowledgments

I would like to acknowledge the LCnano community, which is funded by the Environmental Protection Agency (EPA grant number RD835558001), for outstanding collaborations during the past three years. I would like to thank Dr. Westerhoff for his guidance and desire to explore the nanotechnology realm with me during my PhD career.

References

1. Sanz-Rodriguez, F., Martínez Maestro, L., Rocha, U., García Solé, J., Jacinto, C., Carmen Iglesias-de la Cruz, M., and Juarranz, A. (2012). Optimum quantum dot size for highly efficient fluorescence bioimaging. *J. Appl. Phys.*, **111**(2), 235131–235136.
2. Nick, S. T., Bolandi, A., Samuels, T. A., and Obare, S. O. (2014). Advances in understanding the transformation of engineered nanoparticles in the environment. *Pure Appl. Chem.*, **86**(7), 1129–1140.
3. Chen, Z., Forman, A. J., and Jaramillo, T. (2013). Bridging the gap between bulk and nanostructured impact of surface states on the

electrocatalytic and photoelectrochemical properties of MoS_2. *J. Phys. Chem. C*, **117**(19), 9713–9722.

4. Kulagin, N., Goroshkova, L., and Hieckmann, E. (2012). Change in properties of nano and bulk $SrTiO_3$ crystals. *Can. J. Phys.*, **90**(7), 683–691.
5. Saafan, S. A., Assar, S. T., Moharram, B. M., and El Nimr, M. K. (2010). Comparison study of some structural and magnetic properties of nano-structured and bulk Li–Ni–Zn ferrite samples. *J. Magn. Magn. Mater.*, **322**(6), 628–632.
6. Kreyling, W. G., Semmler-Behnke, M., and Chaudhry, Q. (2010). A complementary definition of nanomaterial. *Nano Today*, **5**(3), 165–168.
7. Popma, J. R., Heugens, E. H. W., Rietveld, A. G., Oomen, A. G., Cassee, F. R., Meent, V, D., and Wijnhoven, S. W. P. (2012). Considerations on the EU definition of a nanomaterial: science to support policy making. *Regul. Toxicol. Pharm.*, **65**(1), 119–125.
8. Cao, G. (2004). *Nanostructures and Nanomaterials: Synthesis, Properties and Applications*, 1st Ed. (Imperial College Press, London, England).
9. Gregorczyk, K., and Knez, M. (2016). Hybrid nanomaterials through molecular and atomic layer deposition: top down, bottom up, and in-between approaches to new materials. *Prog. Mater. Sci.*, **75**, 1–37.
10. Roco, M. C. (2011). Nanotechnology: from discovery to innovation and socioeconomic projects. *Chem. Eng. Prog.* **107**(5), 21–27.
11. Roco, M. C., Mirkin, C. A., and Hersam, M. C. (2011). Nanotechnology research directions for societal needs in 2020: summary of international study. *J. Nanopart. Res.*, **13**(3), 897–919.
12. Roco, M. C. (2011). The long view of nanotechnology development: the national nanotechnology initiative at 10 years. *J. Nanopart. Res.*, **13**(2), 427–445.
13. Gottschalk, F., and Nowack, B. (2011). The release of engineered nanomaterials to the environment. *J. Environ. Monit.*, **13**(5), 1145–1155.
14. Losert, S., Hess, A., Ilari, G., von Goetz, N., and Hungerbuehler, K. (2015). Online characterization of nano-aerosols released by commercial spray products using SMPS–ICPMS coupling. *J. Nanopart. Res.*, **17**(7), 1–14.
15. Tromp, P. C., Oomen, A. G., Marvin, H. J. P., Rietveld, A., Oegema, G., Bouwmeester, H., and Kramer, E. (2012). Presence of nano-sized silica

during in vitro digestion of foods containing silica as a food additive. *ACS Nano*, **6**(3), 2441–2451.

16. Al-Kattan, A., Wichser, A., Vonbank, R., Brunner, S., Ulrich, A., Zuin, S., and Nowack, B. (2013). Release of TiO_2 from paints containing pigment-TiO_2 or nano-TiO_2 by weathering. *Environ. Sci. Process. Impacts*, **15**(12), 2186–2193.
17. Gondikas, A. P., von der Kammer, F., Reed, R. B., Wagner, S., Ranville, J. F., and Hofmann, T. (2014). Release of TiO_2 nanoparticles from sunscreens into surface waters: a one-year survey at the old Danube recreational lake. *Environ. Sci. Technol.*, **48**(10), 5415.
18. Dahm, M. M., Evans, D. E., Schubauer-Berigan, M. K., Birch, M. E., and Deddens, J. A. (2013). Occupational exposure assessment in carbon nanotube and nanofiber primary and secondary manufacturers: mobile direct-reading sampling. *Ann. Occup. Hyg.*, **57**(3), 328–344.
19. Hicks, A. L., Gilbertson, L. M., Yamani, J. S., Theis, T. L., and Zimmerman, J. B. (2015). Life cycle payback estimates of nanosilver enabled textiles under different silver loading, release, and laundering scenarios informed by literature review. *Environ. Sci. Technol.*, **49**(13), 7529.
20. Wilson, M. J. (1999). The origin and formation of clay minerals in soils: past, present and future perspectives. *Clay Miner.*, **34**, 7–25.
21. Bargar, J., Bernier-Latmani, R., Giammar, D., and Tebo, B. (2008). Biogenic uraninite nanoparticles and their importance for uranium remediation. *Elements*, **4**, 407–412.
22. Buseck, P., and Pósfai, M. (1999). Airborne minerals and related aerosol particles: effects on climate and the environment. *Proc. Natl. Acad. Sci. U. S. A.*, **96**, 3372–3379.
23. Cavalli, F., Facchini, M., Decesari, S., et al. (2004). Advances in characterization of size-resolved organic matter in marine aerosol over the North Atlantic. *J. Geophys. Res.*, **109**, 21425.
24. Adegboyega, N., Sharma, V., Siskova, K., Vecerova, R., et al. (2014). Enhanced formation of silver nanoparticles in Ag+-NOM-iron (II, III) systems and antibacterial activity studies. *Environ. Sci. Technol.*, **48**, 3228–3235.
25. Yin, Y., Liu, J., and Jiang, G. (2012). Sunlight-induced reduction of ionic Ag and Au to metallic nanoparticles by dissolved organic matter. *ACS Nano*, **6**, 7910–7919.
26. Yucel, M., Gartman, A., Chan, C., and Luther, G. (2011). Hydrothermal vents as a kinetically stable source of iron-sulfide-bearing nanoparticles to the ocean. *Nat. Geosci.*, **4**, 367–371.

27. d'Almeida, G. A., and Schutz, L. (1983). Number, mass and volume distributions of mineral aerosol and soils of the Sahara. *J. Clim. Appl. Meteorol.*, **22**, 233–243.

28. Lungu, M., Neculae, A., Bunoiu, M., and Biris, C. (2015). *Nanoparticles' Promises and Risks: Characterization, Manipulation, and Potential Hazards to Humanity and the Environment* (Springer InternationalSwitzerland), xiv, 355 p.

29. Shi, Z., Shao, L., Jones, T. P., and Lu, S. (2005). Microscopy and mineralogy of airborne particles collected during severe dust storm episodes in Beijing, China. *J. Geophys. Res.*, **110**, D01303.

30. Yano, E., Yokoyama, Y., Higashi, H., Nishii, S., Maeda, K., and Koizumi, A. (1990). Health effects of volcanic ash: a repeat study. *Environ. Health*, **45**, 367–373.

31. von der Kammer, F., Ferguson, P. L., Holden, P. A., Masion, A., Rogers, K. R., Klaine, S. J., Koelmans, A. A., Horne, N., and Unrine, J. M. (2012). Analysis of engineered nanomaterials in complex matrices (environment and biota): general considerations and conceptual case studies. *Environ. Toxicol. Chem.*, **31**, 32.

32. Wiesner, M. R., Lowry, G. V., Jones, K. L., Hochella, M. F. Jr, DiGiulio, R. T., Casman, E., and Bernhardt, E. S. (2009). Decreasing uncertainties in assessing environmental exposure, risk, and ecological implications of nanomaterials. *Environ. Sci. Technol.*, **43**, 6458.

33. Keller, A., McFerran, S., Lazareva, A., and Suh, S. (2013). Global life cycle releases of engineered nanomaterials. *J. Nanopart. Res.*, **15**(6), 1–17.

34. Hume, S. L., and Jeerage, K. M. (2013). Surface chemistry and size influence the release of model therapeutic nanoparticles from poly(ethylene glycol) hydrogels. *J. Nanopart. Res.*, **15**(5), 1–16.

35. Cho, E., Holback, H., Liu, K., Abouelmagd, S., Park, J., and Yeo, Y. (2014). Nanoparticle characterization: state of the art, challenges, and emerging technologies. *Mol. Pharmaceutics*, **10**(6), 2093–2110.

36. Baalousha, M., and Lead, J. (2015). *Characterization of Nanomaterials in Complex Environmental and Biological Media* (Elsevier, Amsterdam).

37. Lobos, J., and Velankar, S. (2014). How much do nanoparticle fillers improve the modulus and strength of polymer foams? *J. Cell. Plast.*, **1**, 1–32.

38. Dastjerdi, R., Montazer, M., and Shahsavan, S. (2009). A new method to stabilize nanoparticles on textile surfaces. *Colloids Surf. A*, **345**(1), 202–210.

39. Faure, B., Salazar-Alvarez, G., Ahniyaz, A., Villaluenga, I., Berriozabal, G., De Miguel, Y. R., and Naturvetenskapliga, F. (2013). Dispersion and surface functionalization of oxide nanoparticles for transparent photocatalytic and UV-protecting coatings and sunscreens. *Sci. Technol. Adv. Mater.*, **14**(2), 23001.

40. Faria, A. C. L., Bordin, Angelo Rafael de Vito, Pedrazzi, V., Rodrigues, R. C. S., and Ribeiro, R. F. (2012). Effect of whitening toothpaste on titanium and titanium alloy surfaces. *Braz. Oral Res.*, **26**(6), 498–504.

41. Gouda, M. (2012). Nano-zirconium oxide and nano-silver oxide/cotton gauze fabrics for antimicrobial and wound healing acceleration. *J. Ind. Text.*, **41**(3), 222–240.

42. Lee, S., Laldawngliana, C., and Tiwari, D. (2012). Iron oxide nano-particles-immobilized-sand material in the treatment of Cu contaminated waste waters. *J. Chem. Eng.*, **103**, 195–196.

43. Azad, M., Nasrollahi, S. A., and Firooz, A. (2014). Zinc oxide in sunscreen products. *Dermatol. Cosmet.*, **5**(1), 41–48.

44. Godlewski, M., Guziewicz, E., Kopalko, K., Łuka, G., Łukasiewicz, M. I., Krajewski, T., and Gierałtowska, S. (2011). Zinc oxide for electronic, photovoltaic and optoelectronic applications. *Low Temp. Phys.*, **37**(3), 235–240.

45. Buffle, J., Wilkinson, K. J., Stoll, S., Filella, M., and Zhang, J. (1998). A generalized description of aquatic colloidal interactions: the three-colloidal component approach. *Environ. Sci. Technol.*, **32**(19), 2887–2899.

46. Zhou, W., Qi, S., Tu, C., Zhao, H., Wang, C., and Kou, J. (2007). Effect of the particle size of Al_2O_3 on the properties of filled heat-conductive silicone rubber. *J. Appl. Polym. Sci.*, **104**(2), 1312–1318.

47. Boutard, T., Rousseau, B., Couteau, C., Tomasoni, C., Simonnard, C., Jacquot, C., and Roussakis, C. (2013). Comparison of photoprotection efficiency and antiproliferative activity of ZnO commercial sunscreens and CeO_2. *Mater. Lett.*, **108**, 13–16.

48. Wong, A., Wijnands, S. F. L., Kuboki, T., and Park, C. B. (2013). Mechanisms of nanoclay-enhanced plastic foaming processes: effects of nanoclay intercalation and exfoliation. *J. Nanopart. Res.*, **15**(8), 1–15.

49. Kim, J., Shashkov, E. V., Galanzha, E. I., Kotagiri, N., and Zharov, V. P. (2007). Photothermal antimicrobial nanotherapy and nanodiagnostics with self-assembling carbon nanotube clusters. *Lasers Surg. Med.*, **39**(7), 622–634.

50. Nowack, B., David, R. M., Fissan, H., Morris, H., Shatkin, J. A., Stintz, M., and Brouwer, D. (2013). Potential release scenarios for carbon nanotubes used in composites. *Environ. Int.*, **59**, 1–11.

51. Martinet, C., Kassir-Bodon, A., Deschamps, T., Cornet, A., Le Floch, S., Martinez, V., and Champagnon, B. (2015). Permanently densified SiO_2 glasses: a structural approach. *J. Phys.*, **27**(32), 325401.

52. Mutsuga, M., Sato, K., Hirahara, Y., and Kawamura, Y. (2011). Analytical methods for SiO_2 and other inorganic oxides in titanium dioxide or certain silicates for food additive specifications. *Food Addit. Contam.*, **28**(4), 423–427.

53. Liu, J., and Hurt, R. H. (2010). Ion release kinetics and particle persistence in aqueous nano-silver colloids. *Environ. Sci. Technol.*, **44**(6), 2169– 2175.

54. Sayle, T. X. T., Molinari, M., Das, S., Bhatta, U. M., Möbus, G., Parker, S. C., and Sayle, D. C. (2013). Environment-mediated structure, surface redox activity and reactivity of ceria nanoparticles. *Nanoscale*, **5**(13), 663–673.

55. Borm, P., Klaessig, F. C., Landry, T. D., Moudgil, B., Pauluhn, J., Thomas, K., Trottier, R., and Wood, S. (2006). Research strategies for safety evaluation of nanomaterials, part V: role of dissolution in biological fate and effects of nanoscale particles. *Toxicol. Sci.*, **90**, 23–32.

56. Murdock, R. C., Braydich-Stolle, L., Schrand, A. M., Schlager, J. J., and Hussain, S. M. (2008). Characterization of nanomaterial dispersion in solution prior to in vitro exposure using dynamic light scattering technique. *Toxicol. Sci.*, **101**, 239–253.

57. Li, Y., Zhang, W., Niu, J., and Chen, Y. (2012). Mechanism of photogenerated reactive oxygen species and correlation with the antibacterial properties of engineered metal-oxide nanoparticles. *ACS Nano*, **6**(6), 5164–5173.

58. Xiu, Z., Zhang, Q., Puppula, H., Colvin, V., and Alvarez, P. (2012). Negligible particle-specific antibacterial activity of silver nanoparticles. *Nano Lett.*, **12**(8), 4271–4275.

59. Stumm, W. (1997). Reactivity at the mineral-water interface: dissolution and inhibition. *Colloids Surf. A*, **120**(1), 143–166.

60. Rubasinghege, G., Lentz, R. W., Scherer, M. M., and Grassian, V. H. (2012). Simulated atmospheric processing of iron oxyhydroxide minerals at low pH: roles of particle size and acid anion in iron dissolution. *Proc. Natl. Acad. Sci. U. S. A.*, **107**, 6628–6633.

61. Liu, J., Sonshine, D. A., Shervani, S., and Hurt, R. H. (2010). Controlled release of biologically active silver from nanosilver surfaces. *ACS Nano*, **4**(11), 6903–6913.

62. Pokhrel, L. R., Dubey, B., and Scheuerman, P. R. (2013). Impacts of select organic ligands on the colloidal stability, dissolution dynamics, and toxicity of silver nanoparticles. *Environ. Sci. Technol.*, **47**(22), 12877–12885.

63. Hotze, E., Phenrat, T., and Lowry, G. (2010). Nanoparticle aggregation: challenges to understanding transport and reactivity in the environment. *J. Environ. Qual.*, **39**, 1909–1924.

64. Hahn, M., D. Abadzic, and C. O'Melia. (2004). Aquasols: on the role of secondary minima. *Environ. Sci. Technol.*, **38**, 5915–5924.

65. Barbot, E., Dussouillez, P., Bottero, J.-Y., and Moulin, P. (2010). Coagulation of bentonite suspension by polyelectrolytes or ferric chloride: floc breakage and reformation. *Chem. Eng. J.*, **156**, 83–91.

66. Wu, W., Giese, R., and van Oss, C. (1999). Stability versus flocculation of particle suspensions in water-correlation with the extended DLVO approach for aqueous systems, compared with classical DLVO theory. *Colloids Surf. B*, **14**, 47–55.

67. Wouterse, M., Velzeboer, I., Meent, D., Koelmans, A. A., and Quik, J. T. K. (2014). Heteroaggregation and sedimentation rates for nanomaterials in natural waters. *Water Res.*, **48**(1), 269–279.

68. Li, Z., Greden, K., Alvarez, P. J. J., Gregory, K. B., and Lowry, G. V. (2010). Adsorbed polymer and NOM limits adhesion and toxicity of nano scale zerovalent iron to E. coli. *Environ. Sci. Technol.*, **44**(9), 3462–3467.

69. Badawy, A., Scheckel, K., Suidan, M., and Tolaymat, T. (2012). The impact of stabilization mechanism on the aggregation kinetics of silver nanoparticles. *Sci. Total Environ.*, **429**, 325–331.

70. Buffle, J., Wilkinson, K. J., Stoll, S., Filella, M., and Zhang, J. (1998). A generalized description of aquatic colloidal interactions: the three-colloidal component approach. *Environ. Sci. Technol.*, **32**(19), 2887–2899.Qi, Y., Du, N., Zhang, H., Wang, J., Yang, D., and Yang, Y. (2012). Nanostructured hybrid cobalt oxide/copper electrodes of lithium-ion batteries with reversible high-rate capabilities. *J. Alloys Compd.*, **521**, 83–89.

71. Keller, A., Wang, H., Zhou, D., et al. (2010). Stability and aggregation of metal oxide nanoparticles in natural aqueous matrices. *Environ. Sci. Technol.*, **44**(6), 1962–1967.

72. Dalai, S., Pakrashi, S., Kumar, R., Chandrasekaran, N., and Mukherjee, A. (2012). A comparative cytotoxicity study of TiO_2 nanoparticles under light and dark conditions at low exposure concentrations. *Toxicol. Res.*, **1**, 116–130.

73. Lyon, D., and Alvarez, P. (2008). Fullerene water suspension (nC) exerts antibacterial effects via ROS-independent protein oxidation. *Environ. Sci. Technol.*, **42**(21), 8127–8132.

74. Cronholm, P., Karlsson, H. L., Hedberg, J., Lowe, T. A., Winnberg, L., Elihn, K., Wallinder, I. O., and Möller, L. (2013). Intracellular uptake and toxicity of Ag and CuO nanoparticles: a comparison between nanoparticles and their corresponding metal ions. *Small*, **9**(7), 970–982.

75. Parsons, J., Lopez, M., Gonzalez, C., Peralta-Videa, J., and Gardea-Torresdey, J. (2010). Toxicity and biotransformation of uncoated and coated nickel hydroxide nanoparticles on mesquite plants. *Environ. Toxicol. Chem.*, **29**(5), 1146–1154.

76. Preister, J. H., Ge, Y., Mielke, R., Horst, A., et al. (2012). Soybean susceptibility to manufactured nanomaterials with evidence for food quality and soil fertility interruption. *Proc. Natl. Acad. Sci. U. S. A.*, **109**(37), 2451–2456.

77. Lee, W., An, Y., Yoon, H., and Kweon, H. (2008). Toxicity and bioavailability of copper nanoparticles to the terrestrial plants mung bean (Phaseolus radiatus) and wheat (Triticum aestivum): plant agar test for water-insoluble nanoparticles. *Environ. Toxicol. Chem.*, **7**(9), 1915–1921.

78. Kashiwada, S., Ariza, M. E., Kawaguchi, T., Nakagame, Y., et al. (2012). Silver nanocolloids disrupt medaka embryogenesis through vital gene expressions. *Environ. Sci. Technol.*, **46**, 6278–6287.

79. George, S., Lin, S., Ji, Z., Thomas, C. R., Li, L., Mecklenburg, M., et al. (2012). Surface defects on plate-shaped silver nanoparticles contribute to its hazard potential in a fish gill cell line and zebrafish embryos. *ACS Nano*, **6**, 3745–3759.

80. Unrine, J. M., Tsyusko, O. V., Hunyadi, S. E., Judy, J. D., and Bertsch, P. M. (2010). Effects of particle size on chemical speciation and bioavailability of copper to earthworms (Eisenia fetida) exposed to copper nanoparticles. *J. Environ. Qual.*, **39**, 1942–1953.

81. Gottschalk, F., Sonderer, T., Scholz, R. W., and Nowack, B. (2009). Modeled environmental concentrations of engineered nanomaterials (TiO_2, ZnO, Ag, CNT, fullerenes) for different regions. *Environ. Sci. Technol.*, **43**(24), 9216–9222.

82. Velzeboer, I., Quik, J. T. K., van de Meent, D., and Koelmans, A. A. (2014). Rapid settling of nanoparticles due to heteroaggregation with suspended sediment. *Environ. Toxicol. Chem.*, **33**(8), 1766–1773.

83. Liu, H. H., and Cohen, Y. (2014). Multimedia environmental distribution of engineered nanomaterials. *Environ. Sci. Technol.*, **48**(6), 3281–3292.

84. Praetorius, A., Tufenkji, N., Goss, K. U., Scheringer, M., von der Kammer, F., and Elimelech, M. (2014). The road to nowhere: equilibrium partition coefficients for nanoparticles. *Environ. Sci. Nano*, **1**(4), 317–323.

85. Montano, M., Ranville, J., Lowry, G., Blue, J., Hiremath, N., Koenig, S., and Tuccillo, M. (2014). Detection and characterization of engineered nanomaterials in the environment: current state-of-the-art and future directions report. U.S. Environmental Protection Agency, Washington, DC, EPA/600/R-14/244.

86. Irin, F., Shrestha, B., Cañas, J. E., Saed, M. A., and Green, M. J. (2012). Detection of carbon nanotubes in biological samples through microwave-induced heating. *Carbon*, **50**(12), 4441.

87. Doudrick, K., Herckes, P., and Westerhoff, P. (2012). Detection of carbon nanotubes in environmental matrices using programmed thermal analysis. *Environ. Sci. Technol.*, **46**(22), 12246–12253.

88. Bertsch, P., and Hunter, D. (2001). Applications of synchrotron bases x-ray microprobes. *Chem. Rev.*, **101**, 1809–1842.

89. Jawor, A., and Hoek, E. M. V. (2010). Removing cadmium ions from water via nanoparticle-enhanced ultrafiltration. *Environ. Sci. Technol.*, **44**(7), 2570–2576.

90. Nazar, M. F., Shah, S. S., Shah, A., Eastoe, J., and Khan, A. M. (2011). Separation and recycling of nanoparticles using cloud point extraction with non-ionic surfactant mixtures. *J. Colloid Interface Sci.*, **363**(2), 490–496.

91. Hendren, C., Lowry, G., Unrine, J., and Wiesner, M. (2015). A functional assay-based strategy for nanomaterial risk forecasting. *Sci. Total Environ.*, **536**, 1029–1037.

Chapter 7

Categorizing Nanomaterials for Health and Environmental Risk Assessment

Jo Anne Shatkin,[a] James D. Ede,[a] and Christie Sayes[b]
[a]*Vireo Advisors, LLC, Boston, MA 02205, USA*
[b]*Department of Environmental Science, Baylor University, Waco, TX 76798-7266, USA*
jashatkin@vireoadvisors.com, jede@vireoadvisors.com, csayes@baylor.edu

7.1 Introduction

Over decades of evaluating chemical substances, categories have been developed that relate (i) physical properties, (ii) structure, or (iii) known relationships between functional groups and specific health endpoints or environmental behavior such as persistence or ozone depletion. As we look toward the classification of nanomaterials, studies to date suggest the relationships that are well defined for chemicals are not broadly predictive of the behavior of many nanoscale materials [1, 2]. In particular, it has been observed that small changes in some physical and chemical properties can drastically change the toxicity profile of a nanomaterial [3, 4]. Despite significant investment to identify the main physical

Physicochemical Properties of Nanomaterials
Edited by Richard C. Pleus and Vladimir Murashov

ISBN 978-981-4774-80-2 (Hardcover), 978-1-351-16860-1 (eBook)
www.panstanford.com

and chemical attributes responsible for the change in toxicity, it remains a challenge to predict toxicological outcomes on the basis of measuring physicochemical properties [5]. Recognizing this, many efforts by international organizations are instead focused on identifying ways to categorize manufactured nanomaterials as a way to advance knowledge, risk management, and decision making and, ultimately, reduce the health and environmental impacts of new nanoscale substances. In this chapter, we discuss recent efforts toward categorizing nanomaterials for health and environmental risk assessment.

7.2 What Is Categorization?

Categorization is the act of sorting and organizing things according to a group or class. Classifying an object gives it an identity that is recognizable and distinguishable. In other words, categorization schemes are intended to organize a group of objects. These objects can be living (such as animals or plants), inorganic (such as substances or materials), processes (such as information flow or quality control/quality assurance), or techniques (teaching/learning or instrumental analyses). In scientific disciplines, categorization is often accomplished by identifying similar attributes (e.g., properties, features) of individual entities within a field of study. For example, one of the most recognizable biological categorization schemes is the taxonomic rank of life: domain, kingdom, phylum, class, order, family, genus, and species. In this context, a taxonomist determines the classification identifiers of a biological specimen. Taxonomists determine relationships among and between objects within a large group; biological taxonomists classify organisms according to their physical or cellular characteristics; military taxonomists classify weapons, equipment, organizations, strategies, and tactics within combat theater; and economic taxonomists classify products, companies, policies, and industries within a society.

The practice of categorization is not unique to the aforementioned fields. Other scientific fields of study, including astronomy, mathematics, psychology, and computer science, benefit from constructing a taxonomic or hierarchical structure within the discipline. In chemistry, a key example is the periodic table, which groups elements by a defining property. Chemical categorization schemes have developed over time to improve the health and environmental management of substances; these schemes group substances on the basis of characteristics that relate to overall risk such as toxicity, physical hazard, persistence, and others. Table 7.1 provides examples of categorization schemes used to classify chemical substances on the basis of toxicity or other related properties.

Table 7.1 Categorization schemes used for chemical substances

Scheme	Categorization approach	Basis for classification (e.g., toxicity, waste management)	Ref.
UN Globally Harmonized System	Physical, chemical and toxicity characteristics.	Used to communicate the potential hazard of chemical	[6]
US EPA Hazardous Waste Identification	Ignitability, corrosivity, reactivity, or toxicity	Used to determine whether materials meet the definition of "hazardous" for disposal or waste management	[7]
US EPA Organophosphate Pesticide Re-registration	Similar toxicological mechanism	Used to determine the relative potency factor for pesticide re-registration cumulative risk assessment	[8]
NRC Dioxin Potency Factor	Similarity of chemical structure in a mixture	Used in estimating health risks at Superfund sites from exposure to dioxins on the basis of relative toxicity related to chemical structure	[9]
Clean Production Action's GreenScreen	Classification of chemicals based on 18 human and environmental health endpoints	Used to assign hazard levels to chemicals for risk assessment	[10]

Classification schemes group substances into categories. Ideally, a category clarifies the relationships among entities within a data population, that is, their similarities and differences are highlighted. The rationale for classifying entities into categories is that the practice enables conclusions to be drawn or decisions to be made more quickly. In the classification of chemicals, one of the most widely recognized approaches is the Globally Harmonized System (GHS) of Classification and Labelling of Chemicals [6]. Under this system, chemicals are grouped into categories by their relative hazard for a variety of physical, chemical, and toxicity attributes. Grouping into specific categories generates symbols, signal words, and hazard statements that are then used to communicate the hazard associated with a product for those manufacturing, handling, transporting, or using it. By grouping and subsequently communicating the hazard associated with chemicals, the GHS serves to enhance the protection of human health and the environment [6].

7.2.1 Benefits of Categorization

Categorization schemes aid in the transfer of knowledge (such as teaching students, collaborating with peers, and communicating with other professionals) by

> "reducing the complexity of the environment, identifying objects, perceptions, ideas and events, reducing the necessity of constant learning, providing a basis for instrumental activity), creating order and relationship categories, predicting outcomes based on category properties, and extending categories by adding fictive or predicted objects" [11].

Transferring knowledge is a critically important component of the scientific process. It is often understudied, undervalued, and underused. This important component can inhibit the successful implementation of a new or refined technology or process. By extension, technological progress is then hindered and the value of the gained knowledge is potentially mitigated.

The impacts of nanomaterials, and their adoption into technologies, have not been mitigated, but some would argue that its progress hasn't been as impactful as it could have been. In recent years, categorization was proposed as a method to increase the translation of advances in nanomaterials by means of standardized nomenclature, ontological frameworks, and grouping methodologies to allow for generalization. Categorization has been adopted to varying degrees for nanomaterials in patenting, pharmaceutical applications, nomenclature, and health and safety subdisciplines with varying degrees of acceptance.

7.2.2 Selecting the Appropriate Categorization Scheme

Selecting the appropriate categorization scheme is a difficult challenge. The resultant categories must be useful to the taxonomist as well as the larger community that will use the scheme. The categorization must also be valid in order to ensure complete adoption by all stakeholders related to the larger group. There are established procedures commonly used to determine whether categories are valid and appropriate:

- Test the sensitivity and accuracy of the categorization scheme using a sample group.
- On the basis of experience and other similar taxonomic ranks, test which scheme best fits the object being grouped.
- Test the scheme using expert consensus.
- Test the scheme by personal intuition.

7.3 Why Categorize?

7.3.1 The Need for Nanomaterial Categories

Manufactured nanomaterials represent a relatively new class of materials with considerable complexity. Currently, there is generally a lack of predictive knowledge about how physicochemical characteristics of these materials relate to toxicity [5]; further, subtle changes in these physicochemical properties, or the environment matrix surrounding the nanomaterial, can influence its toxicity [1, 12]. For commercialization of nanomaterials to proceed, an understanding of the risks associated with them is required. However, given the number of nanomaterials being produced, the testing of every material is not feasible. Categorization of nanomaterials offers a way to group similar substances so that risk information from one substance can begin to be used to predict risk types for related but less studied substances. Such schemes can aid regulators in their continuing efforts to assess the risks associated with nanomaterials, and having an agreed-upon grouping for nanomaterials will aid regulators and commercial producers alike, improving processes for these materials to get safely to market.

It is generally agreed that grouping manufactured nanomaterials is helpful during risk analysis [13]. Researchers, industry, risk analysts, and regulators can use categorization to identify nanomaterials with particular characteristics indicating the need to conduct more detailed testing and analysis for specific types of effects. If the nanomaterials have an appropriate basis for categorization, then newly collected data and analyses would add to the knowledge base of not only the particular material of interest but also that entire category.

The risk management community can use categories to determine next steps for regulating or mitigating the risks of particular substances. One early example in the development of categorization tools is the development of control banding approaches in nanomaterial manufacturing environments. As we discussed, several classification approaches for nanomaterials are derived from occupational exposure assessment approaches developed for fiber and particle inhalation exposures during manufacturing.

In terms of health risks, categorization has already been shown to mitigate toxicity or detrimental environmental effects, for example, in the classification of persistent, bioaccumulative, and toxic chemicals (PBTs). These apply broadly to a diversity of health and environmental risk assessments from chemical, microbial, physical, and other hazards to screening level analysis, life cycle risk assessments, and assessments (cumulative assessments) in support of regulatory decisions, for example, assessments of drinking water contaminants, waste sites, air pollutants, workplace safety, new chemicals, management of existing chemicals, safety of foods, and food ingredients.

Clearly, data categorization can be beneficial toward conducting analyses within a reasonable time period and without excessive costs by learning from related substances. Categorization is a powerful approach toward making informed decisions under uncertainty. This is a strong driver within the categorization movement and should be considered as not only a benefit but also a need.

7.3.2 Consequences of Not Categorizing Nanomaterials

Without an adopted classification scheme specifically designed for manufactured nanomaterials, there is a potential for lack of standardization in measurement techniques. Standardized sampling techniques would be difficult to develop. Regulation of this group of materials would be challenging to develop and implement, as would supply chain management, particularly across geographies with differing approaches. Nonetheless, while lack of categorization does not halt a technology or material class from developing into market maturity, it does slow the pace of reaching maturity. Advocates of classification systems, especially new systems designed for new industries or technologies, argue that without classification, there would be less identification, definition, composition, and delimitation among industry participants [14].

7.3.3 Implications of Miscategorization in Nanoscience

To miscategorize is to identify or divide individual components into categories incorrectly. One consequence that results from a miscategorization scheme for nanomaterials is adding bias in measurements. Since nanotechnology is primarily application of science revolving around materials of a particular size, measuring characteristics, performance, and effects is central to the success of any categorization scheme—and by extension—the success of the technology in general. A second consequence is adding bias in observations. Adding biases to a categorization effort creates only a partial perspective that will not be translatable to every potential user of the scheme. The most common roadblocks to a successful categorization scheme in nanoscience include:

- Use of only one person's taxonomy
- No ability to change the categorization scheme

- Superimposition of "matter" over "process" or vice versa
- Too many or too few subcategories
- Limited correlations of categories to safety (e.g., if by property or chemistry)

7.4 Categorization for Health and Environmental Risk Assessment

Efforts in categorization for health and environmental risk assessment were initially developed for chemical substances before the advent of manufactured nanomaterials. A variety of frameworks have been devised to date for chemicals (Table 7.1); however, two main techniques have been described for the development of chemical categorization: the analog and the category approach. The Organization for Economic Co-operation and Development (OECD) has released guidance on categorization that describes these two main techniques [15, 16].

For the analog approach, grouping is based on a small number of chemicals. Often grouping using the analog approach consists of just two chemicals: the analog and the target chemical. Here, chemical substances are assessed on an individual basis; the selection of a chemical analog with known endpoint information is used to predict the same endpoint for a target substance that is considered similar on the basis of the grouping criteria using the principles of read-across [15]. Under the category approach, chemicals are grouped on the basis of similar physicochemical, toxicological, or ecotoxicological properties. Unlike the analog approach, a large number of substances are considered and assessments are made by evaluating the category as a whole. This makes the analysis of trends across endpoints possible, and trend analysis can be applied for filling data gaps in addition to read-across techniques [15].

The analog and category approaches are the two main methods for the grouping of chemicals and are used to determine the equivalence between a novel and a known substance. If two materials are deemed equivalent through grouping, a concept of read-across can be used to fill data gaps. Techniques for filling these data gaps vary based on the approach used for grouping but include the read-across method, trend analysis, and quantitative structure–activity relationships (QSARs) [16]. The read-across method fills data gaps by using surrogate data from a similar substance (analog approach) or category (category approach). If the category approach is adopted, trend analysis can also be utilized to fill data gaps for unknown substances. Here, predictive changes in properties of members of the same category are analyzed; these trends are used to predict the properties (i.e., fill data gaps) for new substances in the same category. Similarly, QSARs can be utilized to help fill data gaps when chemicals are grouped. A quantitative relationship between chemical structure or physicochemical properties and an effect or activity is made. This quantitative relationship is then used to fill data gaps for unknown substances on the basis of their chemical structure or physicochemical properties [16]. Ultimately, read-across concepts (i.e., read-across method, trend analysis, and QSAR) reduce the need to test every chemical for every endpoint and result in considerable efficiencies in terms of time and money, while addressing recent calls to reduce animal testing, limiting extensive testing to the most hazardous materials.

7.4.1 Categorization of Nanomaterials for Risk Assessment

Categorization offers a technique to aid in the health and environmental risk assessment of manufactured nanomaterials. In the assessment of nanomaterials, as with all substances, risk is determined by the hazard of a substance (i.e., its potential to cause harm), as well as its use and exposure (i.e., the likelihood of release and actual extent of exposure to that substance). If grouping principles are applied to categorize nanomaterials, data gaps can be filled by estimating these properties from similar substances using the read-across concepts described before. Further, the criteria used for grouping of nanomaterials can be selected to achieve a variety of goals related to risk assessment, including screening and priority setting, classification and labeling, and filling of regulatory information requirements [15]. However, several challenges in applying the grouping concepts currently used for chemicals also apply for nanomaterials [15].

The grouping of nanomaterials is a more complex endeavor compared to the grouping of conventional chemicals, which relates, at least in part, to measurement challenges. For grouping to aid in risk assessment, frameworks need to assess and categorize nanomaterials by criteria that relate to risk. The majority of nanomaterial-grouping frameworks to date acknowledge an ultimate goal of forming categories for nanomaterials on the basis of physicochemical properties as they relate to hazards in order to group nanomaterials on the basis of risk potential [13]. Such an approach would allow novel materials to be rapidly and efficiently evaluated for risk by characterizing their physicochemical properties, categorizing them, and using read-across to quickly ascertain hazards. However, such frameworks are not yet possible. Measurement challenges and the diversity of particle-related properties so far tested have not resulted in a clear consensus on properties of nanomaterials that relate to adverse biological outcomes [16]. Studies attempting to investigate such correlations have identified over a dozen physicochemical properties of nanomaterials that could contribute to their hazard, including chemical composition, size, shape, aspect ratio, surface charge, redox activity, dissolution, crystallinity, surface coatings, and state of agglomeration or dispersion [4, 17]. Determining correlates between physicochemical properties and adverse biological effects is complex [5]. Interdependent relationships exist between various physicochemical properties, isolating and testing these properties for correlates to adverse outcomes is difficult, and there is a lack of reliable, high-throughput, cost-effective physicochemical characterization methods to reliably link properties to effects.

Difficulties in the grouping of nanomaterials for risk assessment also stem from uncertainties surrounding their use and exposure. These are key determinates of risk. The challenges of measuring and characterizing nanomaterials in environmental and biological matrices also contribute, which are important to understand their fate, transport, and potential for exposure. Furthermore, the physicochemical characteristics described before change over the life cycle of a nanomaterial, varying with time and when introduced to new environments and ultimately influencing their behavior and fate [15].

The uncertainties surrounding nanomaterial hazard, use, and exposure led the OECD Working Party on Manufactured Nanomaterials (WPMN) to conclude in its 2014 report on the guidance and grouping of Chemicals that "at present, it seems premature to develop guidance on grouping specifically for nanomaterials" [15].

However, since the WPMN conclusion in 2014, significant strides have been made in our understanding of nanomaterials that relate to both their hazard and exposure, which have led to the development of some classification schemes. Although knowledge gaps exist, stakeholders can and need to utilize the information we have now to move the field forward, avoid a "paralysis by analysis," and build a strong database to inform on assessing risks of new materials [18]. Accordingly, categorizations of nanomaterials should be based on the best-available evidence, take into consideration uncertainties, and be continually re-evaluated as new data are generated. An overview of some of the current approaches to nanomaterial categorization is discussed next.

7.5 Proposed Approaches for Grouping Nanomaterials

7.5.1 Approaches to Grouping for Regulatory Risk Assessment of Nanomaterials

Currently, the regulation of nanomaterials in countries around the world falls under existing legislation for chemicals and products in specific use categories (e.g., foods, cosmetics). Government agencies in many countries have released guidance documents for analyzing the hazards and completing risk assessments for nanomaterials under existing rather than new frameworks (e.g., the US Environmental Protection Agency [EPA]; Environment and Climate Change Canada) [19, 20]. A part of this effort is the formation of categories to aid in regulatory risk assessment of nanomaterials.

One of the major efforts in categorization of nanomaterials for regulatory risk assessment was recently completed by the Regulatory Cooperation Council Nanotechnology Initiative (RCC-NI). The

RCC-NI was an effort to align future regulation of nanomaterials in Canada and the United States; part of the deliverable for this initiative was development of a joint nanomaterial classification scheme to be used for regulatory purposes in both countries [21]. Toward that end, while several parameters were identified in the report (e.g., exposure, use, mode of action [MoA], physicochemical properties), the initial RCC-NI classification scheme used similarities in chemical composition as the basis for grouping (Table 7.2). The RCC-NI proposed seven categories for nanomaterials on the basis of chemical composition: carbon nanotubes; inorganic carbons; metal oxides and metalloid oxides; metals, metal salts, and metalloids; semiconductor quantum dots; organics; and others [21]. Although not part of the grouping criteria per se, the report highlights physicochemical properties of nanomaterials within each of these categories that might be used to identify similarities between materials and evaluate their potential as analog substances for read-across. Under this grouping, hybrid nanomaterials (those nanomaterials composed of multiple chemical compositions) would fall under multiple chemical categories and are not part of the proposed classification scheme. A major goal of this approach for the grouping of nanomaterials was to identify nanomaterials that require unique considerations in risk assessment, and subsequently select appropriate analog substances to allow read-across information [21].

Subsequent efforts of the RCC-NI led to the development of a particle screening assessment framework that begins to integrate specific physicochemical properties of nanomaterials in regulatory decision making [22]. The RCC-NI particle screening assessment framework aims to use physicochemical characteristics (e.g., particle/fiber size, shape, aspect ratio, solubility, composition, surface chemistry) and routes of exposure (e.g., oral, dermal, inhalation) to categorize nanomaterials to focus on potential human health concerns and suggest additional testing requirements for the risk assessment of nanomaterials. The RCC-NI integrates nanomaterial categorizations into a tiered flowchart, incorporating cut-off parameters for grouping and linking categories to additional testing for the risk assessment of nanomaterials. The framework is meant to be iterative, incorporating new knowledge as it emerges to further identify concerns or additional testing required for the risk assessment [22].

Table 7.2 Proposed approaches for grouping nanomaterials

	Proposed categories	Parameters for grouping	Category based on
Regulatory Risk Assessment			
Regulatory Cooperation Council	1. Carbon nanotubes 2. Inorganic carbon 3. Metal oxides and metalloid oxides 4. Metals, metal salts, and metalloids 5. Semiconductor quantum dots 6. Organics 7. Other	• Similarities in chemical composition • Mirror traditional classification schemes used by regulators for chemicals	Classes of nanomaterials that require nanospecific consideration in risk assessment
Human Health Risk Assessment			
British Standards Institute	1. Fibrous 2. CMAR 3. Insoluble 4. Soluble	Physicochemical characteristics of nanomaterials (aspect ratio, solubility) and potential toxicity (CMAR)	Toxic effects that have been reported in conventional (non-nano) analogs
German Federal Institute for Occupational Safety and Health	1. Soluble nanomaterials 2. Biopersistent nanomaterials with toxicological properties 3. Biopersistent nanomaterials without toxicological properties 4. Biopersistent, fibrous nanomaterials	Physicochemical characteristics, biopersistence, and toxicological properties	Toxic effects that have been reported in conventional (non-nano) analogs

(Continued)

Table 7.2 (*Continued*)

	Proposed categories	Parameters for grouping	Category based on
National Institute for Occupational Safety and Health	1. Higher-solubility nanomaterials 2. Poorly soluble, low-toxicity particles 3. Poorly soluble, high-toxicity particles 4. Fibrous particles	Physicochemical characteristics of nanomaterials (aspect ratio, solubility) and potential toxicity	• Potential MoA classes that relate to toxicity of nanomaterials • MoA for category 1: Toxic ions reaching systemic tissue • MoA for category 2: Toxicity based on total deposited particles in respiratory tract • MoA for category 3: Reactive properties, in addition to deposition in respiratory tract • MoA for category 4: Biopersistence, incomplete clearance, interference with cell division, genotoxicity

	Proposed categories	Parameters for grouping	Category based on
European Centre for Ecotoxicology and Toxicology of Chemicals	1. Soluble nanomaterials 2. Biopersistent, high-aspect-ratio nanomaterials 3. Passive nanomaterials 4. Active nanomaterials	Nanomaterial functionality: intrinsic properties, system-dependent properties, biophysical interactions, and toxicological properties	Groupings based on toxicological MoA
Environmental Risk Assessment			
NanoImpact Net	1. Carbon 2. Mineral based 3. Organic 4. Composites/hybrids	• Chemical composition of nanomaterials • Specifically mentions integration of physicochemical criteria for grouping as knowledge becomes available on how these characteristics relate to environmental risk	• Similarities in chemical composition • Evolution from chemical frameworks currently used
US Army Corps Engineering Research and Development Center	1. Materials that are nanostructured in bulk form 2. Materials that are nanostructured on the surface 3. Materials that contain nanoparticles	Physicochemical characteristics of nanomaterials (e.g., size, shape, composition)	Aims to categorize nanomaterials by likelihood of release and exposure routes of nanomaterials

CMAR, carcinogenic, mutagenic, asthmagenic, or reproductive toxin; MoA, modes of action.

7.5.2 Approaches to Grouping for Human Health Risk Assessment of Nanomaterials

Several categorization frameworks have been developed to inform human health concerns related to occupational exposures to nanomaterials. These frameworks draw on a relatively longer history of occupational safety and health practices compared to chemicals management in postmanufacturing environments (e.g., in consumer products). Furthermore, similar principles relating to the physical structure of particles and fibers were easily adapted for nanoscale materials, which were previously managed as fine or ultrafine particles or fibers. In particular, several nongovernmental standards organizations and national authorities released some of the earliest frameworks for categorization of nanomaterials to aid in occupational health and safety risk assessment, including the British Standards Institute (BSI), the German Federal Institute for Occupational Safety and Health (BAuA), and the National Institute for Occupational Safety and Health (NIOSH) in the United States (Table 7.2).

The BSI proposed four categories in its guide to safe handling and disposal of manufactured nanomaterials (Table 7.2) [23]. This grouping framework employs physicochemical properties of nanomaterials as category criteria (solubility and aspect ratio) that relate to known toxicity in conventional (non-nano) materials to allow read-across, with the assumption that nanomaterials have a greater hazard on the basis of mass than non-nanoscale forms of the same material. The four categories are fibrous; carcinogenic, mutagenic, asthmagenic, or reproductive toxin (CMAR); insoluble; and soluble. The fibrous category is described as insoluble nanomaterials with a high aspect ratio, and CMAR is described as nanomaterials whose bulk form is classified as CMAR. The latter two categories are based on their exclusion from fibrous and CMAR categories and their solubility: insoluble or poorly soluble or soluble and neither fibrous nor CMAR [23].

The Committee on Hazardous Substances (AGS) under the German BAuA released Announcement 527 (2013) outlining recommendations and guidance for risk assessment to protect the health and safety of workers during use or production of manufactured nanomaterials [24]. In its assessment of health hazards of nanomaterials, the BAuA concluded that, at a minimum, an assessment should be charged with considering both effects based on chemical composition and biopersistence. As part of this guidance, four categories were proposed for the grouping of nanomaterials to aid in the occupational risk assessment with an emphasis on inhalation exposure (Table 7.2). Similar to the BSI, the categories are based on toxic effects (either known for nanomaterials or the microscale form) as well as two physicochemical parameters: solubility and aspect ratio. The four proposed categories are soluble nanomaterials, biopersistent nanomaterials with specific toxicological properties, biopersistence nanomaterials without specific toxicological properties (i.e., granular biopersistent particle [GBP]), and biopersistent fibrous nanomaterials [24]. In the BAuA framework, solubility is used as a measure of biopersistence and specific criteria are given for classifying according to solubility, adopting definitions in the *European Pharmacopoeia*. Similarly, aspect ratio is used to categorize nanomaterials as fibrous, and criteria are adopted according to the World Health Organization (WHO) fiber criteria. These categorizations are used by the BAuA as a starting point for deciding on specific protocols for occupational risk assessment, for determining occupational exposure limits (OELs), and for implementing occupational exposure measures such as engineering controls and personal protective equipment [24]. The BAuA also integrated these groupings into a tiered flowchart, incorporating cut-off parameters for grouping and linking categories to protective measures to be used in occupational risk assessment of nanomaterials [24].

NIOSH also laid out a categorization framework for occupational risk assessment of nanomaterials (Table 7.2). In the proposed approach, risk categories for nanomaterials are based on toxicological MoA [25]. Physicochemical properties, including solubility, size, shape, surface reactivity, and surface area, are used as parameters on the basis of how they influence the biological response of nanomaterials through different MoA. An objective of the proposed grouping is then to develop benchmark substances (i.e., reference materials that have been thoroughly evaluated and tested with standardized protocols) within each category to use as an analog substance to quantitatively fill data gaps and derive

OELs for new nanomaterials that are similarly grouped via read-across techniques [25]. Focusing on inhalation exposure, four risk-based categories were proposed on the basis of MoA to group nanomaterials: higher-solubility particles (MoA based on release of toxic ions); poorly soluble, low-toxicity particles (MoA based on deposition of inhaled GBP); poorly soluble, high-toxicity particles (MoA based on inhaled reactive particles); and fibrous particles (MoA based on biopersistence, incomplete clearance, cytotoxicity, and genotoxicity) [25].

The European Centre for Ecotoxicology and Toxicology of Chemicals (ECETOC) Nano Task Force proposed a Decision-making Framework for the Grouping and Testing of nanomaterials (DF4nanoGrouping) [26]. Similar to the previously described approaches, it aims to categorize nanomaterials by their MoA that results in apical toxic effects with a focus on exposure via inhalation (Table 7.2). However, unlike other categorization frameworks for human health risk assessment that relate one or a few physicochemical properties to group nanomaterials on the basis of their risk (so-called intrinsic properties that are independent of the biological environment), DF4nanoGrouping aims to categorize nanomaterials using a functionality-driven and exposure-based grouping concept.

Functionality under the DF4nanoGrouping framework incorporates a variety of grouping parameters including intrinsic physicochemical properties, system-dependent properties (characteristics that change on the basis of the biological environment such as agglomeration), uptake, biopersistence, and biodistribution, as well as toxicological outcomes. Exposure under DF4nanoGrouping is also used as a qualifier to assess risk and includes consideration of the manufacture, release, and route of exposure. These parameters are used in three tiers to assign nanomaterials to one of four main categories: (i) soluble nanomaterials; (ii) biopersistent, high-aspect-ratio nanomaterials; (iii) passive nanomaterials; and (iv) active nanomaterials [26]. For these groupings specific criteria and cut-off values are listed and additional subgroupings may be performed [27]. While the objective of the DF4nanoGrouping framework is similar to others (i.e., group nanomaterials by their toxicological MoA), this framework attempts to incorporate a broader suite of parameters for grouping that more accurately reflect the complexity of nanomaterial hazard assessment across its life cycle. Practical in focus, the initial tier seeks to define whether a material meets the definition of a nanomaterial and, if so, then categorize it. However, beyond the initial tiers, the framework is aspirational, as it proposes, for example, using Adverse Outcome Pathway analysis for MoA classification, which is currently only in early stages of development.

Additional categorization frameworks have been proposed to aid in human health risk assessment for exposures beyond inhalation and occupational exposures. As discussed in a review by Arts et al. (2014), a major motivation for these alternate categorization frameworks is to address concerns related to exposure from nanomaterials being incorporated into cosmetics and hygiene products [28]. Grouping frameworks for nanomaterials in cosmetics include a proposal by the International Cooperation on Cosmetics Regulation (ICCR) Working Group on Safety Approaches for Nanomaterials in Cosmetics [29], the NanoDiversity Evaluation Scheme™ [30], and NanoCosmetics Tool [31].

7.5.3 Approaches to Grouping for Environmental Risk Assessment of Nanomaterials

Grouping of nanomaterials for environmental risk assessment involves considering alternate exposure scenarios that impacts the physicochemical properties and life cycle parameters used for grouping criteria. To inform environmental exposure and hazards, categorizations consider properties of nanomaterials that affect their fate and behavior in the environment and their potential toxicological consequences on organisms. However, in a NanoImpactNet environmental workshop examining potential frameworks for the categorizations of nanomaterials, it was concluded that while strides have been made in understanding the characteristics of nanomaterials that contribute to these environmental effects, they are still not fully understood [32]. At least in 2010, insufficient information was available to construct categories based on such parameters.

As a starting point for the grouping of manufactured nanomaterials for environmental health considerations, an expert workshop suggested a grouping framework based on chemical composition (Table 7.2). It was noted that chemical composition alone was not sufficient in the grouping of nanomaterials and that additional physicochemical parameters of nanomaterials also needed to be utilized in forming categories; however, as it is not clearly understood which characteristics of nanomaterials relate to environmental hazard, the report concluded that additional work is required to derive criteria that can be used to generate these categories to inform on the environmental risks of nanomaterials [32]. As a starting point for classification in environmental risk assessment, three categories were proposed: carbon-based, mineral-based, and organic and composite/hybrid nanomaterials. Subcategories of each of these groupings were proposed on the basis of relevant physicochemical properties; proposed parameters included surface chemistry, aspect ratio, and redox activity, but no consensus emerged. While a starting point, the proposed categorization requires additional studies to determine the criteria that can be used for further categorization beyond chemical composition that relate to environmental behavior [32].

A current effort to categorize nanomaterials for environmental risk assessment is underway by the US Army Engineer Research and Development Center (ERDC) [18]. NanoGRID is proposed as a tiered strategy for environmental risk assessment of products or technologies containing nanomaterials with the goal of directing safety testing in a step-wise progression to concentrate on collecting the most relevant data for risk assessment, while eliminating unnecessary testing. Under this approach, testing is concluded at any one of the five tiers once sufficient risk information has been gathered for assessment. Differently from other frameworks, NanoGRID first focuses on the potential for release and exposure to a nanomaterial or nano-enabled technology [18].

Categorization of products incorporating nanomaterials occurs in tier 1 of NanoGRID and is an important step in the determination of risk and subsequent testing (if any), which assesses whether a nanospecific approach to risk assessment is necessary. If specific classification criteria are not met, the material is judged to not require further evaluation in the framework. The parameters are used for an initial grouping into one of three main categories: (i) materials that are nanostructured in bulk form (bulk), (ii) materials that are nanostructured on the surface (surface), or (iii) materials that contain nanoparticles (Table 7.2) [18]. Subsequent subgroupings are then completed for each main category, and are outlined in Table 7.3. This approach aims to categorize nanotechnologies by likelihood of release and exposure routes of nanomaterials; such groupings feed directly into tier 2 in assessing release potential of nanomaterials. For example, category 1 materials have a low likelihood of release of nanomaterials into the environment as they represent solid materials that are unlikely to release their fused nanostructures; as such, in the NanoGRID framework, further testing may not be required for nanospecific hazards. In contrast, categories 3C and 3D represent nanomaterials suspended in liquid or air and may have a higher likelihood of release into the environment, depending on use. Here, further evaluation is required to assess risk, and the material proceeds through the framework [18]. Again, the initial focus on exposure and release, as well as environmental pathways, is unique among proposed risk categorization frameworks for manufactured nanomaterials.

Categorization is an important first step of the larger NanoGRID framework that aims to provide a testing strategy for environmental risk assessment. Once categorization is complete (tier 1), tier 2 is a worst-case determination of the nanomaterial release potential under scenarios of its intended use. If release is likely, tier 3 considers how the properties of the released nanomaterial impact behavior and fate in the environment, and specific testing is conducted to measure the forms and concentrations. Under tier 4, the hazard of the released nanomaterial is determined with targeted biological testing under relevant exposure conditions (previously determined in tier 3). If risk has not been adequately assessed through tiers 1–4, additional information is collected in tier 5 with a case-specific investigation (Table 7.4) [18]. The ERDC's NanoGRID categorization and testing framework offers a significant advance over previous methods for environmental risk assessment of nanomaterials and injects the important concept of exposure and potential release evaluation prior to ecological toxicity testing.

Table 7.3 Proposed categories and subcategories in the NanoGRID framework

Category 1: Materials that are nanostructured in bulk form, for example, nanocrystalline metallic alloys and nanoporous materials	
1A	Solid materials with average grain sizes in the 1–100 nm range in all three spatial dimensions Fused into a single solid Composed of only one phase and material type
1B	Solid materials with average grain sizes in the 1–100 nm range in all three spatial dimensions Fused into a single solid Composed of multiple phases and/or multiple materials (e.g., nanoporous materials)
Category 2: Materials that are nanostructured on the surface, for example, nanoscale structured surfaces and films	
2A	Single-phase materials with a nanoscale-structured surface Nanostructures that range from 1 to 100 nm and extend in two dimensions
2B	Nanoscale films made up of two materials Nanostructures that range from 1 to 100 nm and extend in one dimension
2C	Nanoscale-structured surface made up of two materials Nanostructures that range from 1 to 100 nm and extend in two dimensions
Category 3: Materials that contain nanoparticles, for example, quantum dots, fullerenes, nanotubes, and nanowires	
3A	Nanoparticles bound to the surface of another solid structure
3B	Nanoparticles that are suspended in a solid
3C	Nanoparticles that are suspended in a liquid
3D	Airborne nanoparticles

7.6 Analysis

Manufactured nanomaterials represent a huge diversity of chemically and structurally unique materials; this diversity, coupled with a variety of physicochemical properties, exposure scenarios, and life cycle considerations, means that many approaches to grouping nanomaterials for risk assessment are critically important to advancing risk analysis and risk management. What existing concepts for grouping nanomaterials have in common is focusing on particular aspects of the nanomaterials life cycle, from production to disposal [28]. Several proposed categorization frameworks focus on occupational exposure of nanomaterials during their production; few seek to group nanomaterials on the basis of environmental exposure during their use, disposal, and release. Most categorization schemes incorporate a tiered or stepwise approach, and some envision future evaluations based on science that does not yet exist. The focus in the ECETOC framework on intrinsic and extrinsic physicochemical properties; biophysical interactions; exposure, use, and release; and toxicological effects reflects the broad diversity of categories developing from several large research consortia [28]. This is a significant advance for nanomaterials over earlier frameworks basing manufactured nanomaterial categories on chemical form.

Table 7.4 Tiered approaches utilized in NanoGRID and DF4nanoGrouping

	NanoGRID	**DF4nanoGrouping**
General summary	A progressive testing strategy, with specific goals for each tier. Tier 1: Define and characterize Tier 2: Release potential Tier 3: Environmental persistence Tier 4: Hazard assessment (biological testing for acute and chronic toxicity) Tier 5: Material-specific investigation	A three-tiered grouping strategy to categorize nanomaterials into one of four main groups (based on MoA) using intrinsic material properties, extrinsic material properties, biopersistence, uptake, and cellular and apical toxic effects
Proposed categories	• Materials that are nanostructured in bulk form • Materials that are nano-structured on the surface • Materials that contain nanoparticles	• Soluble nanomaterials • Biopersistent, high-aspect-ratio nanomaterials • Passive nanomaterials • Active nanomaterials
Tier 0	Tier 0: Collect basic information.	Tier 0: Is it nano?

(*Continued*)

Table 7.4 (*Continued*)

	NanoGRID	DF4nanoGrouping
Tier 1	Tier 1: Is it nano? Define and characterize: Technology category determination by physical and chemical property evaluation • Materials that are nanostructured in bulk form (bulk) • Materials that are nanostructured on the surface (surface) • Materials that contain nanoparticles (particles)	Tier 1: Use intrinsic material properties to assign nanomaterials to group 1 (soluble nanomaterials) or do preliminary assignment to groups 2–4. Threshold value for assignment to group 1: water solubility > 100 mg/L Preliminary assignment of nanomaterials to group 2, 3, or 4 on the basis of other listed intrinsic properties: use, release, and route of exposure qualifier analysis
Tier 2	Tier 2: Release Evaluate potential for release by properties and use categories, first assuming 100% release; then by scenario-based screening/ testing to environmental receptors (air, water, soil) under realistic conditions.	Tier 2: Use functionality properties to corroborate assignments to group 2, 3, or 4. Functionality properties include system-dependent material properties, biophysical interactions, and in vitro effects. Threshold values for assignment to group 2: aspect ratio < 3:1; length > 5 μm; diameter < 3 μm; biopersistence (dissolution rate < 100 mg/L or pulmonary half-life ≥ 40 days) Threshold values for assignment to group 3: toxic component < 0.1%; surface reactivity < 10%; Mn_2O_3 reactivity in cytochrome c or FRAS assay; dispersibility AAN > 3; no cellular effects at < 10 μg/cm^2 If material not assigned to group 1, 2, or 3, then assigned to group 4: use, release, and route of exposure qualifier analysis

	NanoGRID	DF4nanoGrouping
Tier 3	Tier 3: Fate Evaluate potential for release through testing and persistence/bioavailability in environmental media. Analyze properties, transport, and fate information and develop studies, as necessary.	Tier 3: Assign confirmatory groups and subgroups on the basis of in vivo short-term testing. Short-term inhalation study (in vivo) used to confirm assignment to group 3 or 4: use, release, and route of exposure qualifier analysis • If low toxicity (e.g., NOAEC > 10 mg/m^3), group 3 assignment confirmed • If high toxicity (e.g., NOAEC < 10 mg/m^3), group 4 assignment confirmed.
Tier 4	Tier 4: Hazard Ecological organism acute and chronic toxicity testing in relevant media	
Tier 5	Tier 5: Class specific Where warranted, material and site-specific testing	

NOAEC, no observed adverse effect concentration.

Clearly, categorizing manufactured nanomaterials for risk assessment is a developing practice based on emergence of new knowledge, and the proposed frameworks here will no doubt continue to evolve as our knowledge of key relationships between properties and behavior develops. For now, each proposed categorization approach adopts key risk assessment principles of decision making under uncertainty. This means the current approaches are starting points for the grouping of nanomaterials; they will need to be continually reassessed, updated, or reclassified as new information emerges.

7.6.1 Regulatory Approaches to Categorization

A number of risk assessment approaches for the categorization of nanomaterials acknowledge an ultimate goal of grouping nanomaterials by physicochemical properties as they relate to hazards. In 2016, the WPMN published a report surveying the present use and development of "grouping, equivalence, and read-across on the basis of physicochemical properties" (GERA-PC) of nanomaterials by regulators in human and environmental hazard assessment [16]. On the basis of survey results from eight OECD member countries, regulators worldwide agreed that regulatory implementation of GERA-PC was not possible until more reliable data were available [16]. According to respondents, the development of a categorization framework for nanomaterials on the basis of physicochemical properties was hindered by both scientific (e.g., lack of comprehensive and reliable data sets with standardized testing methods) and technical challenges (e.g., sample preparation and material characterization). This led to the conclusion by several countries that, currently, a:

> "lack of scientific knowledge limits the confidence/applicability of this [GERA-PC] classification scheme for hazard classification" [16].

Given that most regulators acknowledge that categorization of nanomaterials by GERA-PC is not yet possible, most preliminary categorizations of nanomaterials in a regulatory context take a similar approach to chemicals: categories are based on chemical composition. The benefit to regulators in adopting this approach is clear: it integrates well into current chemical frameworks that are also based on chemical composition and can be used to identify analog substances for nanomaterials, allowing read-across information to be used in risk assessment for regulatory purposes. However, several reports have concluded that the use of chemical composition alone for the grouping of nanomaterials is insufficient given their complexity, and additional physicochemical parameters should be used for grouping [33].

Under the proposed RCC-NI categorization, grouping of nanomaterials on the basis of chemical composition alone doesn't allow for selection of useful analogs for read-across information.

Although the RRC-NI report does highlight several intrinsic physicochemical properties within each category to assess potential analogs for similarity, these parameters are generally described and not directly used for grouping [21]. This represents a significant initial effort, but as more data become available, future iterations of this grouping framework might evolve to include additional intrinsic and system-dependent physicochemical characteristics as parameters to define categories. More explicit guidance (e.g., cut-off values for each characteristic) on how physicochemical characteristics might be used as parameters would also facilitate grouping by either the analog or the category approach, allowing read-across information to be used in a regulatory risk assessment context. Another major drawback of this approach is in grouping hybrid nanomaterials; materials composed of several different chemical compositions are difficult to group by chemistry, and the RCC-NI report acknowledges that currently, it is not possible. Given the number of emerging nanomaterials, which will likely be engineered with increasing complexity over time, hybrid materials will need to be addressed in future categorization frameworks.

Subsequent efforts by the RCC-NI have moved this effort forward and begun to integrate specific physicochemical properties of nanomaterials in decision making. The RCC-NI particle screening assessment framework aims to use the physicochemical characteristics of nanomaterials (specifically size, architecture, aspect ratio, solubility, composition, and surface chemistry) to focus on potential human health concerns and suggest additional testing requirements for the risk assessment of these materials [22].

7.6.2 Approaches to Categorization for Human Health Risk Assessment

The occupational exposure frameworks each apply a similar approach to categorization of nanomaterials. The BSI, BAuA, and NIOSH approaches focus on inhalation as the route of exposure and utilize two predominant physicochemical characteristics as parameters for grouping, solubility and shape (aspect ratio), to create categories based on MoA and toxicological effects. While the specific categories vary slightly for each approach, the BSI, BAuA, and NIOSH each propose four similar categories for nanomaterials: fibrous, soluble, insoluble with low toxicity, and insoluble with higher toxicity. These proposed categories are based on known toxic effects in conventional (non-nano) analog substances and draw upon known toxicological MoA for respirable particles for which there is a wealth of knowledge in occupational exposure settings.

The goal of each of these proposed occupational exposure frameworks is to derive OELs to inform the occupational health and safety management of nanomaterials. However, the basis for deriving OELs varies with each approach. The BSI proposed to use its groupings to apply read-across to conventional materials to derive OELs for nanomaterials, acknowledging that nanomaterials likely represent a greater hazard than non-nanoscale forms of the same material on the basis of mass. In its guidance document, the BSI was one of the first institutes to suggest benchmark exposure limits (BELs) for nanomaterials: 0.01 fibers/mL for fibrous nanomaterials, 10% of the OEL for non-nanoscale forms in the CMAR category, 6.6% of the OEL for non-nanoscale forms in the insoluble category, and 50% of the existing OEL for non-nanoscale forms in the soluble category [23]. The proposed approach by NIOSH suggested using the framework to develop benchmark materials for each category, allowing read-across to new nanomaterials that are similarly grouped, to quantitatively fill data gaps and derive OELs [25]. However, Kuempel et al. (2012) acknowledged the significant effort associated with thoroughly evaluating and testing benchmark materials [34]. Since OELs have only so far been derived for select few nanomaterials, hazard and control-banding approaches remain as NIOSH's most common recommendation [35].

These frameworks represent some of the earliest efforts to group nanomaterials and focused on inhalation exposure in an occupational setting. In comparison, DF4nanoGrouping for human health risk assessment incorporates a broader suite of parameters for grouping that better reflects the complexity of manufactured nanomaterials. It includes considerations from across the life cycle of nanomaterials and aims to moves beyond consideration of occupational exposure [26]. However, similar to previous approaches, DF4nanoGrouping also focuses predominantly on inhalation exposure. There is a need for risk frameworks to start incorporating other routes such as dermal and oral exposure of nanomaterials in grouping. In addition, Arts et al. (2015) acknowledged that the current grouping concept does not take physical hazards such as flammability into account and may be a consideration for future frameworks.

7.6.3 Categorization for Environmental Endpoints

Different from the approaches discussed before, grouping nanomaterials on their potential for environmental risk considers properties of nanomaterials that affect their likelihood of release, environmental exposure routes, and fate and behavior in the environment. This can result in significantly different groupings compared to approaches used for regulatory or human health considerations. Initial concepts in grouping nanomaterials for environmental risk assessment suggested chemical composition as a main parameter for categorization, while acknowledging additional parameters must be incorporated. Recently, the NanoGRID framework has been proposed and represents a more comprehensive approach that integrates the grouping of nanomaterials with a tiered assessment strategy for environmental risk assessment [18]. A key benefit of this approach is that it focuses characterization protocols on those most essential for evaluating hazard and offers a rationale for grouping nanomaterials on the basis of ecotoxicity testing strategies. In addition, the step-wise progression in the framework means that testing is concluded once sufficient information has been gathered to characterize risk, thereby reducing unnecessary testing. However, similar to the other grouping frameworks, this approach is hindered by limited knowledge about how physicochemical properties of nanomaterials relate to adverse biological and ecological outcomes and the complexity of interactions in natural environments.

7.7 Conclusions

Manufactured nanomaterials represent a class of materials with tremendous potential to improve a vast number of technological sectors. Regulators and producers alike recognize that sound health and environmental risk assessment of nanomaterials is required to get these materials safely to market. However, we currently lack predictive knowledge about the hazards and exposures of many materials in this diverse class of substances, suggesting that individual testing of materials currently is often warranted to adequately assess health and environmental risk, and today, most assessments are on a case-by-case basis.

Categorization offers pathways to improve the health and environmental risk assessment of nanomaterials. If grouping principles are applied to categorize nanomaterials, data gaps for a material can be filled by estimating these properties from similar substances using the read-across concepts described before. The benefits of categorization include resource, time, and cost savings resulting from focused and efficient testing to characterize risk as possible. In addition, categorization offers a moral incentive, addressing recent calls to reduce animal testing.

Current approaches to the categorization of nanomaterials for risk assessment all acknowledge an ultimate goal of grouping nanomaterials by physicochemical properties as they relate to hazard; however, this is hindered by the complexity and lack of agreement about how these parameters relate to potency and hazard. While several groups have agreed that more research is needed to understand these principles, fill data gaps, and inform on nanomaterial grouping, progress continues to be made and investment in continued development of categorization approaches is critical.

There is a need to apply the information we have now to move the field forward, avoid a "paralysis by analysis," and help inform risk assessments. Such hesitations in developing and adopting categorization frameworks for nanomaterials represent its largest barrier to success. No single framework will address every risk assessment scenario, and over time our knowledge about the risks of nanomaterials (in terms of hazard, use, and exposure) will improve. Accordingly, categorizations should be based on the best-available evidence, take into consideration uncertainties, and be constantly re-evaluated as new data are generated.

The occupational exposure frameworks discussed here advance concepts for nanomaterials that have long been applied for chemical substances. Beyond these, several of the frameworks reflect this notion that the field is still evolving, and more recent grouping concepts such as DF4nanoGrouping and NanoGRID are integrating more parameters and factors as data emerges to better predict the hazards and risks of nanomaterials. It has also become apparent that on the basis of the incredible number of considerations when assessing the risk of nanomaterials, no single grouping framework will suffice for all classes of nanomaterials in all situations. These frameworks represent the most current approaches to categorization of nanomaterials and offer significant improvement over dated classification schemes based on chemical composition alone. The field is progressing, and results are emerging for developing categorization approaches that better reflect the complexities in assessing the risks of nanomaterials.

References

1. Nel, A. E., Madler, L., Velegol, D., Xia, T., Hoek, E. M. V., Somasundaran, P., Klaessig, F., Castranova, V., and Thompson, M. (2009). Understanding biophysicochemical interactions at the nano-bio interface. *Nat. Mater.*, **8**(7), 543–557.
2. Aillon, K. L., Xie, Y., El-Gendy, N., Berkland, C. J., and Forrest, M. L. (2009). Effects of nanomaterial physicochemical properties on in vivo toxicity. *Adv. Drug Delivery Rev.*, **61**(6), 457–466.
3. Kim, S. T., Saha, K., Kim, C., and Rotello, V. M. (2013). The role of surface functionality in determining nanoparticle cytotoxicity. *Acc. Chem. Res.*, **46**(3), 681–691.
4. Fubini, B., Ghiazza, M., and Fenoglio, I. (2010). Physico-chemical features of engineered nanoparticles relevant to their toxicity. *Nanotoxicology*, **4**(4), 347–363.
5. Rivera-Gil, P., Jimenez de Aberasturi, D., Wulf, V., Pelaz, B., del Pino, P., Zhao, Y., de la Fuente, J. M., Ruiz de Larramendi, I., Rojo, T., Liang, X.-J., and Parak, W. J. (2013). The challenge to relate the physicochemical properties of colloidal nanoparticles to their cytotoxicity. *Acc. Chem. Res.*, **46**(3), 743–749.
6. United Nations. (2013). Globally harmonized system of classification and labelling of chemicals (GHS): fifth revised edition. New York and Geneva.
7. 40 CFR Part 261 Subpart C - Characteristics of hazardous waste.
8. U.S. Environmental Protection Agency. (2006). Organophosphorus cumulative risk assessment.

9. U.S. Environmental Protection Agency. (2010). Recommended toxicity equivalence factors (TEFs) for human health risk assessment of 2,3,7,8-tetrachlorodibenzo-p-dioxin and dioxin-like compounds.
10. Clean Production Action. (2013). *GreenScreen®* for safer chemicals chemical hazard assessment procedure v1.2.
11. Bruner, J. S., Goodnow, J. J., and Austin, G. A. (1977). *A Study of Thinking*; with an appendix on language by Roger W. Brown (R. E. Krieger Pub. Co., Huntington, N.Y.).
12. Verma, A., and Stellacci, F. (2010). Effect of surface properties on nanoparticle–cell interactions. *Small*, **6**(1), 12–21.
13. Godwin, H., Nameth, C., Avery, D., Bergeson, L. L., Bernard, D., Beryt, E., Boyes, W., Brown, S., Clippinger, A. J., Cohen, Y., Doa, M., Hendren, C. O., Holden, P., Houck, K., Kane, A. B., Klaessig, F., Kodas, T., Landsiedel, R., Lynch, I., Malloy, T., Miller, M. B., Muller, J., Oberdörster, G., Petersen, E. J., Pleus, R. C., Sayre, P., Stone, V., Sullivan, K. M., Tentschert, J., Wallis, P., and Nel, A. E. (2015). Nanomaterial categorization for assessing risk potential to facilitate regulatory decision-making. *ACS Nano*, **9**(4), 3409–3417.
14. Monfardini, E., Probst, L., Szenci, K., Cambier, B., and Frideres, L. (2012). Emerging industries: report on the methodology for their classification and on the most active, significant and relevant new emerging industrial sectors. European Cluster Observatory.
15. Organization for Economic Cooperation and Development. (2014). Guidance on the grouping of chemicals, second edition.
16. Organization for Economic Cooperation and Development. (2016). Approaches on nano grouping/equivalence/read-across concepts based on physical-chemical properties (GERA-PC) for regulatory regimes.
17. Oomen, A. G., Bos, P. M. J., Fernandes, T. F., Hund-Rinke, K., Boraschi, D., Byrne, H. J., Aschberger, K., Gottardo, S., von der Kammer, F., Kühnel, D., Hristozov, D., Marcomini, A., Migliore, L., Scott-Fordsmand, J., Wick, P., and Landsiedel, R. (2014). Concern-driven integrated approaches to nanomaterial testing and assessment--report of the NanoSafety Cluster Working Group 10. *Nanotoxicology*, **8**(3), 334–348.
18. Collier, Z. A., Kennedy, A. J., Poda, A. R., Cuddy, M. F., Moser, R. D., MacCuspie, R. I., Harmon, A., Plourde, K., Haines, C. D., and Steevens, J. A. (2015). Tiered guidance for risk-informed environmental health and safety testing of nanotechnologies. *J. Nanopart. Res.*, **17**(3), 1–21.

19. U.S. Environmental Protection Agency. (2015). Chemical substances when manufactured or processed as nanoscale materials; TSCA reporting and recordkeeping requirements. **80**, 18330.
20. Notice with respect to certain nanomaterials in Canadian commerce.
21. Regulatory Cooperation Council - Nanotechnology Initiative. (2014). Final Report - Work Element 2, Priority Setting: Development of a joint nanomaterials classification scheme.
22. Regulatory Cooperation Council, Nanotechnology Initiative. (2013). Particle screening assessment framework.
23. British Standards Institute. (2007). Nanotechnologies, Part 2: Guide to safe handling and disposal of manufactured nanomaterials.
24. BAuA (2013). Announcement 527, announcements on hazardous substances, manufactured nanomaterials.
25. Kuempel, E. D., Roberts, J., Eastlake, A., and Stefaniak, A. (2015). Guidance on nanomaterial hazards and risks.
26. Arts, J. H. E., Hadi, M., Irfan, M.-A., Keene, A. M., Kreiling, R., Lyon, D., Maier, M., Michel, K., Petry, T., Sauer, U. G., Warheit, D., Wiench, K., Wohlleben, W., and Landsiedel, R. (2015). A decision-making framework for the grouping and testing of nanomaterials (DF4nanoGrouping). *Regul. Toxicol. Pharm.*, **71**(2), S1–27.
27. Arts, J. H. E., Irfan, M.-A., Keene, A. M., Kreiling, R., Lyon, D., Maier, M., Michel, K., Neubauer, N., Petry, T., Sauer, U. G., Warheit, D., Wiench, K., Wohlleben, W., and Landsiedel, R. (2015). Case studies putting the decision-making framework for the grouping and testing of nanomaterials (DF4nanoGrouping) into practice. *Regul. Toxicol. Pharm.*, **76**, 234–261.
28. Arts, J. H. E., Hadi, M., Keene, A. M., Kreiling, R., Lyon, D., Maier, M., Michel, K., Petry, T., Sauer, U. G., Warheit, D., Wiench, K., and Landsiedel, R. (2014). A critical appraisal of existing concepts for the grouping of nanomaterials. *Regul. Toxicol. Pharm.*, **70**(2), 492–506.
29. Araki, D., Bose, R., Chaudhry, Q., Dewan, K., Dufour, E., Hirose, A., Lafranconi, M., Montemayor, B., Ratzlaff, D., Rauscher, H., and Suwa, T. (2013). Report of the International Cooperation on Cosmetics Regulation (ICCR) safety approaches to nanomaterials in cosmetics.
30. Anzai, T., Kaminishi, M., Poth, A., Handley, J., and Satoh, T. (2014). Worldwide trend in nanomaterial safety evaluation. *Jpn. J. Environ. Toxicol.*, **15**, 17–29.
31. de Jong, W. H., Delmaar, C., Gosens, I., Nijkamp, M., Quik, J. T. K., Vandebriel, R. J., Van Kesteren, P. C. E., Visser, M. J., Park, M. V. D. Z., and

Wijnhoven, S. W. P. (2015). Description of a nanocosmetics tool for risk assessment.

32. Stone, V., Nowack, B., Baun, A., van den Brink, N., Kammer, F. V. D., Dusinska, M., Handy, R., Hankin, S., Hassellöv, M., Joner, E., and Fernandes, T. F. (2010). Nanomaterials for environmental studies: classification, reference material issues, and strategies for physico-chemical characterisation. *Sci. Total Environ.*, **408**(7), 1745–1754.

33. Kuempel, E. D., Castranova, V., Geraci, C. L., and Schulte, P. A. (2013). Development of risk-based nanomaterial groups for occupational exposure control. *J. Nanopart. Res.*, **14**(9), 1–15.

34. Kuempel, E. D., Castranova, V., Geraci, C. L., and Schulte, P. A. (2012). Development of risk-based nanomaterial groups for occupational exposure control. *J. Nanopart. Res.*, **14**(9), 1029.

35. National Institute for Occupational Safety and Health. (2014). Current strategies for engineering controls in nanomaterial production and downstream handling processes.

Chapter 8

The Regulatory Use of Physicochemical Properties by Environmental Agencies

Jeffery T. Morris* and Maria J. Doa*

Office of Pollution Prevention and Toxics, US Environmental Protection Agency, Washington, DC 20460, USA

Morris.Jeff@epa.gov

8.1 Introduction

This chapter examines the roles that physicochemical (p-chem) properties play in the regulation of nanomaterials as industrial chemicals. While the focus is on nanomaterials' regulation in the US Environmental Protection Agency's (EPA) Office of Pollution Prevention and Toxics (OPPT), also discussed are the EPA's international collaborations on the regulatory implications of nanomaterial p-chem properties. This chapter highlights a number of unresolved issues around the identification, measurement, and application of nanomaterial properties for regulatory science and

*The authors are employees of the US Environmental Protection Agency (EPA). The views expressed in this chapter do not necessarily represent the policies or positions of the EPA or the US federal government.

Physicochemical Properties of Nanomaterials
Edited by Richard C. Pleus and Vladimir Murashov

ISBN 978-981-4774-80-2 (Hardcover), 978-1-351-16860-1 (eBook)
www.panstanford.com

evaluation and presents recommendations for addressing these issues.

P-chem properties govern not only how nanomaterials perform in applications but also how they behave in biological systems and the environment. Understanding how these properties affect nanomaterials' behavior can inform predictions of hazard and exposure. Such predictions are important for evaluating nanomaterials in regulatory programs. The ability to modify a nanoscale particle's size, shape, charge, surface, and other features adds complexity to the role of p-chem properties in nanomaterial evaluation. This is because it can be difficult to determine how much alteration of a particular property will lead to meaningful changes in a nanoparticle's behavior. Take size, for example. For a given type of nanomaterial, would a 10% change in size cause the particle to become more, or less, toxic? Or would it take a 20% or greater change in size to affect the particle's toxicity profile? It is within this context of complexity and uncertainty that we examine how environmental regulators are addressing issues related to the properties of nanomaterials.

8.2 Use of P-Chem Properties for Regulations

The EPA regulates nanomaterials as industrial chemicals under the Toxic Substances Control Act (TSCA) [1]. Within TSCA, there are important distinctions between existing chemicals already on the TSCA chemical inventory and new chemicals that are not on the inventory. A nanomaterial with a molecular identity that is different from that of any chemical substance already on the TSCA chemical inventory is considered to be a new chemical [2]. In 2008, the EPA made a policy decision to consider nanomaterials derived from substances already on the TSCA chemical inventory to be existing chemicals. Exceptions were made for fullerenes, including carbon nanotubes (CNTs), and graphenes. The EPA determined that CNTs and graphenes were distinct chemical substances from graphite and diamond, the two allotropes of carbon that were on the TSCA chemical inventory in 2008.

All new nanomaterials, made either from carbon or from substances not on the TSCA chemical inventory, are evaluated as new chemicals under Section 5 of TSCA. Anyone wishing to domestically produce or import a new nanomaterial under TSCA must submit a premanufacture notice (PMN) to the EPA. Information on p-chem properties is important for the EPA's evaluation of a nanomaterial PMN. As part of its evaluation, the EPA considers health and safety studies in the literature or unpublished studies provided with the PMN. If the EPA's evaluation of the PMN indicates that the commercialization of the nanomaterial may present an unreasonable risk to humans or the environment, the EPA may regulate the chemical, pending the development of data on the hazard, exposure, or other information needed to evaluate the nanomaterial. Such regulation may entail requiring the use of personal protective equipment, engineering controls, or use restrictions (e.g., no release to water) as a condition of approving the PMN.

Once a nanomaterial has undergone PMN review successfully and the company has notified the EPA that manufacture has commenced, the nanomaterial will be placed on the TSCA chemical inventory. At this point, the nanomaterial is an existing chemical, along with other nanomaterials derived from substances already on the TSCA chemical inventory. The EPA administers TSCA Section 5 to ensure that, as with other new chemicals, new nanomaterials are safely introduced into commerce. The EPA expects this to be equally true for nanomaterials. However, it is possible that new information may lead the EPA to re-evaluate under Section 6 a nanomaterial that had been approved under Section 5.

P-chem properties also will play important roles if the EPA evaluates under TSCA Section 6 a nanomaterial made from a substance that is already on the TSCA chemical inventory. Also, should the EPA determine that it must use TSCA Section 4 to require the generation of data on a nanomaterial, clear articulation of what p-chem properties must be measured and what characterization must be done on the test material would be crucial to ensuring that the right form of nanomaterial is tested and that the data generated from the testing will be useful for assessment of the nanomaterial. For example, if the EPA's objective were to estimate the potential of a nanomaterial's toxicity to aquatic species, it would need to understand how the nanomaterial's p-chem properties affect its fate, transport, and transformation in water and sediments so that the test data could inform modeling of the nanomaterial's hazard and exposure potential in a number of aquatic environments sufficient to represent nation-wide potential releases to water. A robust assessment of the nanomaterial in this scenario would necessitate measuring its p-chem properties as produced, as released to water, and as taken up by aquatic organisms.

The measurement of p-chem properties under the given scenario would be difficult but likely would be important if an EPA assessment were to identify risks for a nanomaterial and the EPA attempted to use Section 6 of TSCA to take regulatory action to reduce the risks of the existing nanomaterial. Whereas one standard for EPA action under Section 5 is "may present unreasonable risk to humans or the environment," Section 6 requires making a "presents unreasonable risk" finding. This higher standard means, among other things, that typically there will be less uncertainty in risk assessments to support actions under Section 6 than for assessments that support actions taken under Section 5. Part of achieving greater certainty could be more, and better, measurement of p-chem properties of the nanomaterial as produced, as introduced into the test medium, and as exposed to the target organism.

8.3 Properties of Importance to Regulators

Information on p-chem properties is important for the evaluation of a nanomaterial PMN. For the EPA's new chemical review of nanomaterials, each chemical substance manufactured at the nanoscale is evaluated on a case-by-case basis. The evaluation is based on data submitted for that nanomaterial, including information on its p-chem properties. While a company is required to submit existing health and safety data on a chemical substance in its possession when it submits a PMN, it is not required to generate new data as part of its initial submission. In the absence of data on a new substance, the EPA will use existing data on a close analog or generate estimates based on the p-chem properties of the nanomaterial.

Nanomaterials introduce an added layer of complexity in the regulatory review under TSCA because nanomaterials are frequently engineered to exhibit attributes based on their physical, chemical, and electrical and/or optical attributes. As a result, there are a wide range of p-chem endpoints that the EPA believes are important in assessing nanomaterials under TSCA.

In its review of nanomaterials, the EPA focuses on p-chem properties that provide for the characterization of the following areas: (i) physical identification, (ii) chemical identification, (iii) surface properties, and (iv) p-chem properties relevant for fate and exposure. The EPA considers the following properties to be the most important in characterizing specific nanomaterials in the four areas listed: chemical composition, particle size, particle size distribution, specific surface area, particle shape, zeta potential, dispersion stability, surface reactivity, and surface chemistry. The properties related to these areas inform the health and safety considerations of toxicity, environment fate, and exposure potential and provide a clear way to distinguish among different forms of chemical substances manufactured at the nanoscale. Of course some of these p-chem properties are relevant to more than one area, although the acceptable levels of uncertainly for an endpoint among these areas may vary. Other parameters, such as the wavelength at which light is emitted, may be important to assessing how well the material will function but are less informative to health and safety evaluation.

8.3.1 Physical Identification of the Nanomaterial

The parameters that are important to physical identification and also inform other aspects of regulatory evaluation are particle size and particle size distribution, particle shape, aspect ratio, aggregation/agglomeration, specific surface area, and porosity. These are important characteristics for identifying a material and informing its toxicity, environmental fate, and exposure considerations. The following are important aspects of these parameters.

For particle size, both the mean and the distribution, including the breadth of the distribution, are important. While not always seen in data on particle size provided in the regulatory context, particle size and particle size distribution should be calibrated by standard materials. As with most other p-chem parameters, a decision tree would help identify the appropriate techniques for characterizing particle size and particle size distribution.

Shape is important as a fundamental distinguisher of different nanomaterials. Shape informs the assessment of toxicity. Related to shape is aspect ratio, which is most important in assessing the toxicity of certain nanomaterials, for example, CNTs. Another factor always considered is the number of walls, layers, or shells of a nanomaterial.

Specific surface area is a physical characterization parameter that is important for assessing functionality, reactivity, and toxicity. Specific surface area is the ratio of the surface area to the mass. More precisely, it is the ratio of the area of the surface of a nanoscale material divided by the mass (m^2/kg) or the area of the surface of a nanoscale material divided by volume (m^2/m^3). Increasing the surface area increases the chemical reactivity of a nanoparticle, which may increase its toxicity.

From a regulatory perspective, the ability to distinguish between aggregates and agglomerates is important. The degree and type of aggregation are fundamental determinants in how a material is regulated, since it informs predictions of the nanomaterial's environmental fate and exposure potential. The attributes that can inform regulatory decisions include the number of primary particles in an aggregate, the ratio of aggregates to nonaggregates, and their surface area and size distribution.

8.3.2 Chemical Identification of a Nanomaterial and Any Impurities and By-Products

Basic chemical identification is needed because in addition to any attributes resulting from the engineering of the material, the nanomaterial may be composed of materials that exhibit toxicity whether or not they are part of an engineered material. These include metals such as cadmium or lead, which may reside as contaminants in nanomaterials as a result of the production process.

Surface composition is important to properly characterize the health and safety of a nanoscale material. The reactivity of the nanomaterial will depend, in part, on the composition of its surface. Characterizing the surface is needed to identify functionalization that can be reactive in the body. One example is identifying the presence (including the relative presence) of –OH, -COH, and

–COOH after oxidation of CNTs. In contrast, the absence of surface functionalization for CNTs will also be informative about the toxicity, such as when used in conjunction with aspect ratio.

Crystallinity is a basic attribute that also may be important for understanding the behavior of certain types of nanomaterials and can affect the type of regulatory decision made about a nanomaterial. For example, the regulatory concern level for amorphous silica is different from that for crystalline silica. As another example, studies have shown that titanium dioxide nanoparticles with different crystalline structures may have different toxicological profiles [3].

8.3.3 Surface Properties

A p-chem property important for environmental fate and environmental toxicity is surface charge, a property of materials when suspended in a fluid. The zeta potential, which is related to surface charge, is the electrokinetic potential in colloidal systems. It is measured as the net number of positive and negative charges per unit particle surface area in coulomb/m^2 and is typically measured by electrophoresis.

Surface reactivity provides an indication of the degree to which a nanoscale particle will react with biological systems. The surface reactivity of a nanoparticle is dependent upon factors such as redox potential, which is a measure of the tendency of an entity to lose or acquire electrons, and photocatalytic activity, including the potential to generate free radicals. Reactive oxygen species and free radicals are important in estimating nanomaterial toxicity and developing protocols for toxicity testing.

8.3.4 P-Chem Properties Relevant for Fate and Exposure

In addition to many of the p-chem parameters discussed before, two additional parameters that are relevant for fate and exposure are dispersion stability and dustiness.

Dispersion stability is the ability of a dispersion to resist changes in properties over time and can be defined in terms of the change in one or more physical properties over a given time period. It is applicable in considerations of human health and environmental toxicity.

Dustiness is the propensity of a powder to form airborne dust by mechanical means. A characterization of dustiness is important in considering worker exposure. This is a fundamental consideration for many nanomaterials that the EPA reviews under TSCA.

While the p-chem endpoints for assessing nanomaterials for purposes of TSCA have been identified, the applicability of particular methods and existing test guidelines to specific nanomaterials is not consistently clear. This challenge is recognized by other jurisdictions. Within the Organization for Economic Co-operation and Development (OECD), regulators have initiated the development of guidance for regulators for p-chem characterization and for modified and new test guidelines. This guidance would identify for a specific type of manufactured nanomaterial the type of assessment (e.g., characterization, screening-level risk assessment), the appropriate method(s) to be used for a physical-chemical endpoint for a specific material, and the methods that are not considered appropriate for specific manufactured nanomaterials for a particular purpose (e.g., for use only in screening or need for use in a more robust risk assessment). The OECD is also working to identify if additional test guidelines should be developed or whether existing test guidelines should be modified to address testing requirements specific to nanomaterials.

8.3.5 Challenges with Existing Data

Existing health and safety studies on nanomaterials are sometimes of limited usefulness because, given the complexities of p-chem characterization of nanomaterials, many older health and safety studies (and to a lesser degree in more recent studies), the nanomaterial was not adequately characterized. Adequate characterization of a nanomaterial and consideration of the design of the test (e.g., selected doses, sample preparation to minimize uncertainty/bias) and the selection of the most appropriate methods to characterize the p-chem properties of the nanomaterial are key components of studies that can be used in a regulatory context. There is currently no consensus on the p-chem properties to be measured or the best methods to measure them. However, there is growing consensus that when tests on nanomaterials are performed, there should be a sufficient characterization to allow the dose response to be expressed in the different metrics, that is, number, specific surface area, and mass.

8.3.5.1 Read-across/categorization/prediction

If adequate data are not available to assess the toxicity, environmental fate, and exposure for a PMN nanomaterial, the EPA will use the p-chem properties of the nanomaterial to assess these endpoints. P-chem properties such as specific surface area are of particular importance to inform how the nanomaterial will react in biological systems and the environment and to determine whether there are any appropriate analogs for each of these endpoints. There are challenges in using read-across approaches/categorization based on chemical composition because of the different p-chem properties of different nanomaterials with similar chemical compositions but different physical attributes (e.g., specific surface area). Under TSCA, applying these approaches to nanomaterials is still in its infancy. The EPA groups nanomaterials primarily on the basis of size, shape, and composition. It has started developing groupings within the family of CNTs. The ability to refine this approach will lead to improved assessments and more targeted testing.

8.3.6 Information to Improve Evaluation of Nanoscale Materials

Whether the EPA evaluates a nanomaterial as a new chemical under TSCA Section 5 or as an existing chemical under Section 6, there may be instances where information may need to be collected for the EPA to perform a reasoned evaluation of the nanomaterial. An important component of this information collection is the p-chem properties of the nanomaterial. While the p-chem data available for individual nanomaterials will vary, there are common p-chem parameters that, in general, are useful for nanomaterials. These are the p-chem properties used to distinguish among discrete nanoscale forms of chemical substances that are to be reported. They were chosen in part because they are important in characterizing potential hazards and exposure. These p-chem properties are particle size, zeta potential, specific surface area, dispersion stability, and surface reactivity [4].

8.4 Unresolved Issues

While the EPA has identified a set of p-chem properties that it considers when assessing new chemicals and has proposed a set of p-chem properties to be used to distinguish among different forms of nanomaterials, there is no international agreement on the essential set of nanomaterial properties to measure and report for regulatory evaluation. Internationally, much progress has been made within the OECD's Working Party on Manufactured Nanomaterials (WPMN), as well as in the International Organization for Standardization (ISO) Technical Committee (TC) 229. A current focus within the OECD's WPMN is to identify the appropriate methods to measure the p-chem parameters for specific types of nanomaterials. This will improve the characterization of nanomaterials and the quality of health and safety data. However, this progress has not yet yielded an international agreement on what to measure and how to do the measuring. Ultimately, such agreement will be necessary for the OECD's Mutual Acceptance of Data program to be fully and effectively operational for nanomaterials. For several years there has been some coordination between the WPMN and TC 229 on this issue. This coordination has been useful in shaping and informing the work of both bodies. Nevertheless, given the continued need for resolution on outstanding characterization issues before an international consensus is reached, the point may have been reached where a more formal collaboration between the OECD and the ISO is needed. While there is no existing model for a formal agreement between these two organizations, neither are there obvious legal or administrative barriers to such an agreement. Rather, both entities will have to determine whether they see sufficient benefit in such an agreement to put one in place.

Also of importance to regulators is knowing what percentage of a substance comprises particles in the nanoscale. Such information is important as regulators seek to reach an agreement on how much of a substance must contain nanoscale particles for the substance to be considered a nanomaterial. Currently, the European Union considers 50% nanoscale particles to be the cut-off point. However, the scientific support for choosing 50% is uncertain at best. In fact, it is unlikely that science will provide a clear answer to the question of an appropriate percentage. For effective nanomaterial regulation, a practical, policy-driven solution will need to be found, most likely somewhere between 1% and 50%. Below 1%, in many instances, it may be impossible to measure and quantify the percentage of nanoparticles in a sample. Yet if the cut-off for reporting is significantly above 10%, regulators may not see chemical substances that exhibit unique, nanotechnology-mediated behavior.

Finally, there is no agreement on the relationship between nanomaterial properties and whether a nanomaterial behaves differently from the substance from which the nanomaterial is derived. Reaching an agreement on what properties of nanomaterials may affect the hazard and exposure potential in ways different from the chemical substances from which they are derived can help focus reporting on those nanomaterials on which additional information would be most useful for ensuring human health and environmental protection.

8.5 Conclusions

As national regulators operating within a global scientific, economic, and regulatory context, we believe there are three priorities for advancing and enhancing the use of p-chem and material properties in the regulation of nanomaterials:

- Agreement on what properties inform distinguishing among different CNTs, in particular multiwalled carbon nanotubes (MWCNTs). Because a high percentage of nanomaterials that come through the EPA's new chemicals program are MWCNTs, properties related to them are of the highest priority. The EPA has as an objective of improving the development of a MWCNT characterization of nanomaterials. This will yield higher-quality health and safety data and refine the use of analogs for nanomaterials in regulatory assessments.

- Understanding how key properties influence the results of high-throughput toxicogenomic assays. Twenty-first-century testing approaches, including high-throughput assays, are going to play an increasing role in chemical evaluation, including for nanomaterials. As with traditional testing approaches, understanding what properties affect toxicity is important to understanding the extent to which test results can be generalized beyond the specific test substance. High-throughput approaches have the potential to more quickly and cost-effectively test a large number of variants of particular nanomaterial types (e.g., changes in particle coatings or particle functionalization). However, the ability to run the assays on variants assumes knowledge of whether a variation in a nanoparticle changes key properties of the particle and, if so, whether such changes will affect assay results. These approaches also are going to be an increasingly important part of developing chemical categories—for example, to enable the ability to read-across existing data on MWCNTs to infer environmental behavior to structurally similar CNTs for which data are not available. For traditional chemicals, the EPA for decades has used read-across approaches that employ structure–activity relationship models in order to evaluate new chemical submissions that are accompanied by little or no data. These approaches need to be developed for MWCNTs if the EPA is going to be able to streamline its premanufacture evaluations and limit data requirements to the essential set of information necessary to evaluate a specific MWCNT. At present, in the absence of being able to apply read-across approaches, the EPA must assume that every MWCNT submitted for premanufacture review is toxicologically unique and therefore requires its own data set to inform its evaluation.
- Development of a better understanding of how key properties, for priority nanomaterial types, govern the fate, transport, and transformation of nanomaterials in air, water, soils, and biological systems. Such understanding is crucial to estimating exposure to nanomaterials, which is necessary for making risk-based determinations of nanomaterial safety.

Nanomaterials regulated under TSCA are incorporated into a wide range of industrial uses and consumer products. In many cases, any release of nanomaterials into the environment from such uses and products will lead to transformation of particles as they interact with air, water, soils, or the biological systems of organisms that may be exposed to the released particles. Under TSCA, the EPA may evaluate new nanomaterials at all points in their life cycle: from their manufacture to their incorporation into products and from product use through disposal or recycling. For many nanomaterials, it is likely that, at each of these points in the life cycle, at the point of potential exposure there will be differences in measured properties of the particles to which humans or other species may be exposed. Understanding the hazard and exposure potential of these transformed particles is key to determining whether the use of a nanomaterial regulated under TSCA may or will present risks to humans or the environment.

Clearly, there are other issues related to nanomaterial properties that will need to be addressed before uncertainties in their assessment are reduced to levels on par with those found in traditional chemical assessments. Nevertheless, progress on these three priorities will significantly advance the regulators' ability to assess nanomaterials.

References

1. US Environmental Protection Agency. (2017). Reviewing new chemicals under Toxic Substances Control Act. http://www.epa.gov/reviewing-new-chemicals-under-toxic-substances-control-act-tsca/control-nanoscale-materials-under
2. US Environmental Protection Agency. (2008). TSCA inventory status of nanoscale substances: general approach. http://www2.epa.gov/sites/production/files/2015-10/documents/nmsp-inventorypaper2008.pdf
3. Seitza, F., Rosenfeldta, R. R., Schneidera, S., Schulza, R., and Bundschuha, M. (2014). Size-, surface- and crystalline structure composition-related effects of titanium dioxide nanoparticles during their aquatic life cycle. *Sci. Total Environ.*, **493**, 891–897.

4. US Environmental Protection Agency. (2015). Chemical substances when manufactured or processed as nanoscale materials; TSCA reporting and recordkeeping requirements. 65 FR 18330.

Chapter 9

Physicochemical Properties of Nanomaterials Relevant to Medical Products

Bhaskara V. Chikkaveeraiah,[a] Subhas G. Malghan,[a] and Girish Kumar[b]

[a]*Office of Science and Engineering Laboratories, US Food and Drug Administration, 10903 New Hampshire Avenue, Silver Spring, MD 20993, USA*
[b]*TÜV SÜD America, 10 Centennial Drive, Peabody, MA 01960, USA*
Subhasm7@gmail.com

The use of nanomaterials in medical products continues to evolve to exploit their high specific surface area (surface-to-volume ratio) that imparts high surface reactivity. A large variety of polymeric, metallic, nonmetallic, and lipid-based nanomaterials have found their applications in simple products like dental fillers to more complex products like targeted drug delivery for cancer therapy as well as microfluidic devices for early cancer detection. With some exceptions, for most medical products, prolonged physical and chemical stability of the products and accompanying constituent materials in vivo is critical to the products' performance, safety, and

Physicochemical Properties of Nanomaterials
Edited by Richard C. Pleus and Vladimir Murashov

ISBN 978-981-4774-80-2 (Hardcover), 978-1-351-16860-1 (eBook)
www.panstanford.com

efficacy. The stability of a product implies resistance to break up on a molecular or atomic level, which encompasses phenomena such as dissolution, mixing, melting, hydrolysis, corrosion, and degradation. An important aspect of nanomaterials/nanodevices from the standpoint of risk to the patient is the rate and extent of material loss from the device due to molecular breakup, dissolution, or resorption, which can result in harm to the patient and/or ultimately lead to device failure. Though significant advancements are being made to engineer materials at the nanoscale to achieve desired outcomes, there are still substantial gaps and challenges in understanding of how these nanoscale materials affect the patient's health after exposure. Regulatory science research continues to advance the development of our understanding of the physicochemical stability of nanoscale particles, and the rate and extent to which they break up, and determine whether and how the responses induced by nanoparticles differ from those induced by microparticles and bulk forms of the same materials. This chapter focuses on medical devices distinct from the larger universe of drugs, biologics, and foods that constitute the portfolio of regulatory responsibilities of the US Food and Drug Administration (FDA), since it is not practical to address all products in the space provided. The scope of the FDA's regulatory authority is very broad. The FDA regulates a broad range of medical devices using a risk-based paradigm that addresses complicated, high-risk medical devices, like artificial hearts, and relatively simple, low-risk devices, like tongue depressors, as well as devices that fall in between.

9.1 Introduction

Nanoscale materials often have different physicochemical or biological properties compared to their larger microscale and bulk counterparts. Such differences may include altered chemical or biological activity; increased structural integrity; or altered electrical, optical, or magnetic properties. Because of these properties, nanoscale materials have great potential for use in a vast range of consumer and biomedical products. Nanoscale materials may facilitate new developments in products to advance public health, which is of particular interest to the Food and Drug Administration

(FDA). Also, nanoscale materials may present different safety issues than their larger or smaller (i.e., molecular) counterparts because of some of their special properties.

The FDA is generally responsible for overseeing the safety and effectiveness of drugs and devices for humans and animals and of biological products for humans. The agency is also responsible for overseeing the safety of foods (including food additives and dietary supplements), color additives, and cosmetics. The FDA conducts these oversight functions under a variety of laws and regulations, which establish the specific premarket and/or postmarket oversight mechanisms applicable to a particular class of products [1].

Research and development relating to nanotechnology applications promises the development of products having highly integrated, multiple functions. For example, disease diagnosis, noninvasive imaging elements, and drug targeting are being combined in individual nanotechnology products [2]. The FDA anticipates this shift in the nature of products received for review and authorization and develops a transparent, consistent, and predictable regulatory pathway for such products.

The introduction of new technologies often creates new challenges, particularly if the associated products, in addition to the expected benefits, raise concerns about health and environmental risks. Nanotechnology applications hold significant promise in different technological areas and industrial sectors. Many nanotechnology applications are based on novel as well as conventional materials deliberately engineered to be nanostructured, for which the term "nanomaterial" is frequently used. The size range of a few nanometers to 100 nm is of considerable importance where materials' properties change and many interesting phenomena occur. Materials and devices designed by nanotechnology interact with the cells and tissues with a high degree of functional specificity, thus allowing integration between the device and biological molecule, cell, or organism that was not previously attainable [3, 4]. This chapter focuses on applications of nanomaterials, evaluating the products that contain nanomaterials, classification of medical devices for regulatory purposes, and the FDA's approach to regulation of nanotechnology products.

9.2 Applications of Nanomaterials

Nanomaterials are being used in everyday consumer products to make them lighter, stronger, cleaner, less expensive, more efficient, more precise, or more aesthetic. Products containing nanomaterials may improve the quality of life through more efficient target-driven pharmaceuticals, better medical diagnostic tools, cleaner energy production, faster computers, etc. A few materials that are regarded as nanomaterials today have been on the market for a long time. For example, the well-known carbon black was used in industrial production over a century ago as a reinforcing agent for the production of automotive tires [5], and today the annual production of carbon black is over 10 million tons, still mostly for tires. Other nanomaterials in use today are silver, silicon dioxide (SiO_2), titanium dioxide (TiO_2), and zinc oxide (ZnO). Several medical products available today have been developed by incorporating nanomaterials into existing products, for example, by incorporation into solid, viscous, or liquid matrices. Other examples of products containing nanomaterials are cosmetics and personal care products, paints and coatings, healthcare products, food and nutritional ingredients, food packaging agrochemicals, and diagnostic devices. Sunscreen lotions and cosmetics such as skin care and colorant products are widely known to use nanomaterials as one of the key ingredients to enhance their performance [6]. Both titanium dioxide and zinc oxide nanoparticles are used in sunscreens as they absorb and reflect ultraviolet rays but are still transparent to visible light and; hence, the resulting sunscreen becomes more appealing to the consumer and is claimed to be more effective.

The application of nanomaterials is evolving rapidly, especially for uses related to biomedicine. Four nanomaterials are emerging in biomedical applications. These are metal nanoparticles (gold and silver), quantum dots (QDs), particles with magnetic properties, and carbon nanotubes (CNTs). Nanomaterials provide promising platforms for a variety of biomedical applications, including biosensing, imaging, and drug delivery, due to their unique optical, magnetic, and electronic properties (Table 9.1) [7–11]. As most of the properties of nanomaterials are size and shape dependent, the methods of nanomaterial preparation are an active area of research.

Table 9.1 Nanomaterials and their properties employed in biomedical applications

Nanomaterial	Examples	Properties	Biomedical applications
Metal	Ag, Au, Pt	Surface plasmon resonance (SPR), ease of surface functionalization	Targeted drug delivery, biosensors/ diagnostics, imaging
Carbon	CNTs, Fullerene	Chemical stability, superior conductivity, electronic and mechanical properties	Biosensing, drug and gene delivery, therapeutics
Semiconductor/ Quantum dots	CdS, CdSe, ZnS, PbS	Fluorescence	Immunoassays, bioimaging, biosensing
Magnetic particles	Fe_3O_4	Magnetic attraction	MRI, NMR, drug delivery, bioassays

Due to their unique optical, physical, and electrical properties, metallic nanoparticles have been employed in a wide spectrum of biomedical applications such as sensing, imaging, drug delivery, and gene targeting [12–16]. There are reports suggesting that some of these nanoparticles also have significant therapeutic potential such as antibacterial, antimicrobial, and targeted therapeutic effect [17–22].

Carbon nanomaterials (CNs) include nanotubes, fullerenes, and graphene. CNTs are one of the most widely used nanomaterials because of their remarkable physical, chemical, and biological properties. There are two types of CNTs: single-walled (SWCNTs) and multiwalled (MWCNTs). Theoretically, nanotubes are viewed as rolled-up structures of single or multiple sheets of graphene to give SWCNTs and MWCNTs, respectively. These one-dimensional carbon allotropes have a large surface area, high mechanical strength, and excellent chemical and thermal stability. Due to their unique physicochemical properties, CNTs have been employed to explore their potential in biological and biomedical applications (Fig. 9.1)

[23–25]. CNTs can easily be surface functionalized to attach nucleic acids and proteins and hence are emerging as novel components in nanoformulations for targeted delivery of therapeutic molecules [26].

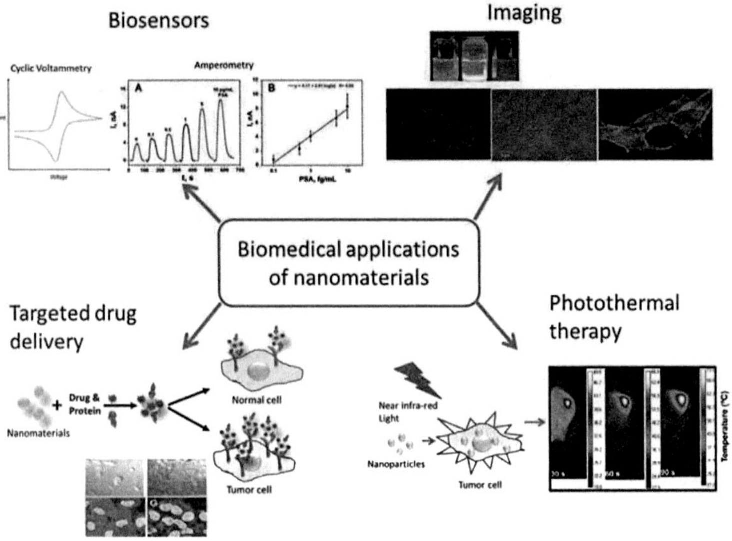

Figure 9.1 Biomedical applications of nanomaterials.

Fullerenes are novel carbon allotropes with a polygonal structure made up of 60 carbon atoms, with a soccer ball–shaped arrangement of 60 carbon atoms per molecule, and show great promise as pharmaceutical agents [27–31]. Fullerenes have numerous points of attachment whose surfaces can easily be functionalized for tissue binding. Many of the fullerene derivatives that are in clinical trials have shown good biocompatibility and low toxicity even at relatively high dosages. Fullerene compounds can be employed as antiviral agents, most notably against human immunodeficiency virus [32], as antibacterial agents (e.g., *Escherichia coli, Streptococcus, Mycobacterium tuberculosis*) [33–35], as photodynamic agents for anticancer therapy [36, 37], and in many other applications. The distinct structural properties of graphene, in particular its high aspect ratio, unique electronic and optical properties, and potential biocompatibility, make it an extremely attractive for biomedical applications such as biosensor development, imaging, drug delivery, bacterial inhibition, and photothermal therapy [11, 38, 39].

QDs are semiconductor nanocrystals with spatially confined excitation states. Coating QDs with another material is crucial for their biological applications to allow their aqueous dispersion and to prevent leakage of the toxic heavy metals. QDs have been widely used in imaging and cell labeling either in vitro or in vivo [40–42]. QDs have also been studied in charge transfer–based biosensors [43], drug delivery [44], and photodynamic therapy [45].

Magnetic nanoparticles provide many exciting opportunities in biomedical applications. The ease of size optimization according to requirement, manipulability by external magnetic force, contrast enhancement in magnetic resonance imaging (MRI), and other such desirable properties of magnetic nanoparticles, has recently been exploited in various applications in the field of biology and medicine, including protein purification, drug delivery, imaging, sensing, and separation [46, 47]. Polymeric nanoparticles such as polysaccharide chitosan–polylactic acid, polycaprolactone, and chitosan nanoparticles have been used as drug carriers [48–50]. The drug is dissolved, entrapped, encapsulated, or attached to a polymeric nanoparticle matrix.

Nanomaterial properties can be exploited by using biological processes or systems to create, order, and investigate new nanoscale materials or devices. Nanomaterial-biological hybrid materials are capable of achieving biomedical advances far more than each individual component alone. Each participant infuses the composite with a unique property or function that is lacking in the other. Thus, nanomaterial bioconjugates have the potential to revolutionize many aspects of science and significant impact in developing biomedical therapeutics and diagnostics [51–53]. Nanomaterial bioconjugation normally occurs via a stochastic process resulting in a distribution of nanomaterials functionalized with different numbers or populations of biomolecules (Fig. 9.2) [54]. Conjugates may consist of nanomaterials both with and without attached biomolecule(s) or, alternatively, a narrow or broad distribution ratio of attached biomolecules.

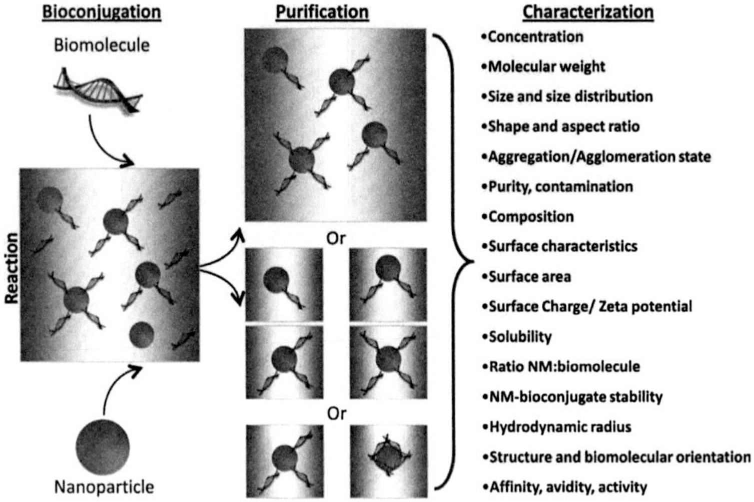

Figure 9.2 Schematic highlighting of issues related to purification and characterization of nanomaterial bioconjugates. Reprinted with permission from Ref. [54]. Copyright (2011) American Chemical Society.

Depending on the conjugation chemistry utilized, there may also be heterogeneity in the orientation of the attached biomolecules. This is especially true when there are multiple groups available when implementing carbodiimide (1-ethyl-3-(3-dimethylaminopropyl) carbodiimide) (EDC) chemistry to form an amide bond between the carboxyls or amines present on proteins and the similar target group present on a nanomaterial [55]. These types of reactions also have a high tendency for cross-linking and forming aggregates. A number of physicochemical properties play important role when characterizing the nanomaterial bioconjugates: nanomaterial size and size distribution, shape and aspect ratio, aggregation/ agglomeration state, purity, chemical composition, surface characteristics, ζ (zeta) potential (overall surface charge), surface area, stability, and solubility (see Fig. 9.2) [56–58]. Bioconjugation adds additional considerations and analyses to this equation, including (i) confirmation of and type of biomolecule attachment, (ii) average ratio of nanomaterial/biomolecule and ratio distribution, (iii) hydrodynamic radius, (iv) structure and orientation of the biomolecule upon attachment, (v) separation distance between the biomolecule and the nanomaterial, (vi) stability of the material during conjugation and of the resulting composite within the nanomaterial environment during the intended application, and (vii) activity of the biomolecule upon attachment.

9.3 Regulatory Aspects

Nanomedicine is one of the most promising fields of application of nanotechnologies. It uses new physical, chemical, and biological properties of nanomaterials in biomedical products, such as medical devices, which provide theranostic advances, but may also be associated with health risks. The FDA's regulatory science priorities are focused on issues relevant to oversight of products subject to its regulations. Identifying whether a product contains nanotechnology or nanomaterials is an important first step. Materials can exhibit new physicochemical properties at nanoscale dimensions, and properties that are attributable to size can be seen or retained even when the material or end-product may not necessarily exist entirely within the nanoscale [59, 60]. Although one definition for "nanomaterial" may offer meaningful guidance in one context, that definition may be too narrow or broad in another. Hence, the FDA is taking a broadly inclusive approach to considering whether FDA-regulated products contain nanomaterials or involve nanotechnology. The FDA has issued draft guidance for industry on this topic [61]. When evaluating whether an FDA-regulated product contains nanomaterials or involves nanotechnology, the FDA will consider the following:

- Whether the material or end product is engineered to have at least one external dimension, or internal or surface structure, in the nanoscale range (~1 to 100 nm) or
- Whether a material or end product is engineered to exhibit properties or phenomena, including physical or chemical properties or biological effects that are attributable to its dimensions, even if these dimensions fall outside the nanoscale range, up to 1 μm

Structures such as agglomerates and aggregates, as well as coated, functionalized, or hierarchically assembled structures are also of interest in this context. This initial broadly inclusive approach may gradually modify over a period of time through experience, using available scientific information (including the agency's own regulatory science research), and public input. Until then, these broad size- and property-related factors are the key factors when considering whether the products might fall within the FDA's purview for nanomaterials, and industry and developers are encouraged to contact the agency early in the development process to get the focused and least burdensome guidance on the regulatory pathway for their product.

Materials exhibit unique physicochemical properties at the nanoscale, which are attributed to their ultrasmall size, high surface-to-volume ratio, physical appearance (shape or morphology), hydrophilic or hydrophobic nature (surface charge), presence of biochemical entities on the surface (functional groups), and aggregation [62]. Due to these unusual physicochemical properties, nanomaterials tend to achieve better functionality, sensitivity, efficiency, and specificity in terms of their biomedical applications [51, 54, 63–67]. Nanomaterials have found significant numerous applications such as imaging, sensing, and targeted drug delivery. Nanoparticles and nanostructures can be easily characterized by several analytical methods such as microscopy, spectroscopy, separation-based, scattering-based, and mass-spectrometry-based analysis. Due to complex nature of nanomaterials and nanostructures, one characterization modality may not be sufficient to adequately characterize the physicochemical properties of nanomaterials. For example, light-scattering-based techniques only provide the hydrodynamic diameter of dispersed nanomaterials and the final measurement favors larger particles more as compared to smaller ones. On the other hand, electron-microscopy-based techniques can only provide electron-dense core diameters of nanoparticles but not the diameter in solution. Each method has its own limitations, and often times it is important to use two independent, orthogonal modalities to more precisely characterize nanomaterials.

9.3.1 Review of Products Containing Nanomaterials

When a new product is submitted for review, whether the product is subject to premarket review (e.g., new drugs, biological products, certain devices, and food and color additives) or not (e.g., cosmetics), the industry is required to ensure that the product satisfies applicable safety standards and complies with other applicable requirements. Substantiation of safety requires scientific evidence. The FDA Nanotechnology Task Force made recommendations for a staged approach to determine whether current tests are adequate to support risk management decisions and where they are not in order to collect more data and update the procedures [68]. The following are of particular importance when nanomaterials are employed in regulated products:

- Routes of exposure of nanomaterials, including inhalation, dermal absorption, and ingestion (e.g., as related to cosmetics and foods); portal-of-entry toxicity (e.g., toxicity to lungs, skin, mucus membranes); and exposure media (e.g., air, water, and food).
- Properties related to absorption, distribution, metabolism, and excretion (ADME) (e.g., related to drugs). Biological interactions may be influenced by size, particle charge or chemical properties, or conditions of exposure; thus, additional analytical techniques may be required for determining physical characteristics (e.g., size or aggregation) not previously assessed for tissue samples collected in ADME studies.
- Particle size, size distribution, surface charge, surface properties, particle interactions (aggregation), particle behavior, purity, stability, and general batch-to-batch variability. The new properties of the products or materials that involve nanomaterials or applications of nanotechnology may require additional product-specific testing and manufacturing controls.

At the FDA, the regulatory science program addresses these questions and involves developing new tools, standards, and approaches to assess the safety, efficacy, quality, and performance of FDA-regulated products in order to help evaluate whether products are appropriate for marketing [69]. The FDA Nanotechnology Task Force recommended and followed through by seeking public input on the adequacy of the FDA's policies and procedures for products that combine drugs, biological products, and/or devices containing nanoscale materials to serve multiple uses, such as both a diagnostic and a therapeutic intended use. The task force also recommends encouraging manufacturers to communicate with the agency early in the development process for products using nanoscale materials, particularly with regard to such highly integrated combination products.

The regulatory science program in the FDA continues to work in areas such as nanomaterial characterization, in vitro and in vivo modeling, and product-focused research. The FDA is coordinating with other US agencies, such as the interagency National Nanotechnology Initiative, to share information and combine resources through collaborative interactions [70]. The agency is also participating in public workshops on such topics as risk assessment and management methods [71] and has formed joint partnerships, including with the National Institutes of Health and the National Institute of Standards and Technology, on establishing a transitional pathway from nanotechnology discovery research to clinical application [72].

9.4 Classification of Medical Devices

A medical device is an instrument, apparatus, machine, implant, in vitro reagent, or other similar article that prevents, treats, mitigates, or cures disease by physical, mechanical, or thermal means (in contrast, drugs act on the body through pharmacological, metabolic, or immunological means). They range from Band-Aid and bedpans to complex programmable pacemakers and laser surgical devices. They also include diagnostic products, test kits, ultrasound products, X-ray machines, and medical lasers. In the FDA, the Center for Devices and Radiological Health (CDRH) regulates medical devices and categorizes them into three classes on the basis of their potential risks. The class to which a device is assigned determines, among other things, the type of premarketing submission/application required for FDA clearance/approval to market [73]. If a device is classified as class I or II, and if it is not exempt, a 510k premarket notification will be required for marketing. All devices classified as exempt are subject to the limitations on exemptions. Device classification depends on the "intended use" of the device and also upon "indications for use." Indications for use can be found in the device's labeling but may also be conveyed orally during sale of the product.

Class I devices are low risk and are not required to have special controls. For example, dental floss, tongue depressors, arm slings, and hand-held surgical instruments are classified as class I devices. Most class I devices are exempt from Premarket Notification 510(k) (see Fig. 9.3).

Class II devices are higher-risk devices and have more regulations to demonstrate the device's safety and effectiveness. For example, condoms, X-ray systems, gas analyzers, pumps, and surgical drapes are classified as class II devices. Manufacturers introducing class II medical devices must submit a 510(k) premarket notification to the FDA. The 510(k) identifies medical device and compares it to an existing medical device ("predicate" device) to demonstrate that the device is substantially equivalent and at least as safe and effective.

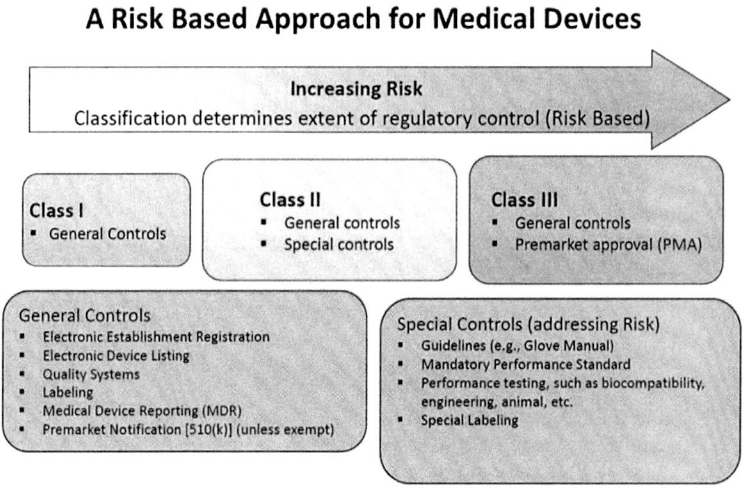

A Risk Based Approach for Medical Devices
Increasing Risk
Classification determines extent of regulatory control (Risk Based)
Class I
▪ General Controls
Class II
▪ General controls
▪ Special controls
Class III
▪ General controls
▪ Premarket approval (PMA)
General Controls
▪ Electronic Establishment Registration
▪ Electronic Device Listing
▪ Quality Systems
▪ Labeling
▪ Medical Device Reporting (MDR)
▪ Premarket Notification [510(k)] (unless exempt)
Special Controls (addressing Risk)
▪ Guidelines (e.g., Glove Manual)
▪ Mandatory Performance Standard
▪ Performance testing, such as biocompatibility, engineering, animal, etc.
▪ Special Labeling

Figure 9.3 Medical device classification.

Class III devices are generally the highest-risk devices and must be approved though the premarket approval (PMA) process by the FDA before they can be legally marketed. For example, implantable devices (devices made to replace/support or enhance part of your body) such as defibrillators, pacemakers, artificial hips, knees, and replacement heart valves are classified as class III devices. Medical devices that are moderate- to high-risk or novel devices for which no "predicate device" exists can be classified via de novo pathways. After classification, a device usually gets its own product code and regulation number. Clinical studies are usually not required for class I and class II medical devices but are often required for class III devices.

Other devices such as a Humanitarian Use Device (HUD) and Orphan Products are also regulated by the FDA. An HUD is a device intended to treat or diagnose a disease or condition that affects fewer than 4000 individuals in the United States per year. The research and development cost could exceed its market returns for such device manufacturers. The HUD provision of the regulation provides an incentive for the development of devices for use in the treatment or diagnosis of diseases affecting these populations. A humanitarian device exemption (HDE) is submitted to the FDA to obtain approval for an HUD. An HDE is similar in both form and content to PMA application but is exempt from the effectiveness requirements of a PMA. The mission of the FDA Office of Orphan Products Development (OOPD) is to advance the evaluation and development of products (drugs, biologics, devices, or medical foods) that demonstrate promise for the diagnosis or treatment of rare diseases or conditions. The OOPD reviews scientific and clinical data submissions from sponsors to identify and designate products as promising for rare diseases and further advances scientific development of such promising medical products. The OOPD provides incentives for sponsors to develop products for rare diseases.

9.5 The FDA's Generalized Approach to Products Containing Nanotechnology Products

As a public health agency, the FDA has long encountered the combination of promise, risk, and uncertainty that accompanies emerging technologies, while using scientific information to make regulatory decisions about products ranging from cosmetics to chemotherapy agents to food packaging. Nanotechnology is not unique in this regard. Materials can exhibit new or altered physicochemical properties at nanoscale dimensions, which can enable the development of novel products. The changes in biological, chemical, and other properties that make nanotechnology applications so exciting also leads to examine whether these changes in properties may have any effects on product safety, effectiveness, or other attributes.

The application of nanotechnology may result in product characteristics that differ from those of conventionally manufactured products, and hence evaluation of safety or effectiveness of those products that include nanomaterials or otherwise involve the application of nanotechnology should consider the unique properties and behaviors that nanomaterials may exhibit. However, the FDA does not categorically judge all products containing nanomaterials or otherwise involving the application of nanotechnology as basically benign or harmful. The FDA will regulate nanotechnology products under existing statutory authorities in accordance with the specific legal standards applicable to each type of product under its jurisdiction.

What makes a final product a nano-enabled product? To classify a product as a nano-enabled product, the material used in that particular device should comply with the regulatory definition of an engineered nanomaterial. Unfortunately at present, there is no universally accepted definition for nanomaterials. Regulatory agencies throughout the world have their own working definitions that they are using for the regulation of such products. Even though there is no internationally agreed upon definition of nanomaterials, working definitions of different agencies do address two important key points in categorizing medical products with nanomaterials. One of them is based on the size of the actual nanomaterial used. It is typically between 1 and 100 nm or is a nanostructure with the internal or surface structure at nanoscale. Second criterion is the acquired "unique properties" of nanomaterials that can be attributable to their size. Such unique properties are absent in the bulk form of same material. Apart from these properties, some regulatory agencies also consider other factors such as agglomerates and aggregates of nanomaterials and certain fraction (such as 10% or more of total material mass) of nanomaterials in the final product. On the basis of these criteria, it is not always clear whether the final medical product contains actual nanomaterials or otherwise involves the application of nanotechnology. As the actual classification of a product as a nano-enabled product depends on the measurement of the size of nanomaterial used, precise physical characterization of the material is important. The research community continues to investigate nanomaterials and their safety and efficacy issues to close the scientific and regulatory gaps to ensure that nanotechnology drives the next generation of biomedical innovation.

In accordance with Executive Order 13563 [74] on improving regulation, as well as with the White House policy statements on regulating emerging technologies [75] and applications of nanotechnology [76], the FDA supports innovation and the safe use of nanotechnology in FDA-regulated products under appropriate and balanced regulatory oversight. By enhancing its scientific expertise and tools necessary to assess the safety and effectiveness of products, the FDA enables the responsible development of products with new and beneficial properties. The FDA intends to ensure transparent and predictable regulatory pathways grounded in the best-available science. According to the published information the FDA's regulatory approach will have the following attributes [77]:

- **The FDA maintains product-focused, science-based regulatory policy**. Technical assessments of the products will be made considering the effects of nanomaterials in the particular biological and mechanical context of each product and its intended use. And the particular policies for each product area will vary according to the statutory authorities. The FDA advises manufacturers to consult with it early in their development process to facilitate a mutual understanding of the scientific and regulatory issues for their nanotechnology products.
- **The FDA's approach respects variations in legal standards for different product classes**. Food additives are considered safe when there is a reasonable certainty of no harm from their intended use [78]. Drugs, by contrast, are evaluated on

the basis of not only their risk profile but also their predicted benefit [79]. These differing legal standards demonstrate how different contexts could lead to different regulatory outcomes, even if two products present the same level of risk. Other products regulated by the FDA are subject to yet different standards for safety or effectiveness. The result may be divergent regulatory outcomes for different product classes and different applications of nanomaterials, even where objective measures of risk are similar.

- **Where premarket review authority exists, attention to nanomaterials is being incorporated into standing procedures**. New drugs, new animal drugs, biologics, food additives (includes food contact substances, such as food packaging), color additives, certain human devices, and certain new dietary ingredients in dietary supplements are subject to premarket review requirements. Premarket review processes for these products require data related to the safety, effectiveness (where applicable), or regulatory status of the products. Individual premarket review procedures include attention to whether the use of nanomaterials suggests the need for additional data on safety or effectiveness, as applicable. Premarket review may also address issues other than safety or effectiveness, for example, product identity verification and manufacturing controls. **Where statutory authority does not provide for premarket review, consultation is encouraged to reduce the risk of unintended harm to human or animal health**. Some FDA-regulated products such as dietary supplements (except certain new dietary ingredients), cosmetics (except color additives), and food (except food or color additives) are not subject to mandatory pre-market review. In these cases, the FDA relies on publicly available or voluntarily submitted information, adverse event reporting (where applicable), and postmarket surveillance activities in order to provide oversight. Where nanotechnology applications are involved, the FDA encourages manufacturers to consult with it before taking their products to market. Such consultation can help the FDA advise companies, review safety information, and design any necessary postmarketing safety oversight.

- **The FDA will continue postmarket monitoring.** The FDA will continue to monitor the marketplace for products containing nanomaterials and will take actions, as needed, to protect consumers.
- **The industry remains responsible for ensuring that its products meet all applicable legal requirements, including safety standards.** Regardless of whether products are subject to premarket review or authorization, manufacturers are required to ensure that their products satisfy applicable safety standards and comply with other applicable requirements. Therefore, the industry must work with current information in product development and continue to monitor products once marketed. The FDA encourages the industry to consult early with the agency to address questions related to the regulatory status or to the safety, effectiveness, or other attributes of products that contain nanomaterials or otherwise involve application of nanotechnology. These early consultations afford an opportunity to clarify the methodologies and data that will be needed to meet the sponsor's obligations. Additional public meetings or workshops may be held to advance regulatory science, identify product-specific data needs, or seek input on specific issues.
- **The FDA will collaborate, as appropriate, with domestic and international counterparts on regulatory policy issues.** The FDA engages in policy dialogue with other US government agencies through the Emerging Technologies Interagency Policy Coordination Committee and other forums, among other things, to contribute to overarching US government policies relevant to nanotechnology and, as appropriate, coordinate its policy activities. The FDA also works with foreign regulatory counterparts to share perspectives and information on the regulation of nanotechnology products and their intended uses
- **For both products that are not subject to premarket review and those that are, the FDA will offer technical advice and guidance, as needed, to help the industry meet its regulatory and statutory obligations.** The FDA prepares

guidance documents for its staff, applicants/sponsors, and the public to describe the agency's interpretation of or policy on a regulatory issue. Guidance documents will emerge over time, and (depending on the product class) will address interpretation of relevant statutory and regulatory standards and provide guidance on the technical data needed to meet those standards. The FDA will tailor guidelines to the unique confluence of the statute governing the product class, the level of scientific knowledge relevant to those applications, and the likely extent of effects on human and animal health.

9.6 Summary

Nanomaterials have unique physicochemical and biological properties compared to their larger counterparts. Due to their small size, shape, structure, charge, and agglomeration, the properties of nanomaterials can greatly influence their interactions with biomolecules. Hence, nanomaterials are used as a promising tool for the development of medical products such as nanomedicines, biomedical imaging and diagnostic biosensors. Regulatory challenges posed by nanomaterials and nanotechnology are many: the diversity of nanomaterials, a lack of data characterizing the materials, and a lack of standardization in nomenclature and metrics. Industries developing nanomaterial products must work with current information in product development and monitor products once marketed. The industry is encouraged to consult early with the FDA, which may afford an opportunity to clarify the methodologies and data that will be needed to meet obligations. Flexible, product-focused, science-based approaches are being used to facilitate innovation and to fulfil the FDA's mission to bring safe and effective medical products to market to safeguard the public health.

References

1. For more information about FDA regulations, including between pre- and post-market approval, review, and notification. http://www.fda.gov/AboutFDA/Transparency/Basics/default.htm.

2. See, for example, descriptions of research and development activities at: www.nrc-cnrc. gc.ca/eng/solutions/collaborative/nint_index. html; www.nano.cancer.gov/about/plan; www.jst.go.jp/EN/research/research3.html.
3. Martis, E. A., Badve, R. R., and Degwekar, M. D. (2012). Nanotechnology based devices and applications in medicine: an overview. *Chron. Young Scientists*, **3**, 68–73.
4. Sahoo, S. K., Parveen, S., and Panda, J. J. (2007). The present and future of nanotechnology in human health care. *Nanomedicine*, **3**, 20-31.
5. Texas State Historical Association, *The Handbook of Texas Online*. https://tshaonline.org/handbook/online/articles/doc01.
6. Vance, M. E., Kuiken, T., Vejerano, E. P., McGinnis, S. P., Hochella, M. F., Jr., Rejeski, D., and Hull, M. S. (2015). Nanotechnology in the real world: redeveloping the nanomaterial consumer products inventory. *Beilstein J. Nanotechnol.*, **6**, 1769–1780.
7. Kamat, P. V. (2002). Photophysical, photochemical and photocatalytic aspects of metal nanoparticles. *J. Phys. Chem. B*, **106**, 7729–7744.
8. Katz, E., and Willner, I. (2004). Integrated nanoparticle-biomolecule hybrid systems: synthesis, properties, and applications. *Angew. Chem. Int. Ed.*, **43**, 6042–6108.
9. Pagona, G., and Tagmatarchis, N. (2006). Carbon nanotubes: materials for medicinal chemistry and biotechnological applications. *Curr. Med. Chem.*, **13**, 1789–1798.
10. Robinson, J. T., Tabakman, S. M., Liang, Y., Wang, H., Casalongue, H. S., Vinh, D., and Dai, H. (2011). Ultrasmall reduced graphene oxide with high near-infrared absorbance for photothermal therapy. *J. Am. Chem. Soc.*, **133**, 6825–6831.
11. Sun, X., Liu, Z., Welsher. K., Robinson, J. T., Goodwin, A., Zaric, S., and Dai, H. (2008). Nano-graphene oxide for cellular imaging and drug delivery. *Nano Res.*, **1**, 203–212.
12. Cao, Y. C., Jin, R., and Mirkin, C. A. (2002). Nanoparticles with Raman spectroscopic fingerprints for DNA and RNA detection. *Science*, **297**, pp. 1536–1540.
13. Daniel, M. C., and Astruc, D. (2004). Gold nanoparticles: assembly, supramolecular chemistry, quantum-size-related properties, and applications towards biology, catalysis and nanotechnology. *Chem. Rev.*, **104**, 293–346.
14. Ghosh, P., Han, G., De, M., Kim, C. K., and Rotello, V. M. (2008). Gold nanoparticles in delivery applications. *Adv. Drug Delivery Rev.*, **60**, 1307–1315.

15. Murphy, C. J., Gole, A. M., Stone, J. W., Sisco, P. N., Alkiany, A. M., Goldsmith, E. C., and Baxter, S. C. (2008). Gold nanoparticles in biology: beyond toxicity to cellular imaging. *Acc. Chem. Res.*, **41**, 1721–1730.

16. Rosi, N. L., Giljohann, D. A., Thaxton, C. S., Lytton-Jean, A. K. R., Han, M. S., and Mirkin, C. A. (2006). Oligonucleotide modified gold nanoparticles for intracellular gene regulation. *Science*, **312**, 1027–1030.

17. Darouiche, R. O. (1999). Anti-infective efficacy of silver coated medical prostheses. *Clin. Infect. Dis.*, **29**, 1371–1377.

18. Huff, T. B., Tong, L., Zhao, Y., Hansen, M. N., Cheng, J. X., and Wei, A. (2007). Hyperthermic effects of gold nanorods on tumor cells. *Nanomedicine*, **2**, 125 –1 32.

19. Li, Y., Leung, P., Yao, L., Song, Q. W., and Newton, E. (2006). Antimicrobial effect of surgical masks coated with nanoparticles. *J. Hosp. Infect.*, **62**, 58–63.

20. (a) Pissuwan, D., Valenzuela, S. M., and Cortie, M. B. (2006). Therapeutic possibilities of plasmonically heated gold nanoparticles. *Trends Biotechnol.*, **24**, 62–67. (b) Boisselier, E., and Astruc, D. (2009). Gold nanoparticles in nanomedicine: preparations, imaging, diagnostics, therapies and toxicity. *Chem. Soc. Rev.*, **38**, 1759–1782.

21. Rojo, J., Diaz, V., de la Fuente, J. M., Segura, I., Barrientos, A. G., Riese, H. H., Bernad, A., and Penades, S. (2004). Gold glyconanoparticles as new tools in anti-adhesive therapy. *ChemBioChem*, **5**, 291–297.

22. Shrivastava, S., Bera, T., Singh, S. K., Singh, G., Ramachandrarao, P., and Dash, D. (2009). Characterization of antiplatelet properties of silver nanoparticles. *ACS Nano*, **3**, 1357–1364.

23. Chakravarty, P., Marches, R., Zimmerman, N. S., Swafford A. D., Bajaj, P., Musselman, I. H., Pantano, P., Draper, R. K., and Vitetta, E. S. (2008). Thermal ablation of tumor cells with antibody-functionalized single-walled carbon nanotubes. *Proc. Natl. Acad. Sci. U. S. A.*, **105**, 8697–8702.

24. Liu, Z., Sun, X., Nakayama, N., and Dai, H. (2007). Supramolecular chemistry on water-soluble carbon nanotubes for drug loading and delivery. *ACS Nano*, **1**, 50–56.

25. Liu, Z., Chen, K., Davis, C., Sherlock, S., Cao, Q., Chen, X., and Dai, H. (2008). Drug delivery with carbon nanotubes for in vivo cancer treatment. *Cancer Res.*, **68**, 6652–6660.

26. Liu, Z., Tabakman, S., Welsher, K., and Dai, H. (2009). Carbon nanotubes in biology and medicine: in vitro and in vivo detection, imaging and drug delivery. *Nano Res.*, **2**, 85–120.

27. Friedman, S. H., DeCamp, D. L., Sijbesma, R. P., Srdanov, G., Wudi, F., and Kenyon, G. L. (1993). Inhibition of the HIV-1 protease by fullerene

derivatives: model building studies and experimental verification. *J. Am. Chem. Soc.*, **115**, 6506–6509.

28. Foley, S., Crowley, C., Smaihi, M., Bonfils, C., Erlanger, B. F., Seta, P., and Larroque, C. (2002). Cellular localisation of a water-soluble fullerene derivative. *Biochem. Biophys. Res. Commun.*, **294**, 116–119.

29. Hetzer, M., Bayerl, S., Camps, X., Vostrowsky, O. Hirsch, A., and Bayerl, T. (1997). Fullerenes in membranes. Structural and dynamic effects of lipophilic C60 derivatives in phospholipid bilayers. *Adv. Mater.*, **9**, 913–917.

30. Schuster, D. I., Wilson, S. R., Kirschner, A. N., and Hirsch, A. (2000). Evaluation of the anti-HIV potency of a water-soluble dendrimeric fullerene. *Proc. Electrochem. Soc.*, **9**, 267–270.

31. Zakharian, T. Y., Seryshev, A., Sitharaman, B., Gilbert, B. E., Knight, V., and Wilson, L. J. (2005). A fullerene-paclitaxel chemotherapeutic: synthesis, characterization, and study of biological activity in tissue culture. *J. Am. Chem. Soc.*, **127**, 12508–12509.

32. Schinazi, R. F., Sijbesma, R., Srdanov, G., Hill, C. L., and Wudl, F. (1993). Synthesis and virucidal activity of a water-soluble, configurationally stable, derivatized C60 fullerene. *Antimicrob. Agents Chemother.*, **37**, 1707–1710.

33. Bosi, S., Da Ros, T., Castellano, S., Banfi, E., and Prato, M. (2000). Antimycobacterial activity of ionic fullerene derivatives. *Bioorg. Med. Chem. Lett.*, **10**, 1043–1045.

34. Tsao, N., Kanakamma, P. P., Luh, T. Y., Chou, C. K., and Lei, H. Y. (1999). Inhibition of Escherichia coli-induced meningitis by carboxyfullerene. *Antimicrob. Agents Chemother.*, **43**, 2273–2277.

35. Tsao, N., Luh, T. Y., Chou, C. K., Wu, J. J., Lin, Y. S., and Lei, H. Y. (1999). Inhibition of group A Streptococcus infection by carboxyfullerene. *Antimicrob. Agents Chemother.*, **45**, 1788–7793.

36. Miyata, N., and Yamakoshi, T. (1997). *Fullerenes: Recent Advances in the Chemistry and Physics of Fullerenes and Related Materials.* Kadish, K. M., and Ruoff, R. S. (eds.), (Pennington, NJ, USA).

37. Tabata, Y., Murakami, Y., and Ikada, Y. (1997). Photodynamic effect of polyethylene glycol-modified fullerene on tumor. *Jpn. J. Cancer Res.*, **88**, 1108–1116.

38. Liu, Y., Yu, D., Zeng, C., Miao, Z., and Dai, L. (2010). Biocompatible graphene oxide-based glucose biosensors. *Langmuir*, **26**, 6158–6160.

39. Yang, K., Zhang, S., Zhang, G., Sun, X., Lee, S. T., and Liu, Z. (2010). Graphene in mice: ultrahigh in vivo tumor uptake and efficient photothermal therapy. *Nano Lett.*, **10**, 3318–3323.

40. Lidke, D. S., Nagy, P., Heintzmann, R., Arndt-Jovin, D. J., Post, J. N., Grecco, H. E., Jares-Erijman, E. A., and Jovin, T. M. (2004). Quantum dot ligands provide new insights into erbB/HER receptor-mediated signal transduction. *Nat. Biotechnol.*, **22**, 198–203.

41. Xing, Y., Xia, Z., and Rao, J. (2009). Semiconductor quantum dots for biosensing and in vivo imaging. *IEEE Trans. Nanobiosci.*, **8**, 4–12.

42. Zrazhevskiy, P., and Gao, X. (2009). Multifunctional quantum dots for personalized medicine. *Nano Today*, **4**, 414–428.

43. Medintz, I. L., Pons, T., Trammell, S. A., Grimes, A. F., English, D. S., Blanco-Canosa, J. B., Dawson, P. E., and Mattoussi, H. (2008). Interactions between redox complexes and semiconductor quantum dots coupled via a peptide bridge. *J. Am. Chem. Soc.*, **130**, 16745–16756.

44. Weng, K. C., Noble, C. O., Papahadjopoulos-Sternberg, B., Chen, F. F., Drummond, D. C., Kirpotin, D. B., Wang, D., Hom, Y. K., Hann, B., and Park, J. W. (2008). Targeted tumor cell internalization and imaging of multifunctional quantum dot-conjugated immunoliposomes in vitro and in vivo. *Nano Lett.*, **8**, 2851–2857.

45. Samia, A. C. S., Chen, X. B., and Burda, C. (2003). Semiconductor quantum dots for photodynamic therapy. *J. Am. Chem. Soc.*, **125**, 15736–15737.

46. Majewski, P., and Thierry, B. (2007). Functionalized magnetite nanoparticles: synthesis, properties, and bio-applications. *Crit. Rev. Solid State Mater. Sci.*, **32**, 203–215.

47. Qiang, Y., Antony, J., Sharma, A., Nutting, J., Sikes, D., and Meyer, D. (2006). Iron/iron oxide core-shell nanoclusters for biomedical applications. *J. Nanopart. Res.*, **8**, 489–496.

48. Makadia, H. K., and Siegel, S. J. (2011). Poly lactic-co-glycolic acid (PLGA) as biodegradable controlled drug delivery carrier. *Polymers*, **3**, 1377–1397.

49. Sailaja, A. K., Amareshwar, P., and Chakravarty, P. (2010). Chitosan nanoparticles as a drug delivery system. *RJPBCS*, **1**, 474–484.

50. Uhrich, K. E., Cannizzaro, S. M., Langer, R. S., and Shakesheff, K. M. (1999). Polymeric systems for controlled drug release. *Chem. Rev.*, **99**, 3181–3198.

51. Agasti, S. S., Rana, S., Park, M. H., Kim, C. K., You, C. C., and Rotello, V. M. (2010). Nanoparticles for detection and diagnosis. *Adv. Drug Delivery Rev.*, **62**, 316–328.

52. Kim, B. Y. S., Rutka, J. T., and Chan, W. C. W. (2010). Nanomedicine. *N. Engl. J. Med.*, **363**, 2434–2443.

53. Rana, S., Yeh, Y.-C., and Rotello, V. M. (2010). Engineering the nanoparticle-protein interface: applications and possibilities. *Curr. Opin. Chem. Biol.*, **14**, 828–834.

54. Sapsford, K. E., Tyner, K. M., Dair, B. J, Deschamps, J. R., and Medintz, I. L. (2011). Analyzing nanomaterial bioconjugates: a review of current and emerging purification and characterization techniques. *Anal. Chem.*, **83**, 4453–4488.

55. Hermanson, G. T. (2008). *Bioconjugate Techniques*, 2nd Ed. (Academic Press, Amsterdam, the Netherlands).

56. Gaumet, M., Vargas, A., Gurny, R., and Delie, F. (2008). Nanoparticles for drug delivery: the need for precision in reporting particle size parameters. *Eur. J. Pharm. Biopharm.*, **69**, 1–9.

57. Powers, K. W., Palazuelos, M., Moudgil, B. M., and Roberts, S. M. (2007). Characterization of the size, shape, and state of dispersion of nanoparticles for toxicological studies. *Nanotoxicology*, **1**, 42–51.

58. Warheit, D. B. (2010). Debunking some misconceptions about nanotoxicology. *Nano Lett.*, **10**, 4777–4782.

59. Lövestam, G., et al. (2010). Considerations on a definition of nanomaterial for regulatory purposes. Joint Resource Centre, European Commission (EC), Luxembourg. https://ec.europa.eu/jrc/sites/default/files/jrc_reference_report_201007_nanomaterials.pdf.

60. Scientific Committee on Emerging and Newly Identified Health Risks. (2010). Scientific basis for the definition of the term "nanomaterial" (EC, Brussels). http://ec.europ a.eu/health/scientific_committees/emerging/docs/scenihr_o_030.pdf.

61. FDA. (2014). Considering whether an FDA-regulated product involves the application of nanotechnology: guidance for industry. http://www.fda.gov/RegulatoryInformation/Guidances/ucm257698.htm.

62. Nel, A., Xia, T., Madler, L., and Li, N. (2006). Toxic potential of materials at the nanolevel. *Science*, **311**, 622–627.

63. Chikkaveeraiah, B. V., Bhirde, A., Malhotra, R., Patel V., Gutkind, J. S., and Rusling, J. F. (2009). Single-wall carbon nanotube forest arrays for immunoelectrochemical measurement of four protein biomarkers for prostate cancer. *Anal. Chem.*, **81**, 9129–9134.

64. Chikkaveeraiah, B. V., Mani, V., Patel, V., Gutkind, J. S., and Rusling, J. F. (2011). Microfluidic electrochemical immunoarray for ultrasensitive detection of two cancer biomarker proteins in serum. *Biosens. Bioelectron.*, **26**, 4477–4483.

65. Moghimi, S. M., Hunter, A. C., and Murray, J. C. (2005). Nanomedicine: current status and future prospects. *FASEB J.*, **19**, 311–330.

66. Sapsford, K. E., Granek, J., Deschamps, J. R., Boenman, K., Blanco-Canosa, J. B., Dawson, P. E., Susumu, K., Stewart, M. H., and Medintz, I. L. (2011). Monitoring botulinum neurotoxin A activity with peptide-functionalized quantum dot resonance energy transfer sensors. *ACS Nano*, **5**, 2687–2699.

67. Sapsford, K. E., Spindel, S., Jennings, T., Tao, G., Triulzi, R. C., Algar, W. R., and Medintz, I. L. (2011). Optimizing two-color semiconductor nanocrystal immunoassays in single well microtiter plate formats. *Sensors*, **11**, 7879–7891.

68. Nanotechnology Task Force Report. (2007). www.fda.gov/ScienceResearch/SpecialTopics/Nanotechnology/NanotechnologyTaskForceReport2007/default.htm.

69. FDA, Nanotechnology regulatory science research categories. www.fda.gov/ScienceResearch/SpecialTopics/Nanotechnology/ucm196697.htm.

70. National Nanotechnology Initiative. http://www.nano.gov/about-nni.

71. NNI, Capstone meeting: risk management methods and ethical, legal, and societal implications of nanotechnology, Arlington, VA, 30–31 March 2010. www.nano.gov/events/meetings-workshops/capstone.

72. FDA Collaborations with National Cancer Institute, (NCI, NIH) and National Institute of Standards and Technology (NIST) on Nanotechnology. www.fda.gov/AboutFDA/PartnershipsCollaborations/PublicPrivatePartnershipProgram/ucm231125.htm.

73. Medical device classification. http://www.fda.gov/MedicalDevices/DeviceRegulationandGuidance/Overview/ClassifyYourDevice/.

74. Executive Order 13563: Improving regulation and regulatory review. www.whitehouse.gov/the-press-office/2011/01/18/executive-order-13563-improving-regulation-and-regulatory-review.

75. Principles for regulation and oversight of emerging technologies: memorandum for the heads of executives departments and agencies. https://www.whitehouse.gov/sites/default/files/microsites/ostp/etipc-memo-3-11-2011.pdf.

76. Policy principles for the U.S. decision-making concerning regulation and oversight of applications of nanotechnology and nanomaterials. https://www.whitehouse.gov/sites/default/files/omb/inforeg/for-agencies/nanotechnology-regulation-and-oversight-principles.pdf.

77. The FDA's approach to regulation of nanotechnology products. http://www.fda.gov/ScienceResearch/SpecialTopics/Nanotechnology/ucm301114.htm.
78. Federal Food Drug and Cosmetic Act (FFDCA) § 409 (21 U.S.C. 348) and 21 CFR 170.3(i).
79. Federal Food Drug and Cosmetic Act (FFDCA) § 505 (21 U.S.C. 355) and 21 CFR 330.10(a)(4)(iii).

Index